THE RAINBOW DIET

THE RAINBOW DIET AND HOW IT CAN HELP YOU BEAT CANCER

Chris Woollams M.A. (Oxon)

Chris Woollams asserts the moral right to be identified as the author of this work.

A catalogue record for this book is available from the British Library.

The Rainbow Diet – and how it can help you beat cancer is compiled and written by Chris Woollams for CANCERactive from the information contained on the charity website and in its research centre Cancer Watch.

This book is written to provide information in line with CANCERactive's agreed Charity Commission remit. CANCERactive does benefit from the proceeds.

First Edition published July 2008
Second Edition published September 2010
Third Edition published February 2013
Reprinted December 2013
Fourth Edition published January 2015
Reprinted with updates March 2016
By: CANCERactive, Registered UK Charity No: 1102413
Registered address: Appletree Cottage, Hay Lane, Fulmer, Buckinghamshire, SL3 6HJ
Contact Telephone Admin: 0300 365 3015

Cover design by Jeremy Baker.

ISBN 978-0-9565391-7-5

Printed and bound in the United States of America by Edwards Brothers Malloy, Inc.

*'Let your food be your medicine
and let your medicine be your food'*

Important Notice

This book represents a review and an interpretation of a vast number of varied sources available to anyone on the subject of diet, healthy eating, and cancer, its prevention and possible cure.

Whilst the author has made every effort to ensure that the facts, information and conclusions are accurate and as up-to-date as possible at the time of publication, the author and publisher assume no responsibility.

The author is neither a fully qualified health practitioner nor a doctor of medicine and so is not qualified to give any advice on any medical matters. Cancer (and its related illnesses) is a very serious and very individual disease, and readers must consult with experts and specialists in the appropriate medical field before taking, or refraining from taking, any action.

This book and the information contained are not intended as an alternative to such specialist advice, which should be sought for accurate diagnosis and before any course of treatment.

The author and the publisher cannot be held responsible for any action, or lack of action, that is taken by any reader as a result of information contained in the text of this book. Such action is taken entirely at the reader's own risk.

This book is dedicated to all the sensible people who know that there is more to life than taking drugs.

(**December 2013**) Leading clinicians have today written a joint letter to David Cameron, the British Prime Minister, urging him to put the Mediterranean Diet at the heart of health policy and to make it centre stage in the fight against dementia.

The letter was signed by experts from Britain, France, the United States, Greece and Italy. It calls for governments to spend more educating adults and children on the benefits of a healthy diet and lifestyle.

Dr. Aseem Malhotra, a top cardiologist at Croydon University Hospital and one of the letter's signatories, said, *"We are not going to overcome the increasing burden of chronic diseases by prescribing more pills. The medical profession has itself been guilty of placing too much emphasis on drugs, the benefits of which are often grossly exaggerated and fuelled by a powerful pharmaceutical industry, who naturally wish to expand the use of their drugs for financial gain"*. He went on to add, *"The evidence base for the Mediterranean diet in preventing all of the chronic diseases that are plaguing the Western world is overwhelming."*

In 2004, I first did a speech about the Rainbow Diet. It followed an extensive review of available research on a great number of diets. I first wrote this book in 2007, some nine years ago. The research was strong then, It is overwhelming now. We even sent a document to the then Health Minister with a detailed plan to build dietary education into schools for pupils, teachers and parents alike. Urged to apply for a Government grant, we were turned down – the reply lied, "It's already being done".

PREFACE

Can one book really change your life? I think The Rainbow Diet can, because I genuinely believe it will give you a much better chance of beating cancer – whether you have it already, or simply want to avoid ever developing it in the first place. Sadly, it is increasingly likely that one in two of us will have to face this hurdle at some point in our lives.

I've written this book because I want people to understand how we are ignoring the foods and their bioactive compounds that have **protected and corrected** us for the last 200,000 years and more. And I want to empower people so that they can easily understand exactly what a 'Good Diet' really entails, and how it differs from the rag bag of advice you glean from the media, much of which has nothing to do with sensible science but is borne out of politics, ignorance, handed-down mythology or the latest 'fad', whether from the hips of a film star or the lips of a 'Diet Expert' who has studied the diet of some distant race living in vastly different circumstances to your own and thinks you should copy it.

In the midst of all this the real truth is that all over the world in the last decade, top scientists have been showing exactly how foods 'work', which ones can help you, and which ones can harm you, often to see their work all but ignored.

Why restrict the message to cancer?

Surely a good diet helps fight all sorts of diseases? This is almost certainly true. In this book you will see that the Rainbow Diet is now known to fight Alzheimer's, dementia, diabetes, epilepsy, while aiding longevity, amongst other benefits. The truth is that since I first came up with the theory in 2005, science has proved me right for cancer, and caught up in areas of other chronic illness too!

However, there are certainly some foods that have been shown to have very specific actions in restricting cancer and I have focused on those a little more than others. And anyway, the last ten years of my life have been devoted to studying cancer. I don't feel I'm on safe ground commenting on heart disease but on cancer I genuinely feel I'm a bit of an amateur expert.

Back in the spring of 2001 my eldest daughter, Catherine (then 22), was diagnosed with a malignant brain tumour. Look up glioma on the internet and basically it says, '*You're dead. No hope*'. When we started our research we found that even the mighty UK medical magazine, *The Lancet*, all but said the drugs were useless.

But, I refused to accept her oncologists offer of, '*Don't worry, we'll give her a good summer*'. I read books and covered the Internet. I rang experts in orthodox and complementary fields. I talked to people at the boundaries of our cancer knowledge. And I found so much – so very much – information out there, most of which UK oncologists simply do not know exists. For example, there is research on natural compounds that had been shown to have real potential with gliomas: Like echinacea, curcumin, Coenzyme Q10, omega-3 and chokeberry.

When it came to having radiotherapy, we found that certain natural compounds could improve the success of the treatment, while others could protect the patient from the possible side-effects. The MD Anderson Cancer Center in Texas were talking about astragalus, St Thomas' Hospital had conducted limited research on the benefits of isoflavones and selenium; other mainstream cancer centers were using vitamin D.

When it came to having chemotherapy there was suddenly a debate engulfing us about taking antioxidants and whether they would negate the effects of the drugs. Was this really true, or another example of handed-down mythology? I know now that there should be no debate – there is good quality research in the USA – from UCLA, from MD Anderson, from Harvard and others. A number of supplements and the right diet can make your chemotherapy far more effective. (These effects are not confined to chemotherapy for brain tumours. There are a number of drugs whose effect is enhanced in clinical trials by vitamins and natural compounds.)

Increasing survival times

I'd given Catherine a 'diet programme' and she was taking lots of supplements. Importantly everything we did was 'with purpose'. We were not just throwing random foods, vitamins and minerals into her with crossed fingers.

After 6 months – the maximum time the doctors had predicted she would live – a scan suggested she was 'All Clear', but with the scarring of the brain tissue no one could be truly certain. Every three months she returned for a further scan, and each was 'clearer'. After two years one of St Thomas' Hospital's top doctors suggested I write down what we had found out. And my first book, *'Everything you need to know to help you beat cancer'*, was the result. It sold out after three months!

I was asked to speak at the NHS Conference to a large audience of Doctors; then at the UK Brain Tumour conference. More invitations followed from the USA, Australia, Japan, Russia, Germany and elsewhere.

All the time my knowledge was increasing – I was by now receiving information and newsletters from over 60 cancer centres worldwide. Catherine suggested that we launch a patient-orientated magazine of helpful and highly usable information, and so **icon** (*Integrated Cancer and Oncology News*) was born – at 68 pages in full colour, it is now available free in over 640 UK Hospitals, Cancer Centres and Health Libraries. At least 300,000 people pick up a copy. Its focus is on using complementary therapies to build Integrative Programmes and thus increase your personal odds of beating cancer.

We started a cancer charity – **CANCERactive** – but one with a unique difference: It didn't only tell you about the Orthodox Therapies available, it told you about effective Complementary and new therapies too; and the latest on possible causes that also might be maintaining the disease. Nowadays, I am regularly in touch with top oncologists in the Royal Marsden, MD Anderson, Memorial Sloan Kettering and more.

One of the biggest falsehoods of modern medicine is that there's no research evidence for Complementary Therapies. There is an enormous amount if you know where to look and have a biochemistry degree to sort the wheat from the chaff. Interestingly, the last two years has seen the start of clinical trials in the USA with Calorie Restriction, Ketogenic Diets (almost identical to the Rainbow ideals) and Hyperbaric Oxygen each used to complement drug and radiotherapy treatment. Preliminary research says that they each improve outcomes AND reduce side-effects.

Our Charity (www.canceractive.com), receives an average of 6,200 visitors a day, up from about 3,400 just one year ago! There you can sign up for my free monthly newsletter which brings you the latest information from around the world.

But you no longer have to accept just my word that sceptics and critics talk tosh. In May 2012 the American Cancer Society released a report in which they talked about an 'explosion' of research since 2006; 'overwhelming' evidence that complementary therapies like diet, exercise and weight control could increase survival times and even keep people cancer-free, preventing a cancer returning!

Be clear: There are foods, vitamins and natural compounds which can increase your odds of survival; only the ignorant will now question this.

Good food prevents cancer

But the truth is that the debate should have been terminated years ago. While I am adamant that the changed diet and selected supplements were a vital factor in helping Catherine survive nearly eight times longer than predicted, my views can, of course, be dismissed as 'just anecdotal'.

But an odd thing happened at the Cancer Prevention Conference organised by CANCERactive in 2004. Professor Tony Howell of Christie Hospital, Manchester, one of the UK's top experts in breast cancer and then one of our patrons, explained that his job was to help women prevent breast cancer returning and increasingly he had the drugs to do it.

But we have known for a long time that a 'good diet' is also a significant cancer preventer – oncologists, cancer experts and even the World Health Organisation endorse this. So why are people ignoring this and not telling you accurately what diet to embrace?

Indeed, the reality is even worse. While I can tell you about research on natural compounds that shows they can reduce inflammation, reduce oestrogen levels, kill cancer cells or stop metastasis, cancer patients instead receive NHS booklets on what to eat during chemotherapy featuring little drawings of cheese-burgers, milk shakes and sticky buns!

As you will read, major research studies show people with the highest blood glucose levels survive least and the hormone IGF-1 in cows' dairy makes your cells grow and divide more quickly! Can it really be wise to be feeding the very cells your oncologist is trying to kill off?

The role of the charity

CANCERactive aims to provide top-quality research information that empowers you, even inspires you, to build yourself a personal 'Integrative' programme, choosing the 'best of best', to thus increase your odds of beating this disease. Using Complementary and Integrative Medicine (CIM) doubled survival in breast cancer patients in research at the Block Center in Chicago.

Eat-to-beat cancer

The first edition of my diet foray was a book called, *'The Tree of Life'*; it sold out in seven months. I used the symbol of a tree so people could see easily what roots underpinned the 'diet', what supported it and that the volume of the total diet should be in the highly protective branches.

But life moved on rapidly. A number of the 'revolutionary' points I made in that book are now widely understood to be true.

And I wanted something simple for people to remember easily (rather like the Government's 'five-a-day'). In speeches I coined the phrase '**The Rainbow Diet**' to show the width of nature's gifts to us including the importance of natural pigments (flavenoids, phenols, anthocyanins etc) and other food compounds (like vitamin D and fish oils) for your health.

Then came a centerfold in **icon** in the spring of 2006 entitled *'Over the Rainbow'* – inviting people to take a little daily sunshine, drink clean water and nourish their bodies with a rainbow of vibrant foods. We loaded it onto the website, www.canceractive.com, and it has been one of the five most read pages for seven years now.

So I took the best of *The Tree of Life* and updated it with all the latest scientific research but changed the name. The Rainbow Diet, in its first edition, went considerably further. It developed a

theory, based on a study of all the available research in 2007/8 that rather than diets of deprivation (like the South East Asian diet) so often thrown at us as ideal diets by media and health bodies alike, there was a need for genuinely bioactive ingredients to be included in a real diet plan. A diet of inclusion, not omission. Stop and think for a minute: How can eating not very much help you correct an illness?

You are currently reading the third edition of the Rainbow Diet and I am pleased to say that there is now overwhelming research evidence which turns the theory into fact.

This is a non-guilt diet. If you eat something naughty just make sure you do something to correct it with your next meal. The Rainbow Diet is easy-to-understand and easy-to-use. I also give you an understandable plan – including a shopping list.

The diet is genuinely empowering. Now you really can eat foods that can make a difference, increase your survival and stop a cancer returning, all without making the rest of the family suffer weird meals!

Thank you

So, here we are with 'The Rainbow Diet', a book that has evolved from the 'The Tree of Life'. Along the way, many people have helped me. I should like to thank my friend Larry Brooks for kick-starting the project originally, and Lindsey Fealey for all her hard work. Thanks also to Karen Holden and Jane Reynolds, the team at **icon**, including Malcolm, and Ginny Fraser and Madeleine Kingsley, Brian Mawer and Jeremy Baker for all the proof reading and changes.

Thanks also to Dr. Rob Verkerk for helping me with the water chapter, Alan Hopking for his help with herbs, Roger Coghill for his help on melatonin, the late Gerald Green for his expertise on yeasts and Lawrence Plaskett, Dr. Contreras and Charlotte Gerson for spending so much time with me. And thanks to all the research scientists of Cancer Centres from Harvard to Tokyo, and UCLA to Moscow. Your research does matter – it enables people like me to tell the whole truth about the benefits of food, and I'm sure it saves lives.

CONTENTS

INTRODUCTION – Nourishment and healing   1

SECTION 1 – KNOWLEDGE IS POWER

Chapter 1:   What is cancer – and how could diet
             possibly help?   9

Chapter 2:   Toxic bodies   19

Chapter 3:   Atomic man   27

Chapter 4:   Healthy liver – healthy body   37

Chapter 5:   Cancer – a weighty problem   45

Chapter 6:   A diet for prevention?   51

Chapter 7:   Mending a life   59

Chapter 8:   The French Connection   65

Chapter 9:   A diet for people with cancer?   73

Chapter 10: The appliance of science   85

Chapter 11: Acid and alkaline bodies   99

Chapter 12: Clean water – the only solution   103

Chapter 13: Cutting out the bad guys   113

Chapter 14: Organic food – living food   127

Chapter 15: Deriving the maximum nourishment
             from your diet   137

Chapter 16: Vitamins and minerals in the fight
             against cancer   143

Chapter 17: Herbs in the fight against cancer   165

Chapter 18: Helping hormones   181

SECTION 2 – RE-BUILDING A LIFE

Chapter 19:   Eat-to-beat oestrogen?   189

Chapter 20:   Eat-to-beat inflammation?   207

Chapter 21:   Eat-to-beat insulin?   213

Chapter 22:   Oxygenating your cells   221

Chapter 23:   Eat-to-beat yeasts and microbes   231

Chapter 24:   Natural compounds in the fight
               against cancer   239

Chapter 25:   Eat-to-boost your immune system   281

Chapter 26:   Food for thought   287

Chapter 27:   The Rainbow Diet: Eating a spectrum
               of benefits   291

Chapter 28:   The Rainbow Diet: The shopping trolley   299

Chapter 29:   The Rainbow Diet: The programme   303

Chapter 30:   The Rainbow Diet: A postscript   309

APPENDIX I   Liver Cleanse/Gallstone Flush   319
APPENDIX II Factors with Epigenetic effects   323
INDEX   327

INTRODUCTION
NOURISHMENT AND HEALING

*"An apple a day keeps the doctor away.
Especially if well aimed."*

(Mark Twain)

Mark obviously had his own theories on diet and doctors. When it comes to nutrition he was probably right on both counts.

The common apple contains, for example, large quantities of potassium but little sodium, good quantities of magnesium, cancer protecting flavenoids, quercitin, polysaccharides and the ability to help promote an alkaline cellular environment. Its pips contain 'vitamin' B-17, whilst the whole apple contains pectins, which feed your crucial Lactic Acid gut bacteria.

The common doctor, unfortunately, doesn't know too much about any of this. My GP couldn't name a single antioxidant. When I named six for him to write down, he couldn't even spell lycopene.

But I wouldn't wish to criticise doctors for one moment – they are intelligent, caring people who have trained for seven years, and are dedicated to saving our lives. They deserve all the praise we can give them. The people who train them, the ones who set the syllabus and the examinations, simply do not ask that they learn much, if anything, about food, diet, nutrition, vitamins and minerals.

When talking recently to a newly qualified GP, it transpired that during her seven years training she had spent just one morning on the subject of nutrition – a morning on heart disease.

In the USA, so worried were American Medical Professionals about this very issue that the Physicians Committee for Responsible Medicine (PCRM) distributed a 900 page guide to medical students in the USA and Canada. It covered everything from evidence-based information on the role of nutrition in prevention and treatments, to macro- and micro-nutrients for all stages of life. Oh, that we had this initiative in the UK too.

But in America there is a generally a much greater awareness

1

of the benefits of complementary therapies in increasing survival rates for cancer. Much of the 'explosion' of research into natural compounds has come from America; from Harvard Medical School, the Fred Hutchinson Cancer Center in Seattle, UCLA, MD Anderson – even the supposedly staid Memorial Sloan-Kettering has studied the benefits of curcumin and is in the midst of clinical trials using mushrooms right now. It is important that you remember this when talking to your UK oncologist whose ignorance of the latest dietary research often makes him/her defensive and even hostile to the benefits of bioactive ingredients.

Yet, common contributory factors in heart disease, cancer and diabetes include poor diet (for example high blood sugar levels and high 'trans' fat consumption), being overweight, smoking, too much alcohol and a lack of exercise. Governments, the press and Health Authorities harangue us over our modern hedonistic lifestyles: One recent UK report even told us that 50 per cent of cancers were our own fault.

Is that really fair? If our Government is quite clear that the roots of the three most common, and increasingly prevalent, diseases lie in poor diet, where are the education programmes on nutrition for school children and for doctors? If our families are not educated in what foods can nourish and protect them, and our doctors are missing an important chunk of the picture when giving us advice on our health, no wonder we are witnessing a crisis in illness levels. The only education we now receive are press and TV advertisements persuading us to eat pizzas and hamburgers!

Nourishment

The reality of food in the Western world is that the majority of it offers little genuine NOURISHMENT. When Hippocrates talked of food being your medicine, it was in an era when whole foods, grown locally and in season, nourished your body. Now we have refined wheat, refined olive oil, trans-fats, salt, processed foods, preservatives, pasteurised cheese and so on.

Where is the nourishment in all this? Will mass-market, refined foods nourish your cells, boost your immune system and fight a cancer?

The fact is that you are a highly complex 'chemical laboratory' with eight trillion chemical reactions happening every second of your life. Some inevitably go wrong, especially if you are not supplying the correct raw materials to them and/or you have poisons in your body that inhibit them.

The truth is you actually 'get sick' hundreds of times a day. But the reality is that your body and your immune system constantly correct the problem – they constantly heal you. Scandanavian scientists have argued that most people develop cancer up to six times in their lives and never know it. Your body just 'heals' you. But the fact is that the likelihood of someone incurring more moments of illness increases the worse their nourishment. The likelihood that your immune system cannot correct and heal you increases the worse your nourishment.

So just as 'illness' moments are constant, so healing is constant and it is aided and abetted by the foods and natural compounds you consume each day. Whether you have been 'diagnosed' or not.

Diets are about addition not deprivation

The truth is that the health of living organisms is always in harmony with the immediate environment. It was ever thus. Go back a thousand years – you ate and drank from your immediate environment. And the foods you ate provided bioactive ingredients nourishing the body, killing bacteria, boosting the immune system and constantly preventing and correcting illnesses. Even though we were surrounded by quite a hostile, microbe-infected environment, we survived and thrived. Take out the loss of life at birth and infant mortality from the statistics, and life span has hardly changed since biblical times – 'three score years and ten' Even though we have clever surgery, vaccines and less war to keep you alive longer.

But the real issue is still you in your immediate environment; your own personal microclimate. Does it nourish you? Does it provide the bioactive ingredients that can protect and correct? That can HEAL you? For just as we have stopped talking about nourishment, so we have stopped talking about HEALING. Now you are far more likely to read about 'junk food' and 'five-year survival' than the words nourishment and healing.

Using a spectrum of natural compounds to beat cancer

This book is not intended as a detailed scientific tome; it is a normal person's everyday guide to bioactive, natural compounds and how they may protect and heal you. My 'sound bite' as a description of these natural compounds - that are often vibrant, colourful pigments - is the RAINBOW. The intention is that you should nourish your body with a width of natural compounds across each week – all you have to do is 'Eat a Rainbow' of colours.

In this book I'll tell you:

- How you need beneficial bacteria in your intestine, without which you cannot MAKE certain cancer-fighting, cholesterol-fighting or diabetes-fighting compounds from whole foods.
- About mauve pigments that can kill off pre-cancer cells.
- An orange spice that may help prevent Alzheimer's and is increasingly studied as a colon-cancer fighter.
- A white bulb that can stop blood supplies forming to tumours.
- A natural compound in red grapes that seems to make you younger and repair damage to your DNA.
- The bright red factors found in raspberries that can stop HPV infection and heal lesions that can lead to cervical cancer.
- Compounds in olive oil and green tea which, according to one American Cancer Center, *'Can stop leukaemia in its tracks'*.
- Yellow and red pigments in peppers that are claimed to stop breast cancer returning.
- Certain green foods that contain compounds that can take aggressive oestrogen molecules in your body and downgrade them so that they are less harmful.
- A herb that can make the viruses, bacteria and cancer cells more responsive to your immune system.
- And half a dozen foods that can reduce inflammation, the precursor to diseases like arthritis and cancer.

And so much more.

Reds and oranges, and yellows and greens, blues, and indigo and violet – all the colours of the rainbow.

And before anyone jumps in to suggest that foods can't 'cure' cancer, I suggest that they consult the pharmaceutical companies because right now they are trying to concentrate and patent all manner of natural compounds found in herbs and foods, to make drugs they know have these powers.

You could be eating these bioactive compounds right now. But make no mistake: By depriving yourself of these natural compounds in your weekly diet, you are putting yourself in real danger. By making them the focus of your diet they will protect and correct, nourish and heal.

SECTION 1

KNOWLEDGE IS POWER
BUT, WITH CANCER, IT CAN BE THE DIFFERENCE
BETWEEN LIFE AND DEATH

One day you may read vitamin D is a wonder vitamin, the next there's a problem with it. Then melatonin, the sleep hormone, helps defeat breast cancer – but it is illegal to sell it in the UK.

The Government wants you to avoid fats, salt and sugar – yet hospitals produce booklets for patients having chemotherapy telling them to eat cheeseburgers, sugared buns and milkshakes!

Dairy may be harmful if it is a Tuesday, vitamin E if it's a Friday. My doctor says *'You don't need supplements if you eat a balanced diet'* but then he tells me he's never studied nutrition.

The Government and cancer experts tell me to "*Eat five portions of fruit and vegetables a day, don't smoke and stay out of the sun. And remember, 50 per cent of cancers are your own fault because of your lifestyle'*. I wonder what the other 50 per cent are and who is in charge of that! And anyway, isn't sunshine good for me?

No wonder we're all confused.

CHAPTER 1

WHAT IS CANCER – AND HOW COULD DIET POSSIBLY HELP?

My cousin Lindsey Fealey, who was CEO of our charity at the time, was 'manning a stand' for **CANCERactive** at the nurses conference in York a few years back. Two rather plump nurses wandered over. One picked up a copy of the first edition of the *Tree of Life* and briefly flicked through it. A few seconds later she tossed it back towards the table hitting Lindsey in the face, whilst uttering the words, *'How could anyone be stupid enough to think diet could beat cancer?'*

Unfortunately, before we focus on diet, I need to set the scene on cancer. I will try not to bore you but give a short version of what is contained in more detail in *'Everything you need to know to help you beat cancer'*, the best seller and first book I ever wrote, and now in its fourth edition.

Cancer is a modern disease

Cancer is essentially a modern disease. In Asia it is dubbed 'rich man's disease'. An American research study of 7,000 years of skeletons in Croatia showed the first signs in bones dating from less than 150 years ago. Other studies from Manchester and UCLA have confirmed this. We do know that there were illnesses called cancers as long ago as Ancient Egypt, Greece and Rome – aloe vera plants were used to treat skin cancers; Hippocrates actually treated patients with a special soup and enemas. But cancer in any volume was almost unheard of before the Industrial Revolution.

So how do I develop it?

Your body is in a state of constant change. Each day old cells die, new cells replace them, the copying of genetic messages takes place along with billions of chemical reactions. In all this incredibly complex hive of activity, mistakes (mutations) happen and these cause crucial message loss.

However, recent studies on the genome have shown that these 'mutations' are far too random and inconsistent to fulfill this textbook theory of cancer. Indeed, it is becoming more and more likely that cancer is, almost always, a metabolic disease. Biological scientists like Professor Thomas Seyfried of Boston College and even American biologist James Watson (joint discoverer of DNA) have advanced the case. It's an inconvenient truth. Without a core mutation, who needs drugs?

Epigenetics rules. OK?

Your core DNA double Helix is about 1.8 metres long, but very, very thin. It is rolled up into a tiny ball and fits inside each of your cells' nucleus. Holding it in this tight ball are proteins called histones. They are held in place by chemical bonds to the DNA, the product of methylation and acetylation.

If something happens to alter the methylation or acetylation, the histones shift. And this causes a problem. One way this might happen is through 'free-radicals'; you've probably heard the term. Free radicals are destructive; they can rip pieces off the bonds. Another route is through a compound called 'homocysteine'. Prior to illnesses such as cancer and Alzheimer's, levels of homocysteine rise in the body. Homocysteine is known to increase methylation around the core DNA. Conversely, scientists at Oxford have shown B vitamins (and especially folate) can reduce the problem. In a healthy individual, histones only cover a proportion of the genes in the DNA code, allowing little trains to jump on to the gene at a specific point, read and copy a sequence, and then hit the buffers and fall off.

These copies are crucial messages sent out from the nucleus to direct all your bodily processes. If the histones shift, certain sequences can no longer be read, and crucial messages are lost. For example, a message might be lost that tells the cell to divide slowly; or one may be lost that suppresses tumours. This is the principle behind cancer.

Calling these changes to the bonds that hold histones in place 'mutations' is actually just sloppy science. No mutation in the core DNA has occurred. In fact, cancer is rarely a genetic disease;

it is primarily a metabolic disease, caused by metabolic changes around the genetic code.

Right now, scientists are hard at work on the whole process looking at how drugs might reverse the process, by directly attacking the changed bonds, or affecting the methylating or acetylating enzymes that caused the changes.

This is the science of Epigenetics ('epi' meaning 'outside'). It started in about 1994/5 but has exploded since 2010. If you read the many research papers from scientists studying the new breed of developing drugs you will see three recurring themes.

1. The changes to the surrounding bonds of the genome are caused by four factors – poor diet, toxins (environmental and infections), stress and hormones (like oestrogen). Exactly the same 4 Pillars of Cancer that I wrote about in 2005 on our website.
2. The irregular bonds created are TOTALLY REVERSIBLE.
3. As a result, if you have a chronic illness like cancer, YOU ARE NOT DOOMED.

A world of Epigenetics in bioactive natural compounds

And here's the really good news: Since 2006 an enormous momentum has been building around natural compounds. There are scores with epigenetic benefits. As we will see, research shows that vitamin D, which actually acts more like a hormone in the body, is a great illness preventer. And there are also studies which show it can CORRECT abnormalities surrounding the core genetic code. A quick Google Search will find you research studies by expert scientists that Sulphoraphanes (from broccoli, kale, cabbage and sprouting seeds) in a concentrated form will correct some of the epigenetic changes that lead to breast cancer, prostate cancer and leukaemia.

I will be talking about this in detail later. Suffice it to say that I have found over 60 bioactive compounds with significant research on their epigenetic benefits. There is probably a core of about 20 to 25 bioactive compounds you will want to know about.

The role of the immune system

It is a recurring problem in cancer patients that their immune system is weak. In fact this weakness may have allowed the cancer to take hold in the first place. A second problem is that it often doesn't recognize the cancer cell as 'foreign'. The Science of Epigenetics explains this easily. Genes that make immune boosting proteins have been blocked and thus turned off. But some natural compounds – for example those in certain herbs – help turn them back on again.

Breakthrough thinking – stem cells

In November 2014 Professor Wang and his team at British Columbia presented another 'non-mutation' theory about cancer. They even claimed that the text books 'would need to be rewritten'.

When conducting research on stomach cancer, Wang noted that, as usual with cancer and chronic illnesses, first you get chronic inflammation. At this point repair stem cells rushed from the bone marrow to repair the problem in the stomach lining. Except, instead of converting to new stomach wall cells, the stem cells became 'stuck', under the influence of oestrogen, in their rapidly dividing 'primitive' state. A message telling them to convert normally, seemed to have gone missing.

Worse was to come. In 2012 three studies were published simultaneously in the journals *Science* and *Nature* confirming the existence of cancer stem cells 'at the heart of all cancers'. The cells were even separated out by CRUK. But, as of today, there is no drug in the world that kills cancer stem cells. They may knock the tumour back by 50, 60 or 70 per cent. But they will not kill it off completely.

However, in 2012 research from Dr. Young S. Kim at the National Cancer Institute in Bethesda showed that, while a poor diet encouraged the tumour to regrow, certain bioactive food compounds had the potential to stop the regrowth. We will cover which compounds later in the book.

Oestrogen

The effect of oestrogen in cancer is not confined to stem cells. Every cell in your body has receptor sites on its surface. Chemical messages arrive at these sites and activate events inside the cell. Certain receptor sites receive messages from the oestrogen family of hormones. One family member, called oestradiol, is made from your fat stores and is very dangerous and can cause havoc inside the cell. Fortunately, it has 'safer sisters'; one, oestrone, is about forty times less powerful and certain natural compounds have been shown to be able to degrade oestradiol into its safer sisters.

Many cancers have now been observed to be 'oestrogen' driven. It fuels the fire in most breast cancers, many stomach and bowel cancers, non-small cell lung cancers, most prostate cancers and many womb cancers.

Plants have similar hormones, called phytoestrogens, which are thankfully far, far less aggressive still than human oestrogen and are actually known to be able to bind to these same receptor sites and thus block oestradiol from creating its havoc. It's yet another example of the role diet can play to protect and correct.

Low magnesium/high sodium

The havoc that oestradiol causes in the cell includes increasing levels of sodium, decreasing levels of potassium, power and oxygen and making your cells more acid. But you don't need oestrogen; you can cause this yourself. A poor diet involving too much sodium and not enough magnesium or potassium would be a start.

A downward spiral takes place. Less and less energy is produced and yet more acidity with sodium salts. When the level of energy production falls below a certain figure (think of your cells as little batteries) the *p53* repair gene switches off, but the genes that make the cell divide rapidly (*ras* genes) need far less power and still operate. Cells with no repair system but dividing uncontrollably in the absence of oxygen? A cancer in the making.

Minerals can show epigenetic benefits too!

Your cancer is as individual as you are

There are many ways your healthy messaging process can be interrupted. Not just are there different 'types' of cancer (breast, colon, prostate etc), but beyond this there may be many ways you can develop a breast cancer or a brain tumour. Already orthodox medicine has acknowledged that there are oestrogen positive, or progesterone positive, or HER-2 positive, or stem cell breast

13

cancers but even that might not be enough. A 2012 study discovered that there were twelve types of breast cancer, concluding we don't have the treatments yet! One American study looked at over 1,400 cases of breast cancer and found they were all histologically different. And if that is the state of play with breast cancer, sadly we are a long way off any such understanding and treatment for other cancers.

Your cancer is as individual as you are. Of course, there are 'more common' formations, but I really can't agree to 'one size fits all', and this is one of the reasons, I don't think that there will ever be a single wonder drug. And oncologists already know this too.

Cancer is a whole body disease

However, there are some common factors to cancer. For example, if you take the blood of a cancer patient and look at it under a microscope you will usually see two things: First, that the red cells are clumped together, indicating lowered levels of oxygen; and secondly, that the white cells are static, indicating a weakened immune system.

Also, the liver of cancer patients is almost always toxic, not damaged but debilitated, poisoned by the effects of the cancer and its causes. And your liver controls your whole body – from its ability to be detoxified, to the strength of the immune system to the energy production systems.

This is important because it suggests that whilst a cancer tumour may well be localised, the conditions that caused it and its effects are present throughout the body. Cancer is a disease of the whole body – and you have to treat it as such.

Cancer cells are different

There are certain features known about cancer cells that you might find helpful to know up-front.

Cancer cells produce their energy by a process of fermentation 'burning' glucose and sometimes glutamine (an amino acid) in the cytoplasm of the cell, rather than burning pyruvate in the presence of oxygen in the power stations (mitochondria). This process is very inefficient and so cancer cells need increasing supplies of glucose to grow. Experts such as Professor Thomas Seyfried of the

Boston College have noted that in the absence of glucose, healthy cells are flexible and simply switch to burning fats (ketosis), whereas in the absence of glucose and glutamine, inflexible cancer cells wither and die.

Research from Johns Hopkins *(Journal of Clinical Oncology)* confirmed that cutting glucose could benefit colon cancer patients, while researchers Onodera, Jin Min Nam et al *(Journal of Clinical Investigation, Jan 2014)* have gone further and shown glucose actually CAUSES cancer.

Seyfried is adamant that cancer is a metabolic disease (caused by poor metabolism) and is therefore reversible. You can start by not feeding it refined common sugar and carbohydrates, and lowering protein consumption whilst increasing good fat consumption – something officially called the Ketogenic Diet, but which has been the basis of the Rainbow Diet for 8 years.

Meanwhile drugs companies have scientists studying the unique enzymes and proteins of the energy processes in cancer to try to interrupt their actions, but nature has proven it already knows the answers.

Cancers are very acid at their centres. Acid bodies and lowered oxygen encourages their spread. Certain foods increase blood oxygen, and others are very alkalising.

Cancers like iron and this is why, even before taking drugs, cancer patients can be anaemic. The last thing you should do is take iron supplements. You'll be supporting the cancer.

Finally, heat is known to kill cancer cells – localised hyperthermia seems capable of killing them. But there are foods that can create the same conditions inside the cancer cell.

So – how can anyone think diet could help beat cancer?

I hope you can now see that any cancer – your cancer – might have come about in any number of ways. It is as individual as you are. And it is also a systemic, all-over-body disease.

And as I went through the options could you see how diet might play a role?

As I go through this book I will show you how a good diet and natural bioactive compounds can help by:

- Providing important factors to perfect DNA copying
- Providing important factors to correct DNA mis-copying
- Avoiding excesses of factors that increase free-radicals
- Providing more antioxidants to neutralise free-radicals
- Removing the toxic chemicals and heavy metals from your body and cells
- Boosting your immune system and helping it 'see' rogue cells
- Keeping your cells and immune system alkaline
- Avoiding parasitic and microbial infection
- Minimising pathogens in the blood stream
- Reducing inflammation – a precursor of many cancers
- Preventing a blood supply to the developing tumour
- Lowering aggressive oestradiol levels
- Keeping blood and cellular oxygen levels up
- Strengthening your liver, and therefore your immune system
- Increasing your pancreatic enzyme production
- Killing cancer cells
- Increasing survival rates through epigenetic effects

These are just 17 examples – it could have been more! The fact is that science has shown, rather unsurprisingly I suppose, **there are natural compounds that can have a significant effect in each of the many cancer stages.**

Please be clear – this statement is very different to claiming a food or a natural compound is a 'cure' for cancer. No natural compound, to my knowledge, can be honestly said to work on **all of the development stages** of cancer. But then certainly no drug should claim this either. For example:

- There is good research that isoflavones and garlic can stop the blood vessels developing that are needed for the tumour to grow bigger. But there is little evidence they can attack and kill a cancer cell or stop it firing off secondaries.
- There are a number of compounds – from salicylin to omega-3 – which can reduce inflammation, but there is little evidence they can help the immune system recognise a rogue cell and kick it out.

Cancer isn't an item – it's a process

And that leads me to another important conclusion that can be drawn from this little look at the life and times of a cancer. I have shown how there can be many 'types' of cancer which have developed in different ways. But more than that, a cancer can be present in any number of stages – rogue cell, tumour formation and metastasis being just three.

So you should not think of cancer as a 'single item' – it is a complex, multi-step, multi-stage process. It's not an ant you can tread on. It's a complex chain of events and you need a width – a package – of activities that can tackle it.

I gave you only a taster above. John Boik, formerly of the MD Anderson Cancer Center in Texas, estimates that there are 20 stages of cancer – and you may have any number of them in your body at any one time.

Just as I don't think that there will ever be a 'magic bullet' to kill all the different 'types' of cancer, I don't think there will be one to kill the cancer in all the many stages it might be in within your body. It is simply too much to ask of one drug, one natural compound or one herb. But I do genuinely believe you could select a number of natural compounds and herbs each of which tackled different stages of the cancer formation and existence and so worked synergistically to tackle the whole job. And by the end of this book I sincerely hope you will agree.

Boik's theory is contained in his book called '*Natural Compounds in Cancer Therapy*'. There he looked at over 4000 major research studies on natural compounds – and that was in 2001. There would be ten times that number nowadays!!

From this body of evidence he assigned various natural compounds (including foods, herbs and supplements) against the twenty stages, in terms of their proven scientific abilities.

Now, I'm not going to frighten you in this book with the biochemistry of how each foodstuff fights each step. I'm not a professor talking to scientists at a symposium. I'm a knowledgeable layman trying to help people who want to beat cancer build a picture of what foods should be in their diet. And that's what I will do.

17

But I think that the crux of this whole chapter is an understanding that cancer is:

- A disease that can have many drivers – it's as individual as you are.
- A disease that can have many stages – it's a process not an item.

And natural compounds have been proven in history (and increasingly in the latest research) to be able to tackle each and every facet of both of these.

Yes, I am 'stupid enough to think that diet could help beat cancer'. You are not doomed – it is reversible.

"I believe cancer can be cured, today – if not 'cured' then held in remission permanently"

I didn't make this statement, although I have long held it to be true. One of America's top oncologists, Henry S. Friedman MD, did and it's on the home page of The Preston Robert Tisch Cancer Center website!

CHAPTER 2
TOXIC BODIES

We receive a vast number of telephone calls, e-mails and enquiries into the **CANCERactive** offices from people newly diagnosed with cancer. In 95 per cent of cases, it takes about two minutes, often less, to see what is wrong – what caused the cancer: Most people are both **Toxic**, and **Nutritionally Deficient**.

Some aspects of 'Toxicity' may be caused by poor diet. Obviously, addressing the issue of poor diet is the prime purpose of this book and we will cover it in due course. But there are other causes of toxicity which I need to cover here, especially as I'm sure most people would assume diet had no role to play in helping overcome these 'non-diet induced problems' – and they'd be wrong!

Much of this toxicity is down to this modern world of ours – and it's getting worse.

Drugs

Some people in the medical profession like to tell you that modern drugs have all been through extensive clinical trials to prove their efficacy and safety. Sadly, they are deluded. Only about 15 per cent of the drugs available in the UK today have been through a clinical trial. Even then, the latest clinical trials quantify the benefits but rarely quantify the side-effects. The great white hope of more tightly targeted drugs with fewer side effects also seems an illusion. The Lancet Oncology magazine reported on the problems of high levels of side-effects when testing new monoclonal antibodies in 2007. We've all read of 'Elephant man' drug tests and deaths caused by Vioxx, with associated scandals. We are not deluded.

More worrying is the increasing quantity of drugs consumed. While a single drug may have been through a clinical trial, rarely, if ever, have combinations. Someone on heart medication may be taking others to prevent nausea and side-effects. They then get a cold and cough and take paracetamol, antibiotics and cough mixture. According to Dr. Stern at the New York Presbyterian

Hospital, it is not uncommon for people over 65 years of age to take more than 10 drugs at one time. He should know. So alarmed was he at the increasing level of hospital admissions he joined other doctors in coining a new disease, 'Polypharmacy' – illness due to a cocktail of drugs.

Polypharmacy currently accounts for 28 per cent of all hospital admissions in the US. These have more than tripled in the last seven years – as has the death rate from the disease. It is now the number one cause of death in Florida ahead of heart disease and cancer.

Drugs are tested on fit, healthy young to middle aged people. Two thirds of them are used by the over 65 age group whose biological systems are weaker and less able to deal with the toxins.

But don't think this is something beyond your own personal world. US Medical websites claim cancers like kidney cancer can be caused by painkillers. In **icon** we covered research that showed taking paracetamol with coffee can cause liver damage! How many times have you seen someone do that?

The truth is that all drugs are toxic; all drugs have (even minor) side-effects. And this includes the contraceptive pill, HRT (the alarming figures are on our website) and synthetic vitamin pills too.

Worryingly, three quarters of the applications to **CANCERactive** for Personal Prescriptions come from people who have had an illness for six or more years and have been taking a cocktail of drugs – for diabetes, thyroid, intestinal problems etc. Did they ever think to go to a naturopath or nutritionist? Do they and their doctor understand that taking drugs for six years may merely be covering up an underlying problem which could have/should have been addressed? Ignoring it while adding immune weakening drugs just makes matters worse.

We had one lady develop oesophageal cancer – she'd been on a stomach drug for 10 years. On the web it said quite clearly that the drug 'should not be prescribed for more than six months'. We asked her doctor what he thought might have caused her cancer. His reply? *"Just bad luck"*.

Finally, a recent study showed that 524 drugs available in the

USA had actually been manufactured in China – a country that has had more than its fair share of criticism over poor quality controls. Many more are made in other 'cheaper' production countries. Questions asked of the American drug approval organisation, the FDA, produced a response that less than three per cent of overseas drug production was monitored or safety checked. One wonders what percentage of UK administered drugs are safety checked, or have their production monitored, or their factories visited?

Chemicals

One million tonnes of chemicals were made in the world in 1946. Now the figure is 500 million tonnes. Apart from drugs and pesticides, where does it all go?

In *'Everything you need to know to help you beat cancer'* I go into more detail. But the answer starts with your home. The atmosphere in an American home has been shown to be more toxic than standing in Times Square, New York.

Household cleaners, bleaches, bathroom toiletries, shampoos, hair dyes, perfumes and so on contain chemicals that can disrupt your hormones, or chemicals that can poison you and are actually banned in some countries of the world. A number of these chemicals are proven carcinogens. Then there are glues for carpet and ceiling tiles, and gases from chipboard or old lead paint. According to the US Environmental Protection Agency 1500 hazardous substances are found in the average American home.

In 2007, Euro MEPs voted in favour of banning certain everyday chemicals like formaldehyde – it is already banned in Sweden and Japan. However, the Commissioners were lobbied by vested interests and did not ratify the bill, instead forming a regulatory board (REACH) which estimates a 15 year time frame before full regulation!

Europe is not alone in this stalled legislation. There are 80,000 chemicals registered in the USA, 15,000 in daily use but Federal Law does not require chemical companies to even review potential hazards! In 2005 there were 35 bills against hazardous chemical in the US legislature – all failed. California has

21

announced it is going to 'go it alone' in terms of regulating chemicals in the state. The latest news involved finding hermaphrodite fish (fish with both sexual organs) off the coast, thought to be the result of chemical waste passing down the rivers. Enough is enough, says California. We'll see.

There are several studies from the World Wildlife Fund showing that of 78 harmful chemicals, most of us now have between 25 and 49 in our bodies. And it is getting worse. Another of their studies reviewed levels in grandparents and grandchildren, finding twice as many in the youngsters.

The most hazardous chemicals are called dioxins. Later I will tell you about a natural compound that can prevent their damage and even remove them from your body!

Pesticides, fertilisers and herbicides

To complete the picture on chemical danger, there are pesticides, fertilisers and herbicides. We know that farmers have higher rates of certain leukaemias and myeloma; and incidence of leukaemia is increasing in homes next to golf courses in Australia. Children in households using garden and household pesticides have higher rates of certain cancers and there's even a link to flea collars! IARC have pointed a finger at nitrates and nitrites in fertilisers – with links to stomach, oesophagael and brain cancers.

In the UK Government Ministers responsible for pesticides and safety (DEFRA) requested a Royal Commission on Environmental Pollution. Despite conclusions that criticised existing policies, the Government has refused to recognise health risks as a result of spraying agricultural crops. Pesticides were not even mentioned in the 2004/5 White Paper on cancer.

Campaigners are now considering taking the UK Government to the High Court. However, the UK Government view is in direct contrast to that of Europe, who on 12th July 2006 stated that *'Long term exposure to pesticides can lead to serious disturbances to the immune system, sexual disorders, cancers, sterility, birth defects, damage to the nervous system and genetic damage'*. If that's not cause for concern, then I'm not sure what is!

Of course, there is much you can do with the foods and liquids you consume to avoid and correct the dangers of pesticides.

EMFs

The mobile phone and brain tumour controversy may well be reaching its end game as the WHO/Interphone worldwide study saw some researchers in some countries jumping the gun, and publishing their research in advance of the total results. All those researchers are saying there could well be problems with long term (over 10 years) usage. Australian experts are the latest to agree with experts in Sweden and Norway on this matter.

But more worrying is the bigger picture – the toxicity in our bodies caused by 'electrosmog'. 1500 phone masts have actually been pulled down in Taiwan, such were the health concerns. They are not the only country waking up to the threat. Worse, WiFi has absolutely no proper research on its safety, and small scale studies have even indicated that it might be more dangerous than direct beams from phone masts. Yet hotels, airports, apartment blocks, offices, the London Underground and even schools and hospitals rush to install it.

Computer screens, TVs in your bedroom and natural fault lines emit these EMFs and there are now clear research links (for example, between power cables and child leukaemia) with cancer.

As we will see later, these effects may not be direct genetic changing effects, but more likely effects causing a weakening of the immune system. One way this can happen is through melatonin depletion. Melatonin is a hormone most normally produced about 90 minutes after you fall asleep. It puts you into a deeper sleep. Its levels affect various other hormones, regulating oestrogen levels and the level of IGF-1, a hormone that increases cell division. And it is a powerful antioxidant. Now IARC have endorsed US research that shows melatonin depletion is carcinogenic.

EMFs are known to cause melatonin depletion. The good news is that poor melatonin levels can be addressed by diet.

Negating the damage - the amazing role diet can play

The question you must be asking yourself is, 'With all this going on around me what chance have I got?'

The answer is, 'A really good one'.

It is true SOME toxins cause genetic damage but, as I said, only a very few cancers come about in this way. This **Direct** attack produces rogue DNA, but most such changes usually result in gobbledegook messages being produced, which will be mopped up by your immune system.

In far more cases the toxins don't change the actual DNA structure but disrupt the chemical messages that it directs – for example, certain proteins or hormones. This may result in certain essential chemicals being over- or under-produced. And this is what has a huge and damaging effect on the body.

But diet can address the root cause and the excesses or deficiencies caused.

Pie in the sky? I can tell you that there are a number of natural compounds that can make a difference and can compensate for these imbalances – the research is very new.

For example, the Dana-Faber Cancer Institute have stated that there is no reason why the effects of cancer cannot be reversed. In cloning experiments with mice and melanoma, they concluded that, **whilst the body could not re-alter rogue DNA to make it normal again, the effects could be turned off and neutralised.** Thus, they concluded, **malignancy was not the inevitable effect of a cancer cell.**

Some people may feel cancer runs in their family and they have little chance of beating it. Firstly, it is true that you may have an hereditary genetic issue, but again this is not as widespread as some people suggest. It occurs in less than seven per cent of the population, although it is true that people with these problems seem to be particularly affected by toxins and chemicals. However, a Swedish Epidemiology study showed that identical twins who lead different lifestyles can have very different risk levels – so there is much you can do with your diet to minimise the risks.

By far largest group of people have not been 'Directly' genetically poisoned anyway. With these people toxins have an **Indirect** effect in the cancer process, for example, by weakening the immune system, by poisoning the cells, or by feeding dangerous hormones which may stimulate and maintain it. And all of these really can be addressed and corrected by a good diet.

Where the changes are not structural, the great majority of the toxins can be eliminated from your body, and diet can have a significant effect. For example:

- Pesticide research with children shows that switching to an organic diet 'washed' out key pesticides within 5 days.
- Heavy metals that are cumulative can be tackled by changes to the diet. Selenium is known to replace certain heavy metals from tissues; chlorella and spirulina can displace others.
- Beneficial bacteria have been shown in clinical trials to break down toxic oestrogenic and nitrosamine compounds, and aid natural fibrous compounds to bind to heavy metals to aid their excretion.
- Dangerous oestrogenic products – both human and chemical – have been shown in research to be broken down and neutralised by certain natural compounds like indoles
- Where toxins have caused mineral imbalances in the cells leading to acid cells, high potassium, high magnesium and low sodium diets have been shown to return cells to their healthy and alkaline states.
- Even dangerous chemicals like dioxins have been shown to have their effects neutralised by certain natural compounds, as we shall see.

So even where external factors like chemicals or EMFs may have significantly contributed to your cancer, research shows there are many things you can do in your diet to increase your personal odds of survival.

This is nothing new. Your body, its immune system and its little helpers, the beneficial bacteria in your intestine, have spent 200,000 years helping you kick out unwanted toxins using certain everyday foods as catalysts or carriers. For example, when beneficial bacteria break down oestrogenic chemicals they use plant indoles to help them cause destructuring, and plant lignans to carry the by-products out of the body. One question you might ask yourself is, *'Do I eat enough of the everyday foods that contain indoles and lignans, and do I have enough beneficial bacteria to complete the job?'*

Indeed, do you eat enough of the foods that provide the bioactive compounds that can protect you from the toxic world in which you live, or heal you when the toxins have caused a problem?

CHAPTER 3
ATOMIC MAN

Can you really change your cells?

The fully healthy body works in a state of balance and harmony. The unhealthy body is in a state of imbalance and disharmony.

This balance and harmony is both internal – through all your hormone, nervous and enzyme systems, from your brain right to the power stations in your breast or prostate cells – and external – in your inter-relationship with your localised, immediate environment, like the air you breathe, the water you drink, the flowers and the foods growing in your back garden.

Some civilisations believed that an illness in one person was a reflection of the strength of the whole tribe. Modern governments would do well to reflect on this.

At least 99 per cent of you and me is air, although, to look at each of us, I admit it is hard to imagine. Every molecule in your body is made of atoms and these are simply electrons spinning around a nucleus of neutrons and protons. Both electrons and neutrons are infinitesimally small particles, and between them, relatively speaking, are huge spaces or air masses. Think in terms of the earth, the sun and the moon, and you will understand the massive air gaps relative to the small 'solid' masses in an atom.

Atoms attract and repel other atoms. They are little electronic forces each with their own magnetic field. Too many of one atom might completely overwhelm the presence of another and prevent it from doing its job. It might simply displace it from its position in a molecule, and thus might stop the molecule working properly and helping other molecules work properly.

Building the correct molecules with the correct atoms makes for a body in harmony and balance with all its systems working perfectly. Obtaining the right numbers of atoms for your body is very important. Insufficient of the right ones, or too many of the wrong atoms will lead to illnesses.

This is not just a mathematical and practical issue. It is an energetic issue. If you have the wrong atoms and molecules in your breast cells you will also experience the wrong electronic and magnetic forces in those tissues. Since the Russian scientist Kirlian, we have been able to see the damage caused to our electronic fields around our body by excesses or deficiencies of minerals, and by illnesses. Interestingly, US scientists showed that our electronic fields (or auras) around our body 'become sick first'. And this is already being used in a variety of new diagnostic tools.

These electronic forces are very powerful. They affect and are affected by all manner of external atoms and their electronic fields. Recent research showed that little lizards climb up walls because each of their toes has a thousand minute hairs under them. The molecular fields of these hairs actually interact with the molecular fields of the atoms in the wall and 'hold' on. They are released by a nervous impulse sent from the brain when the animal wants to move. Such electronic interactions can make and break hundreds of times per second.

So where are the limits of your body? Certainly the electronic forces of the cells in your body, do not stop at your skin and the influence on your body by radiation from a mobile phone, power cables, WiFi, microwaves and X-rays is easy to understand.

Everyone has the power to change

It is easy to see how you might poison your metabolism quite quickly. But it is also easy to see how your recovery is equally possible. Clearly you have the power:

- **To change your own internal atoms.**
- **To control how many 'good' atoms you have.**
- **To stop negative external influences, and to build positive ones.**

Every day you exchange millions of atoms with your environment, every time you breathe, eat or drink, and even through your skin. So much so that **every 90 days the great majority of the body's tissues have atoms that are completely new to the body.**

You are 'Atomic Man' – a truly bionic being.

Four atoms in the health of your cells and immune system

The sodium-potassium balance

Common table salt is refined sodium chloride, as is about 90 per cent of sea salt. It doesn't matter whether it comes from the sea or from the mountains – it is sodium chloride.

You may hear the word 'salts'. These are something completely different. All manner of compounds like the carbonates, nitrates, bicarbonates and sulphates of many minerals like magnesium, calcium and manganese are 'salts'. Himalayan and Dead Sea salts, when pure, contain over 20 per cent of these other important mineral salts.

While salt contains sodium, not all sodium is consumed in salt. We ingest sodium as 'table' salt (sodium chloride), 'preservative' salt in meats and other foods (sodium nitrate, sodium nitrite); or 'taste-enhancing' salt (like monosodium glutamate).

Whichever way we take our sodium, the average individual in the West consumes much, much more than they need. So much more that it is making them ill. As animals in the wild, hundreds of thousands of years ago we ate virtually no salt. Indeed, we had to go to a salt 'lick' just to get some. In Roman times through to the Middle Ages salt was still a rarity and had become a currency to barter with. Hence the origin of the word salary from the Latin word *'salarium'*; *'sal'* being the word for salt. Salt had its place, but largely as a preservative for food stored for the winter months. From all this I could easily construct an argument that the maximum sodium intake should be around one gram per day in the cold climate of the UK. Yet the Food Standards Agency (FSA) still says six grams for adults and three for children, with no detailed rationale given. Worryingly, eight grams is a more usual Western consumption, whilst the average New Yorker consumes about eight kilogrammes per year or over twenty grams per day! And that is an average figure!

In February 2004 the US Institute of Medicine published a report stating that healthy 19–50-year-olds should consume 1.25 grams of sodium per day, much nearer to the figure I have suggested. Even allowing for the weight of the chloride or nitrite, this would yield an upper 'salt' limit of around 5 grams maximum. They note that 95 per cent of American males and 75 per cent of American females exceed this figure.

icon reported on new Japanese research that showed people who ate 12–15 grams of 'salt' per day on average doubled their risk of stomach cancer (*British Journal of Cancer*, February 2004).

Excess sodium has a devastating effect on all cellular membranes and inhibits the correct flow of essential elements into the cell. To that end it affects everything from your brain cells, to your immune cells, and virtually all the normal and healthy metabolic processes in every cell of your body.

It is impossible to talk about sodium without talking about potassium – they are opposing forces. Potassium is essential to the healthy workings inside your cells. Without it the cell becomes imbalanced and unhealthy. The easiest way to think of this is that sodium should largely work outside the cell, while potassium works inside the cell. Too much sodium stops potassium getting into a cell and, worse, actually causes the kidneys to expel it from the body as a whole.

If excess sodium moves inside the cell, it will prevent the proper action of potassium and will result in serious harm. Excess sodium poisons cells and particularly their power stations. Over thousands of years, our power stations, or mitochondria, have evolved to use potassium. It could have been anything – that's evolution for you – but it has turned out to be potassium. This is what makes them run smoothly, and potassium hydroxide, one of the main waste products produced, is alkaline.

If sodium displaces the potassium in the power stations, they will still work, but just not as well. The chemical reactions falter, the cell works inefficiently. Sodium waste products are produced and these are more acid than the potassium ones so the system becomes more acidic and yet more poisoned, drawing in less oxygen and producing less power, and the next cycle produces even more sodium salts and makes the cell even more acid, drawing in even less oxygen and producing even less energy. It's a vicious downward spiral and the cell is on its way to being a typical oxygen-free, restricted reaction, low-powered cancer cell.

If you want healthy cells your dietary intake of these two atoms should significantly favour potassium, about five to one over sodium. If you consume a gram of sodium today, can you really consume five of potassium? I doubt it. Just look at these figures for guidance.

Prime sources of **stressful sodium** are (approximately in milligrams):

Salt (1 teaspoon)	2000
Cheese, processed (100 gms)	1200
Cheese spread (100 gms)	1100
Stock cube (1)	1030
Bacon (1 rasher)	1000
Chicken nuggets (6)	1000
Corned beef (100 gms)	1000
Soy sauce (1 tablespoon)	1000
Gravy and sauces (100 gms)	1000
Cornflakes (100 gms)	1000
White bread (4 slices)	900
Baking soda (1 teaspoon)	820
French fries, salted (1 portion)	750
Cheddar cheese (100 gms)	600
Sausage (1 medium)	500
MSG (1 teaspoon)	500
Baked beans, canned (100 gms)	500
Pie casing (1)	500
Cottage cheese (100 gms)	450
Soup, canned	450
Fish, canned	450
Peanuts (100 gms)	420
Fish fingers (100 gms)	400
Spaghetti hoops, canned (100 gms)	400
Biscuits (100 gms)	375
Baking powder (1 teaspoon)	350
Crisps (2 packets)	350
Butter or margarine, salted (2 tablespoons)	250
Bread (1 slice – white, brown, wholemeal)	250

So you can see stressful sodium is found in certain categories of foods: preserved meats and sausages, condiments (from tomato ketchup to soy sauce), canned foods, breakfast cereals, bread (white or wholemeal), biscuits and cakes, all baked flour products, fast food, crisps and peanuts. Worst are preserved foods and processed foods, while a Chinese meal can give you a whopping 14 gms of the stuff.

Obviously fish, particularly shellfish, contain sodium (but nowhere near the levels of bread or fast foods) and even beer and fizzy soft drinks contain quite high levels of sodium to enhance the taste!

An excess of sodium is debilitating. Apart from its potential disruptive and even cancer-inducing effects inside the cell, it affects the water balance of the body and causes stress, fatigue and even depression.

Perky potassium is highly corrective of this. Apart from its control of the energy production in our cellular power stations, it affects crucially our protein and DNA synthesis. It helps in brain function, nerve transmission and muscle tone and is anti-ageing, whilst excess sodium ages tissues.

So it's not just about cutting sodium consumption. It is about consuming the right quantities of potassium, too. If cells are depleted of potassium, pathological change occurs with damaging acidic metabolites being produced, and the cell is on its way to disease and even death. Furthermore a lack of potassium inside a cell causes sodium to fill in the vacuum and sodium increases the metabolic acidity, further causing degenerative disease and cell death. A real double-whammy.

Perky potassium can be found in (approximately, in milligrams):

Lentils (100 gms)	1400
Potato, baked with skin (medium)	1250
Broad beans and peas (100 gms)	1200
Muesli, homemade (100 gms)	1000
Potatoes (250 gms)	800
Nuts (100 gms)	700
Banana (medium)	450

Fish, fresh (100 gms)	450*
Vegetables, green leaf (100 gms)	350
Meat, lean organic (100 gms)	350
Orange (medium)	300
Rice, brown (100 gms)	250
Carrots (100 gms)	250
Apple (medium)	200

* Depends on the fish – can vary from 150–450

In all of the above foods, sodium levels are negligible (even in fish where it is approximately 100 mgs per 100 gms). Potassium is found in vegetables and fruit, nuts and fish, brown rice and lean organic meat (beware non-organic red meat which often has sodium salts added to it to give it better colour). Parsley and garlic, those two French staples, are also good sources.

A simple rule of thumb is also that fresh food is low in sodium and high in potassium, whilst preserved, refined and prepared foods are the opposite.

The calcium-magnesium balance

One of the biggest and worst dietary hoaxes portrayed to the Western world over the last fifty years is that osteoporosis is caused by a deficiency of calcium so we must drink more milk to correct it. **This is completely inaccurate**, not borne out by the scientific evidence, and just a successful end product of Milk Marketing Board PR campaigns.

People in the West have the highest levels of blood calcium in the world – thanks to dairy. And the lowest levels of bone and tissue calcium – thanks to dairy.

Let me explain. **Dodgy dairy** provides high levels of blood calcium, but this inhibits the body's uptake of zinc (crucial in helping vitamin C with its cellular and anti-cancer activities), iron (crucial for maintaining the correct oxygen levels in blood and cells), and magnesium.

The last one is significant. The daily calcium requirement for good health is just less than one gram. Amounts in excess of this will actually cause magnesium depletion.

If you inhibit the uptake of **magnificent magnesium** you cannot absorb calcium into your cellular tissues or bones. Unsurprisingly in a population awash with cows' dairy, 2004 American research has shown that 40 per cent of adults are magnesium deficient.

Apart from magnesium, calcium also needs vitamin D to deliver it into the bones. Vitamin D is generated by the action of sunlight on your fat layers under the skin. Apart from this as a source, there are very small amounts in oily fish, and very, very low levels in dairy.

Magnesium is needed for vitamin D synthesis in the body. Low magnesium levels mean low vitamin D levels. So, too much dairy means high blood calcium, low magnesium and low vitamin D levels as a result. And low vitamin D levels mean low calcium absorption into bones and, worse, vitamin D deficiency is now clearly linked to a number of cancers from colon and breast cancers to brain tumours. Not surprisingly vitamin D supplementation is now being given as part of cancer therapies at a number of worldwide cancer centres.

Traditional healthy diets, from China to the Kalahari, or Greece to the Eskimos incorporate **no magnesium-depressive** cow's milk. Rather, they are magnesium-rich. Magnificent magnesium-rich.

Best foods for magnesium are nuts, pulses, melons, mango, fresh sweetcorn, jacket potato, bananas, green leaves, whole grains like millet, oats, buckwheat or wheatgerm and brown rice – a similar list to that of potassium.

If you cut all dairy from your diet this instant, you could still get your daily calcium requirement from 150 gms of spinach, or from a few almonds, or any of green beans, broccoli, leeks and an orange; or dried apricots, whole grains and wheatgerm. It's really quite easy to get your daily dose of calcium. Ordinary folk in South East Asia and China don't touch dairy – and they have no osteoporosis.

But this book is about cancer and diets – importantly in the context of cancer, magnesium is also crucial to your cells because it works a little pump which sits in your cell membranes. This pump actually pumps sodium out of the cell and potassium in. Without it, sodium drifts back in to poison the cells, whilst potassium drifts out.

Magnesium is also crucial in the efficient working of your mitochondrial power stations. It prepares the fuel for burning. Without it – for example, if you are on a slimming diet – you might have terrible cravings for food when in reality you have ingested more than enough calories. Without magnesium to prepare the food you ingested and turn it into the right sort of fuel, your cells will go hungry.

Magnesium levels are also lowered by:

- Refining our foods – which removes magnesium from the grain.
- Stress and excess physical activity – which burns up magnesium in the energetic process.
- Tea, coffee, alcohol – alcohol reduces magnesium levels significantly.
- High sugar, carbohydrate and fat diets – which are nutritionally empty yet require magnesium for energy production.

It is not recommended that you supplement long term with magnesium. And calcium supplements that are neither organic, nor combined with magnesium can cause more harm than good. The answer is good nourishing foods – like those listed above.

Finally, magnificent magnesium is crucial to a healthy liver; a healthy liver is your crucial organ of detoxification for the whole body, and the neutraliser of nasty free-radicals. Having a healthy liver is vital if you want a healthy body.

Atomic Man?

So, by eating potassium and magnesium-rich foods and limiting your intake of sodium and calcium, you will see that you have the ability to alter the power levels in your cells, your total body energy and even the electrical forces in and around your body.

This 'ability' is a product of the minerals you consume daily. Each and all of them has an 'electronic influence' whether positive – like boron, selenium, zinc or iron – or negative like chlorine, cadmium or mercury. Minerals thus have epigenetic benefits; some help maintain the integrity of your DNA code by their presence in the 'soup' around your core double helix; others hinder.

The universe is energy. Even the Queen is 100 per cent energy. You are indeed Atomic and Bionic Man (or Woman!)

CHAPTER 4
HEALTHY LIVER – HEALTHY BODY

In the UK and America few of us pay any attention to our livers. We know we have one but we don't know too much about it. Worse, we mistreat it. Day in, day out.

Yet the people of China or Italy look to their livers at the first sign of illness. The routine health check I had in Beijing consists of a doctor looking into your ears and eyes, and then at your tongue. The state of the tongue will tell you much about the state of your intestines and liver; the colour of your eyes will tell you the levels of toxins present.

In France and Italy the feeling of being a bit 'rundown' is normally met with a shrug and the explanation 'une crise de foie' – a crisis of the liver. A little too much alcohol perhaps; even something they ate; and occasionally a bit of an infection. The locals will avoid fat for a few days and eat more vegetables like artichokes, fruits like melon and drink water. Why, they even have bottled waters that are well suited to reviving a flagging liver! The brand Hepar in France is magnesium-rich and sells itself on its benefit to your liver.

By contrast, I cannot remember the last time a doctor in the UK looked at my tongue, nor the last time someone said they were feeling 'a bit livery'. Whatever happened to Andrews Liver Salts?

But your life depends on your liver. It is the largest organ in your body and a very complex one at that. It has a great many important functions, none more so than its ability to **detoxify the blood**: A healthy liver filters almost two pints of blood per minute, cleaning your system, so it can draw in all the toxins and waste that your cells need to excrete.

The modern world subjects a liver to a huge range of 'poisons' which impair its function: Alcohol, pesticides, chemicals, antibiotics, drugs and external hormones like animal hormones, HRT and the contraceptive pill. Any and all of these poisons can damage the Kupffer cells, which are responsible for breaking down toxic matter, thus impairing the biochemical pathways and reducing the performance of the liver significantly. Oestrogen can be a particularly debilitating agent, preventing the liver from detoxifying fats and generally reducing its effectiveness.

The liver also **helps make some vitamins and hormones** – it plays a role in converting precursors into vitamin D, for example.

It helps in **'energy' control systems**, being involved in providing the correct fuel for your cells from the stores of sugar and carbohydrate.

A healthy liver plays **an important role in the immune system,** being involved with the white cells, and manufacturing substances like anti-histamines, essential to the immune system.

One of the main jobs of a healthy liver is to **produce bile** – about three pints per day. The bile, along with its metabolic agents, the bile salts, works with the liver to metabolise fats and cholesterol and excrete waste. The process involves vast numbers of small bile ducts running throughout the liver and collecting into one common bile duct, which passes directly into the intestine. About half way along this duct sits a balloon-like object, the gall bladder, whose contractions help force the bile, along with its waste products, into the intestine.

A healthy liver also **aids digestion and absorption.** If the bile system is blocked and working inefficiently, the body's system for absorbing vitamins and minerals will be impaired. The bile works alongside enzymes, helpful bacteria and acids in the intestine to break down foods into absorbable parts. Afterwards, up to 95 per cent of the bile acids are normally reabsorbed and carried back to the liver.

Fatty livers

A fatty liver affects more than 50 per cent of adult Americans. Their carbohydrate-rich and fat-rich diets cause a log-jam in the liver.

This is not helped by the increasing number of toxins we 'ingest'. When the liver is damaged by such toxins, it loses its efficiency to clear fats and toxins from the body, and is more likely to become 'clogged up'. If it then cannot process the fats, they will build up in the blood stream and fatty deposits will occur all over the body causing all sorts of health problems.

Worse, fat is an excellent solvent and so those fatty deposits will be toxin-charged, holding free-radicals, hormones and toxins in various parts of the body and creating the environment for a cancer to form.

Gallstones

Gallstones resemble small grains of sand. They are formed by cholesterol and fat collecting around clumps of bacteria, or even pieces of dead parasite (rather like a pearl forms around sand particles, or around dead cells).

You might have none, but it is unlikely. Research showed that some 70 per cent of Americans have gallstones. Because each tends to be very small you may have as many as 3000.

Gallstones multiply the problems of fatty livers by blocking the bile ducts of the liver and preventing the free flow of the unwanted fats, cholesterol and toxins into the intestines.

Another research study in the US showed that 99.95 per cent of cancer patients in American hospitals had gallstones. But then cancer patients, after chemotherapy or radiotherapy treatment, also have a lot of dead cells in their livers.

The liver and cancer

If the liver function is impaired, if it is over-worked or full of fats, or blocked by gallstones, or poisoned by toxins, the whole body becomes less efficient, from the immune system to the removal of toxins from inside your cells.

It's a chain reaction. Your power stations become toxic and they pass the waste into the cell. From there it passes to the lymph and from there into the blood. Finally, the wastes circulate to the liver, are 'treated' and pass into the bile, and from there out into the intestine. Block one step and the toxins find it hard to leave the power stations – the control centre for cancer.

Because the liver is involved in so many functions, there are other repercussions. For example:

- The impairment of the white immune cells' ability to recognise, attack, ingest and then bring the cancer cells for treatment in the liver.

- The impairment of the body's fuel storage system, resulting in lowered levels of stored fuel (glycogen) whilst increasing the fuel loved by cancer cells (glucose).

Cancer cells burn glucose and, sometimes glutamine, in the absence of oxygen.

The end product of this energy production is lactic acid, in itself highly toxic. The only place lactic acid can be detoxified is in the liver and that further increases the workload.

Then, of course, the doctors give you chemotherapy drugs – and the dead cells and the toxins in the drugs will all demand processing space from the liver cells. Radiotherapy, anaesthetics, antibiotics, steroids. Let's load it up and see where the breaking point is!

What steps can we take?

We will take the extreme case, namely that of a cancer patient. People wishing to prevent a cancer can decide for themselves how much of this is relevant to their circumstances.

The start point is that you can do things to flush out your liver – and other things to strengthen it.

The good news is that liver cells re-grow. Where a liver has been cut away, it will regenerate itself. Liver cells can completely detoxify themselves given the right conditions in about 8-12 weeks.

So here goes.

Cleaning out your liver

Some of you may have heard about the Gerson Therapy. It has its fans, and it has its critics. One part of it is the use of coffee enemas. Some oncology experts when criticising the Gerson Therapy in the National Press exposed their ignorance by saying daft things like 'How can anybody expect coffee to cure cancer?' Well Gerson didn't! He used coffee enemas simply because they dilate the bile ducts and help the excretion of more of the waste – especially if there are blockages in the bile ducts. Five freshly prepared coffee enemas per day were in his original therapy, although other therapists have now reduced it to two, saying that preparing them can take a lot of time.

Another option is to use a proper liver flush. An effective liver flush and gallstone remedy is included in the Appendix. This uses a mixture of Epsom Salts, olive oil and fruit juice to clear out the blockages. You mix the Epsom Salts, olive oil and a fruit juice of your own choosing (to make the whole thing palatable) then drink a quarter at 10.00pm, another quarter at 10.30pm. Then you retire for the night. The last two quarters are consumed upon waking, and half an hour later. The effects (!) may last for two days, but people who have used it said it was all over by lunch time. One lady complained that she had excreted masses of small yellowy-green 'bits'. Well, that's the bile-covered gallstones. It worked. The general response amongst all users who tried it has been excellent with talk of more energy and a better feeling of health afterwards.

The simplest version – although possibly not as effective – is to take a dose of Epsom Salts once a month. A tablespoon of Epsom Salts dissolved in lukewarm water tastes foul, but the next morning after a visit to the toilet, you may well have a much cleaner liver.

Strengthening your liver

Epsom Salts contain magnesium sulphate and so provide much needed magnesium. This will help strengthen the liver (remembering that alcohol and caffeine both cause the liver stress and deplete magnesium levels). You should also major on magnesium-rich foods.

Probably the best herbs are milk thistle and dandelion, which strengthen the liver system and cells. Both are better taken as liquid than pills.

Boldo tea strengthens the bile system as does globe artichoke, both promoting the excretion of fatty bile. Beets and radishes also get the juices going, as do green salads, green vegetables, spirulina, chlorella, wheat grass and barley grass.

Stopping the problem in the first place

Cutting fat out of the diet is, of course, one of the key principles seen in a number of anti-cancer diets. But it's not as simple as that. Some fats are bad – from animal fats to 'trans' fats, while some fats are good, like those in olive oil and walnut oil. Even the infamous cholesterol is recognised now to have two forms – a bad and a good. And, be clear, you need the good one!

Diets high in saturated fats, polyunsaturated fat and refined carbohydrates should be avoided as all cause the liver to produce triglycerides, which are particularly stressful to the body. A number of research studies have shown that the cholesterol molecule is too big to get across the gut wall, and is actually re-formed on the other side. The components don't have to come from fats. They can come from carbohydrate too. So carbohydrate can just as easily give rise to your fatty blood and liver problem.

One way of regulating the level of circulating bad fats has been shown to involve the right beneficial bacteria in your intestines.

Beneficial bacteria, which are in reduced numbers in the modern body especially if you are taking prescription drugs, can break certain foods down to form short chain esters. In the blood stream these act to stop bad fats and cholesterol re-forming. We will look at beneficial bacteria in more detail later, but having enough of them in total, and enough of the right strains, are a vital part of your good health, and the fight against cancer.

A diet high in lignans (plant fibre) provides factors that can bind to fats in the blood stream and help expel them from the body. Do you want to lower your (bad) cholesterol? Never mind statins. Start with whole oat porridge in water for breakfast, virgin olive oil, fish oils, garlic, flaxseed and lycopene (tomatoes) in your diet.

Free-radicals provide the spark igniting triglycerides in the liver to become dangerous and aggressive. Vitamin E and selenium work in the liver to neutralise these free-radicals. Turmeric and the B vitamins, especially choline and inositol (found in soya lecithin), will also keep them in check.

Finally, most people live in blind ignorance of the fact that they may well have a parasite. This does not have to be ten feet long. It can be microscopic – a virus, yeast, microbe or a bacterium. Up to 70 per cent of people in the Western world have excessive yeast infections (typical signs are thrush, cystitis, yellow toe nails, bloating). We will deal with this in detail in a later section.

Suffice it to say here that parasites may occupy the liver or, at minimum, produce toxins and even carcinogens the liver has to deal with and which debilitate the immune system. Herbal parasite purges do exist and are usually a mixture of wormwood, slippery elm, Pau d'Arco, black walnut, clove and garlic, plus a number of immune system boosters. Interestingly Pau d'Arco was originally thought to be a 'cure' for cancer until its true action as a yeast and parasite killer was discovered. Wormwood has been found to kill yeasts and parasites but also to have a direct effect on cancer cells *(Professor Lai, University of Washington)*. Wormwood also weakens certain enzymes which help accumulate the high iron levels needed in cancer cells.

Phew!

The final word

Love your liver!

Ignore it at your peril.

Help it, strengthen it, clean it and stop the potential problems at source.

Your diet should be its FRIEND.

CHAPTER 5
CANCER – A WEIGHTY PROBLEM

A bigger health risk than smoking

It may surprise you to know that, according to the statistics, **being obese is a bigger cancer risk factor than smoking.** I could quote you any number of studies but, by and large, smoking increases your risks of cancer by about 25 per cent and being overweight increases your risks by between 40 and 60 per cent depending on how overweight you are.

Erasmus College Rotterdam re-analysed American population data taken over a fifty-year period and concluded if you were forty years old and just four kilograms overweight you reduced your life expectancy by 3 years. At ten or more kilograms the loss was 7 years for women and 5.6 for men.

If you are ten or more kilograms overweight and you smoke, **you chop 13 years off your life expectancy.**

Be clear. 7 kgs is not a big number. By and large people delude themselves. They write to CANCERactive – for example one, a woman with breast cancer who, at 5 feet 2 inches and 73 kgs, described herself as 'a bit chunky'. She should be around 52 kgs.

Furthermore, overweight people pay 12 per cent more visits to the doctor each year and spend 19 per cent longer per year in hospital *(Men's Health UK, 2002)*.

Being overweight has been linked to several cancers like breast, prostate and ovarian cancer. The UK Under Secretary for Health, Hazel Blears, said, *"There are clear links between obesity and our biggest killers – heart disease and cancer."*

We have covered a number of research studies in **icon** on the links between being overweight and cancer risk. *Cancer Epidemiology* (Feb 13 2004) contained a study showing that women who increased weight after the age of 18 increased breast cancer risk. Over 9 kgs and risk goes up by 40 per cent, over 30 kgs and the risks double. The Fred Hutchinson Center in Seattle has directly linked obesity in women with a 20 per cent increase in breast cancer risk – they have yet to look at other cancers.

All is not lost though. North Carolina University has produced a study showing that women who lose their excess weight, even after developing cancer, greatly improve their survival rates. This is totally in line with the American Cancer Society report I told you about that people who actively include weight control in their Integrative Programme do survive longer and even prevent cancer returning

It might be in your genes

Researchers from 77 Institutions in six countries have been analysing the DNA of 90,000 individuals. One in seventeen Britons has a genetic flaw in their FTO gene, discovered in 2007, and this gives them a problem in losing weight. Adults with the flaw are around three and a half pounds heavier and 24 per cent more likely to be obese than those without the flaw. However, since genes come in pairs, those people with a pair of flawed genes and two flawed copies of FTO tend to be more than 7 pounds (3.5 kgs) heavier than those 'flaw-free'. And so, according to lead researcher Dr Innes Barroso, some people will find it harder to lose weight than others.

I haven't got any answers for this – I just thought you should know! Being overweight is not always because you simply eat too much!

The overall problem's getting worse

The Organisation for Economic Co-operation and Development published a report in October 2002 stating that the UK has the second highest level of obesity in the world after the USA. With 21 per cent obesity we follow the USA at 26 per cent. By contrast the Swiss are Europe's best at only 6.8 per cent and the Japanese have a lowly 2.9 per cent.

One third of UK boys under six are overweight or obese, rising to almost 50 per cent by the age of 16. In the USA it is 60 per cent. The picture is worsening.

The European Conference on Oncology in 2005 heard that the UK leads Europe: 25 per cent of England's 13-17 year olds are obese. Next come Greece, Cyprus, Italy and Ireland at 23 per cent, but Germany has only 11 per cent and Holland just 9.

The old description of 'puppy fat' has now been shown to be an error. More than a quarter of schoolchildren are overweight or obese by the age of 11. Worse are girls (29 per cent) and especially black girls (38 per cent). The figure then hardly decreases at all as they age, according to CRUK.

Another study that year showed that the top ten foods of our teenagers are:

Boys	Girls
1 – Pizza	1 – Chocolate
2 – Chocolate	2 – Strawberries
3 – Ice Cream	3 – Fruit Juice
4 – Chocolate Biscuits	4 – Pasta
5 – Fruit Juice	5 – Pizza
6 – Ice Lollies	6 – Ice Cream
7 – Fizzy Drinks	7 – Grapes
8 – Pasta	8 – Ice Lollies
9 – Cakes	9 – Chocolate Biscuits
10 – Crisps	10 – Cakes

Girls eat fruit and vegetables more than boys but the average young person's diet is salt- and sugar-rich, biased towards refined, non-nourishing foods and, not surprisingly, they are already deficient in important minerals like magnesium, and consume virtually no 'greens' which provide essential anti-cancer vitamins like vitamin K.

47 per cent of children in Britain eat no vegetables other than potato in a month and a recent survey showed that half of ten-year-olds could not even recognise certain vegetables like broccoli correctly.

Junk food is so named for a reason. For example, in 2012/13 McDonalds in the USA finally agreed to cut out trans fats, despite having been taken to court twice.

Several studies in 2007 have put fizzy soft drinks in the spotlight. Apart from large quantities of empty sugar, or dubious sweeteners like aspartame, there are increasing concerns over the ingredient E211 (sodium benzoate) which messes up your mitochondria, and scientists say safety limits have been set too high. Then other colourings have been linked with tissue inflammation, and a study from Harvard on 6000 middle aged men and women showed those who drank at least one can a day were 30 or more per cent likely to be obese, have higher blood triglycerides and bad cholesterol.

Sadly, the UK is top of the table for the consumption of junk food in Europe with both our 5-9 and 10-13 age groups consuming more confectionary and fizzy soft drinks. Our next-to-useless Foods Standards Agency merely says this could be a warning that they will be the first generation to live shorter lives than their parents.

So, what's the problem with being overweight?

The problem with being overweight is that it has a number of consequences. For example:

- Fat is a wonderful solvent – and so stores toxins, excess hormones you would rather have excreted.
- Your hormones are more likely to be out of balance.
- Your sugar control and energy production systems are weaker.
- The excess weight puts stresses and strains on key organs, like your thyroid, pancreas and liver.
- While you cannot see it, visceral fat is actually more dangerous than the spare tyre you have round your waist. Visceral fat coats our internal organs like our liver and kidneys, thus holding toxins right up against cells we would like to remain healthy.

Being overweight is also indicative of other 'lifestyle' features:

- A poor diet, higher consumption of poor foods, higher toxicity, nutritional deficiency.
- A lack of sufficient exercise, a sedentary lifestyle, lowered lymph movement, lowered blood oxygen levels.
- A lack of self esteem, inattention towards one's own importance and health.

Being overweight is invariably simply due to an intake of too many calories, and the use of too few. Not only do most overweight people eat too much – they eat badly. And it causes a number of health problems and is linked to diseases like heart disease and diabetes, not just cancer.

The junk diets of the British (when compared, say to the Mediterranean Europeans) make Britons a sick bunch of people. According to a 2006 epidemiology study by Leicester University, the populations of seven out of eleven countries in Europe live longer than us – their women by up to three years more. However, we don't just die younger, we are ill longer. Apparently our women have 60.9 healthy years compared to, say, Italian women at 74.4, Spanish at 70.2 and the EU average at 66.0. Our men fair slightly better at 61.5 healthy years, compared to Italian men at 70.9, Spanish men at 66.8 and an EU average of 64.5 years. The Mediterranean diet, sunshine, attitude to life and happiness were suggested as factors.

Moving further afield, the Okinawans have the highest life expectancy in the World, followed close behind by the Bush people. Two factors are significant. Firstly, unlike Western adults, both have reducing blood pressure as they age, probably due to the lack of sodium salt in their diets. Secondly, they have calorie-restricted diets – the Okinawans consume about 40 per cent less calories than even the Japanese.

Calorie restriction

This is not the first time calorie restriction has been noted as a benefit to life expectancy. The Norwegians had their food supplies dramatically reduced by the occupying German Military during the Second World War, yet their restricted diets of fish and lowered calories resulted in a 35 per cent overall health improvement.

Research studies with rats show that calorie deprivation results in increased longevity: A 10-30 per cent reduction can almost double their life span. Harvard Researchers (**icon** 2 – 2007) have even released a video explaining how cutting the food intake of any organism by 30-40 per cent can increase longevity.

Calorie restriction has a number of benefits:

- The body is slimmer and leaner. Less fat means less stored toxins.
- You will have a reduced metabolic rate. Your power stations are not required to work as hard or burn as much fuel, so less waste products, toxins and free-radicals are produced.
- You will have reduced levels of insulin and IGF-1 production (IGF-1 is a hormone that speeds up cell division). As we will see later, this reduces the risks of both diabetes and cancer.
- The body will exhibit an increase in stress response – increasing

survival hormones and, along with this, its ability to repair DNA and heighten cellular efficiency.

- It stimulates production of a group of hormones called 'sirtuins'. Whilst pharmaceutical companies are working on drugs to stimulate their production, your eat-to-beat cancer strategy can be improved by the knowledge that sirtuins are stimulated by resveratrol, a natural compound found especially in the skins of organic red grapes. It is found in all red grape, raspberry, blueberry and blackberry skins, its primary role being to stop moulds entering the fruit. Unfortunately, the use of pesticides kills the mould and less resveratrol is produced in non-organic fruits, as there is less 'mould attack'.
- There are also scientific studies which show a restriction of calories can stop tumour growth.

So where do you start if you are overweight?

Most people think losing weight involves quite extreme measures such as starving oneself and joining a gym. Try some simple things first:

- Buy only the foods listed in the shopping list part of this book. Eating the right foods is far better than eating no foods!
- Eat a plate of salad vegetables as a starter 30 minutes before your main dinner or lunch. It will reduce the levels of 'hunger hormones'.
- Eat 6 small meals a day, not one or two big ones.
- Don't have carbohydrate and protein on the same plate – it confuses the stomach systems as we will see later, and increases fat stores.
- Don't eat less than two hours before going to bed.
- Yes, and try to take daily exercise. For example, walk briskly for at least 20 minutes every day (or take other forms of exercise, which I will tell you about).

CHAPTER 6
A DIET FOR PREVENTION?

"There is a convincing body of information that proves that there is a strong dietary basis to the development of cancer."
(Jonathan Waxman, Professor of Oncology, Imperial College, London, writing in BMJ 25 November 2006)

The World Health Organisation has said as much too, concluding that 30-50 per cent of cancers are caused by 'Poor Diet', depending upon which report you read. Poor diet is one of the main 'causes' of cancer while a good diet prevents.

So, what is a 'Good Diet' in the context of cancer prevention?

As this book develops you will increasingly realise that diets can, and do, help a great many people beat cancer, whether they have it already, or simply want to prevent developing it in the first place.

But is a good anti-cancer diet the World Health Organisation's mantra of, '*A little bit of everything, based on starchy foods and 5 lots of fruit and vegetables a day*', or is it something else?

Possible diet contenders for the Annual Cancer Prevention award include:

- The Vegetarian Diet
- The South East Asian Diet
- The Macrobiotic Diet
- The Mediterranean Diet
- Newer theories like the Paleo Diet or the Ketogenic Diet

Adding to the confusion

There seems little doubt in some people's minds that some diets, like the Vegetarian Diet or the South East Asian Diet, are associated with lower levels of cancer. They seem excellent 'preventative' diets.

Of course 'diet' is, in itself, a terribly ambiguous word. To the

51

great majority of women, say the word diet and they will answer, "*Which one?*", or "*Oh, no!*" Diet to them is a wearing experience, synonymous with cutting certain, often enjoyable, foods out of their normal daily lives. The French word for diet is 'régime', implying strictness as much as deprivation. Many cancer books will point you immediately in the direction of cutting out meat and maybe even fish too.

Obviously, I know that the Vegetarian Diet involves eating no meat. But people also tell me that's the basis of the South East Asian Diet too, and I know that's not true. I live there.

Is meat eating wrong?

There is clear research that eating too much red meat increases cancer risk.

Too much meat and especially animal saturated fats can increase free-radicals in the body. But, too much protein *per se* can increase risks of cancer *(Tannenbaum)* by increasing free-radicals, causing cellular changes, making your cells and your body too acid and more. (Remember, of course, that meat is not the only protein source in your diet.)

Meat has been shown in several research studies to increase levels of hormones responsible for cellular inflammation in the body.

Furthermore, the meat comes with the animal's own hormones, perhaps injected hormones, toxins and pesticides from the fields, and even colourings to make it look good in the shops. It's a good idea to cut it out, isn't it?

The Oxford Study on vegetarians and their diets concluded that they had 40 per cent less cancer than meat eaters. However, other information has to be factored in, for example: What if I told you that vegetarians are 80 per cent less likely to smoke? Or 60 per cent less likely to drink excess alcohol? For all I know, their increased interest in health might make them more likely to take daily exercise too. They are certainly 40 per cent less likely to be obese. To what degree does all this contribute to their 40 per cent reduced risk of cancer? Diet is merely a part of their whole 'healthier lifestyle' and it may be this which gives them 40 per cent less cancers.

Please believe me I'm not trying to be facetious here. I have received a couple of letters from indignant vegetarians saying that all the evidence points to a meat-free diet being highly protective. But research on organic meat and game shows it to be much higher in levels of inflammation-reducing omega-3. Is all meat really bad for you?

Several of the studies recently have compared the health of non-meat eaters with those eating the equivalent of a 12 oz steak each day! Is a moderate amount of meat bad for you?

I am also concerned about the real possibility of cancer resulting from vitamin and mineral deficiencies. For example, a little over 60 per cent of breast cancer patients seem to have vitamin B-12 deficiency. A Vegetarian Diet could make matters worse. Three quarters of vegetarians are known to be deficient in B-12, as the prime source is meat. (So, if you do decide to become vegetarian after cancer is diagnosed, please take chlorella, an excellent natural source of minerals, enzymes and certain vitamins – like vitamin B-12 and beta-carotene.)

Sally Beare in her book *The Live Longer Diet* studied longevity in various populations, and the Okinawans and the Bush People come top. The former eat fresh fish, the latter a little wild meat, and they both live longer than vegetarians. Vegetarians also don't actually live longer than an equivalent sample of health conscious, meat eating, non-smokers either. One important reason is that they still eat salt and sugar and these are important factors in restricting life-span.

One man's meat

Moreover, one man's meat can really be another's poison. Peter D'Adamo has written a very good book on choosing the right foods for your blood type: *Eat Right for Your Type*. In this book, he tracks how populations moved out of Africa and developed different blood types around the world. These different types actually thrive on different foods, often the foods that surrounded them over many thousands of years. The fittest adapt and grow stronger in tune with their localised, natural environments.

Choosing what is best for you and your personal biochemistry is called 'Metabolic Typing'. It has been taken to a fine art form by experts, like Bill Wolcott in the USA, who use blood tests or hair samples and can tell you that some people have a body biochemistry that thrives on meat eating, while others would do better to avoid it.

So, while I acknowledge that eating meat and animal fats can definitely be an increased risk factor for some people, I am actually not convinced that there is an benefit in giving up meat as part of an Integrative Programme if you already have cancer. Indeed, I have seen not one study that shows becoming vegetarian after you have developed cancer has any effect on increasing survival times. Of course you shouldn't eat too much red meat. But, from a scientific point of view on current research available I can't see what is wrong with eating a little free-range poultry or game. But then I am much more interested in trying to learn what foods we should be building into our diets to try to correct cancer.

The South East Asian Diet

Frankly, a lot of rubbish is talked about the South East Asian Diet, mostly from people who have never been near the place and merely pass on their interpretation of other people's interpretation of someone who visited once. I will try to give you an accurate feeling for the real South East Asian Diet.

I have travelled extensively in the region, from Vietnam, to Cambodia to rural China. I live in Thailand and my wife is Khmer – a vast area that crosses from East Thailand, through Laos and Cambodia. Cancer is almost non-existent and, although I do think that their diet is part of the reason, I think other factors are actually more important.

The Khmer eat soup for breakfast – made from boiling rice with herbs, chopped spring onions, garlic and ginger (or galangal), and a little chicken, pork or fish. Lunch is also soup – possibly the dish known as Tom Yum Kung in the West, a boiled river prawn dish with herbs, galangal, lemon grass, tomatoes and a little coconut milk. Alternatively, if they are out working in the fields, they will take sticky rice with them in little circular 'hampers' plus bits of fish and slices of green mango. Dinner might be 'barbequed' chicken, duck or river fish with vegetables, or Som Tam, a salad dish consisting of shredded green mango, papaya, cucumber, green beans, onions, tomato, herbs and carrot all mixed in a fish sauce with lime juice, chilli and garlic – very spicy. They might even throw in a river prawn or a small river crab.

Only in towns and cities is food fried in woks. In the rural areas it is boiled, or they grill it or bake it in improvised ovens. They never add salt – but do have thyroid problems from a lack of iodine, and sea salt is now extensively farmed along the coast.

They nibble at vegetables and fruit all day – they seem to be eating all the time. Fruit, which is fresh and sweet, is everywhere. Mangosteen, lychees, papaya, bamboo shoots, watermelon, rambutan, durian, pomelo, bananas, pineapple and many more. When Thais come to Europe they complain that our fruit is sour – and it is, because it has been picked unripe to travel and then last longer in our supermarkets.

They eat a lot of chilli (mainly in the evenings) and garlic and spring onions. Frankly, a lot of their vegetables resemble bits of twig and grass, but are fragrant so I guess are more correctly termed herbs.

Chickens run wild everywhere; they do have ducks, pigs and lots of cows, which they eat immediately after killing them; and they fish the rivers and lakes continuously. They eat a lot of fish. So you can see straight away that it is a fallacy that they are vegetarian, or too poor to eat 'meat'. A home can have five cows, three water buffalo and sixty chickens. In China the markets are full of fish, chickens and pork meat. Oh, and dead field rats and gutted, skinned dogs. In the North of Thailand and in Laos and China they eat certain wild birds, snails, whole frogs – not just the legs – and fried beetles and cockroach-like flies. They eat lots of eggs and even snakes.

They do not touch milk, and only recently has soya and sweetcorn milk come in packs to their villages. Interestingly the soya milk is 'reinforced with milk protein' according to the pack.

But, their food has no pesticides. They are scrupulously clean, but they use no make up or perfumes or toiletries. Their stone floors are swept clean and household cleaners and bleach unheard of.

Their natural exercise levels are high. One report about the Chinese showed that their natural exercise consumes 3600 calories per week. You would need to go to the gym and work out for one hour per day to equal this. They walk everywhere (in China they cycle!), they make everything themselves – houses, furniture, fences, etc., and they are fit. My wife's father at seventy six years of age is solid muscle, the sort of physique you see on the front cover of *'Men's Health'*.

They go to bed at eight-thirty at night (it gets dark at six-thirty) and sleep in total darkness. They wake at first light, and get up.

They smoke little, but drink in excess: Beer (every region has its own brand), rice wine and 'whisky' (which is really rum, because it is made from sugar).

They have two or three children – bribery helps get round the rules in China – and wouldn't dream of not breast feeding them for about nine months.

Their life expectancy, in my opinion, is lower than ours because they work so hard, outdoors in the sun and they simply get tired. It is also an issue of statistics – they have greater infant mortality and that reduces the average age of death, compared to the West. However, given that 80 per cent of cancers occur in the over 65 age group in the West, you can also see how many of them might not even be living long enough to develop the disease!

They are the happiest people I have ever come across – any excuse and they are dancing and laughing, being poor is just 'bad luck'. If someone is rich, it is their 'good luck', so jealousy is unheard of. If you have good luck then you share it with your family and friends. And the monks. And then you will come back in the next life luckier still.

Everyone eats 'a bit of dirt' daily. Hands touch cows or dogs and pass bits of chicken to you to eat, or scoop sticky rice up for the children's mouths.

Overall, the cancer rate in Thailand (which has the same population as the UK), is a quarter of ours. But, 'rich person's disease' is growing. The Thai Health Minister has already been on the front page of the national newspapers urging Thais to go back to their historic diets and telling them to avoid the American fast food outlets. He'd be sued if he said that in Britain.

Burger King, McDonalds, Starbucks, and various pizza parlours have arrived. So too has Tesco with its household cleaners and arrays of perfumes and soaps. And also mobile phones and masts, and even WiFi in the towns' hotels. Doctors now dish out antibiotics for everything. Toyota have a showroom in the village. And there is even talk of GM crops. No doubt they'll soon be offered mortgages!

So, please don't be confused. In my opinion, yes, their diets are a contributory factor to their low cancer rates – starting with no frying, the consumption of lots of vegetables and fruit and lean wild meat and fish, but also no salt and no dairy. Lemon grass, galangal and kafir lime leaves – used frequently in their soups – are three of the most potent antioxidant-containing foods known; the active ingredient of lemon grass is almost 300 times more powerful than beta-carotene in carrots. Papaya and bamboo shoots contain good levels of vitamin B-17. But we have natural compounds in our native foods in Europe that are equally potent.

A second area of benefit is that they ingest lots of beneficial bacteria, no antibiotics and drugs, and the coconut (caprylic acid), garlic, onions and chillis kill off yeasts and microbes – their digestive systems and the blood systems work and are 'clean'. (See Chapter 23)

They sleep naturally in the dark – whereas, sleeping in artificial lighting and sleep deprivation due to night shift work are actually being declared known carcinogens by IARC (The International Cancer Agency in Lyon).

Happiness helps build a strong immune system too, as does plenty of all-day exercise, and they have none of the stresses of the Western world to weaken it.

Finally, they are chemical- and pesticide-free. And they are, usually, thin.

Now please tell me that, in Birmingham or Bristol, I should adopt a meat-free South East Asian Diet if I want to beat cancer.

Cancer is a lifestyle disease

The important thing is to be open-minded, rational and to start to learn from this. We might conclude that eating a little wild meat and fish, no dairy, lots of vegetables and fruits can help you prevent cancer – but it's a bit woolly. And it certainly isn't much of a plan.

What I think both the Vegetarian and South East Asian diets do tell us is that you really cannot separate diet from the total lifestyle. To suggest, if you want to beat cancer, that you should just bolt a new diet onto an existing, possibly flawed lifestyle is nonsense.

Cancer is 'rich person's disease' and rich people eat more, are fatter, drive around in cars, using household chemicals and personal toiletries, live on mobile phones, have more stress, sleep poorly (often with street lights outside their windows), do less manual work and so on. When Chinese people go to live in the USA they adopt the US illness rates and cancer statistics very quickly. Cancer is a lifestyle disease.

So if you develop cancer **you need to mend your whole life** – the full width of it. Diet is just one aspect.

CHAPTER 7
MENDING A LIFE

In balance with your environment

One's environment, one's lifestyle, one's diet and one's health are all interlinked, as is one's soul and one's mental attitude to the community at large and the greater universe. A disease in an individual is an affliction on the community, a measure of its failings, and cannot be thought of as separate or confined to the individual.

Is this a crank view? I suggest you read the paragraph slowly and carefully again.

Giraffes have long necks because the ones with short necks couldn't reach the leaves on the trees and died out. Over hundreds of thousands of years these leaves best nourished the giraffes' biochemistry and the biochemistry was built on that nourishment. So too papaya best nourishes someone in the Philippines, an apple someone in Austria, seal meat best nourishes an Eskimo and oats a Scotsman.

But it is not just food that nourishes the biochemistry. Buddhism nourishes the body in Bhutan, yoga in Lahore. Praise might nourish a child in Paris; criticism might depress a cleaner in Cologne.

Naturopathy is an ancient system of healing, which encourages building your immunity naturally by viewing the individual as an integral part of nature's big picture.

Conventional medicine and naturopathy overlap in the study of Psycho-Neuro-Endocrino-Immunology or PNEI. Put simply: Our feelings, emotions and thoughts are connected fundamentally through the nervous, energy and hormone systems to all the workings of our bodies.

And it is easy to see how lifestyle, food and diet can affect the lot – and quite quickly. For example:

- Stress greatly increases your cortisol levels. Doctors normally send patients home to rest for a week. Seattle Medical Centre showed us, in matched research samples, that your first ever yoga lesson can reduce cortisol levels by 25 per cent compared with just a 5 per cent drop after a full week in the stay-homers.

- Meditation causes changes in the hypothalamus, which through the pituitary gland affects the whole body. The New York Presbyterian Hospital has shown us in clinical trials that meditation before surgery can reduce blood loss by 40 per cent.
- Several universities have shown us that depression is related to lower blood oxygen levels. Pennsylvania and UCLA have shown that blood oxygen levels can be raised through exercise. And this can relieve depression.
- Aggressive children can find themselves locked up in state institutions in the USA if their aggression has lead to crime. Several research studies have shown that supplementation with fish oils (omega-3) considerably alters the levels of aggression, through changes to the brain biochemistry

So, just as our diets affect our biochemistry, so our stresses, our depressions, our aggressions can affect it – they are all interlinked.

Of course, some mental states are caused by diet – alcohol would be the most obvious example, but too much, or too little sugar can also cause dramatic effects in some people. Then there are illnesses due to deficiencies or sensitivities. We all understand that we may have food intolerances. Some are extreme: I have a friend who cannot eat shell fish – he goes bright red, can't breathe and has to be rushed to hospital.

Physical factors, mental factors, diet, lifestyle, our historical, local surroundings and the nourishment they provide are all inter-woven.

The Macrobiotic Diet

Between 1896 and 1907 a Japanese army officer was, even then, deeply concerned at the Westernisation of the traditional Japanese diet and he implored the Japanese people to re-embrace their traditional healthy values.

Sagen Ishizuka went 'back to basics' and stated his

fundamental belief that the food we eat not only sustains life, it makes for our basic health and happiness. He set up a clinic and started to treat hundreds of patients with the principles of Yin and Yang, and the traditional Japanese peasant diet. His fame and success brought him the title of the 'anti-doctor,' not because he was against doctors but because his disciples simply didn't need them!

In the 1950s George Ohsawa brought Ishizuka's diet and principles to the West. Later, Michio Kushi consolidated his work and there is a Kushi Institute in London.

And that was how **macrobiotics** started. Sadly, the use of the diet by certain media stars has caused some people to ridicule or trivialise the value of the diet. But it is simple, sensible and sound.

The term itself comes from the Greek: *macro* meaning 'great' or 'long' and *biotic* meaning, 'concerning life'. The original word was attributed to Hippocrates, the father of modern medicine. However the concept of macrobiotics is not focused on diet *per se* but rather the ancient Chinese belief that all life, indeed the whole universe, is a balance of two opposing forces Yin and Yang.

Unlike most modern-day diets, many of which give the feeling of having been created or invented often with slimming in mind, macrobiotics is best described by the phrase 'back to basics' – for your food and for you and your health. A macrobiotic diet is thus just a part of a 'back-to-basics' and balanced overall lifestyle.

Yin elements in the macrobiotic diet are regarded as cold, slow, filling and weak; Yang in contrast is quick, dry and hard. Most disease, and especially cancer, is regarded as having a Yin cause. However for any individual all aspects of their life should be assessed by Yin and Yang principles, not just their diet. Any excess thought to be causing an illness can then be corrected or counterbalanced by providing foods of the opposite force.

The five basic principles of the macrobiotic diet are that:

- Foods are the foundation of health and happiness.
- Sodium and potassium are opposites in food, reflecting opposing Yin and Yang Forces.
- Man's staple food is grain.

- Food should be unrefined, whole and natural.
- Food should be grown locally, ripe and consumed in season.

If you meet with a macrobiotic consultant concerning a cancer do not be surprised if he delves into everything in your past from diet to lifestyle, from illnesses to allergies. To undertake macrobiotics is to try to mend your whole life.

He is likely to recommend a core diet, around which he will introduce specific foods particular to your needs. It should be noted that a fundamental tenet of macrobiotics is that every one of us is an individual and one man's grain may be another man's poison.

The core diet is likely to include:

- Whole grains (e.g. millet, barley, brown rice).
- Vegetables (including pulses and some fruits).
- Seaweed and sea vegetables.
- Fermented soya products (e.g. tofu, shoyu and miso soup).
- Regular consumption of oily fish.
- Monounsaturated oils.
- Japanese low caffeine green tea.

Whenever possible, everything should be fresh, and freshly prepared. Freshly prepared juices may also be recommended, but raw food may not at the outset as, even if vegetables are only blanched, cooked foods supposedly have more 'fire', more energy. Dairy, sugar and meat are likely no-go foods. Organic food predominates and the diet may be extended to include exercise, yoga and even a little meditation.

A change to a macrobiotic diet and lifestyle has helped many people achieve a new health, and it has helped many cancer patients. It does require a little effort and time, but it does not have to be forever. Some people find its corrective action may only be needed for a year or so.

Some argue that the use of grains, whole or otherwise, in a modern world that stores them in silos and finds them developing moulds and carcinogenic aflatoxins, should be cut out, while others argue that this established, hundred-year-old viewpoint places too much emphasis on cooked rather than raw foods. However, I think it is an excellent starting point on our search for the best anti-cancer diet, not least because the Japanese traditionally had such small rates of cancer (pickled food, high salt consumption and smoking is changing all that).

Of course, the macrobiotic diet is not dissimilar to the diet still used by the Okinawans we refered to earlier. Surrounded by a coral sea, their diet has less carbohydrate (and therefore calories) than even the Japanese diet, and small amounts of protein from fish and vegetables. They have an extremely high organic mineral intake, the lowest cancer rates in the world bar none, and an average life expectancy of 81.2 years, the highest in the world.

Some elements of the macrobiotic diet are strongly anti-cancer, like the emphasis towards potassium-rich foods and away from sodium and like the use of green tea and seaweed both of which contain natural compounds that can cause cancer cell death. Whole grains have their vitamins, minerals and fibre content intact; pulses provide protective plant oestrogens, as does the fermented soya. Oily fish contribute small amounts of vitamins E and D, and large amounts of anti-inflammatory omega-3. The avoidance of dairy, sugar and meat is important, too.

Eating locally grown, fresh, ripe fruit and vegetables is a very sensible rule for delivering the most nourishment from your natural foods – how can picking a fruit half ripe, storing it in nitrogen, shipping it across the world, 'ripening' it in the shop window and eating it four weeks after it was picked be expected to bring nourishment to your body? Why, in Britain, do we want to eat lychees, rice and mangoes from China when our ancestors have built their biochemistry with nourishment from apples, pears and potatoes?

In summary, the macrobiotic diet is actually inseparable from a more balanced and healthy life overall. Some elements reduce the risks of developing cancer, while others are genuinely corrective, the whole possible tackling the complete process that is cancer. Do we have anything like this in the West?

CHAPTER 8
THE FRENCH CONNECTION

The following statements are all true:

- The Japanese eat very little fat and suffer fewer heart attacks and cancers than us.
- The Mexicans eat a lot of fat and suffer fewer heart attacks and cancers than us.
- The Chinese drink very little red wine and suffer fewer heart attacks and cancers than us.
- The Italians drink excessive amounts of red wine and suffer fewer heart attacks and cancers than us.
- The Eskimos eat more fat than anyone else in the world, and they have fewer heart attacks and cancers than us.
- The French eat more fat than us, and drink excessive amounts of red wine, and even they suffer fewer heart attacks and cancers than us.

Conclusion? Eat and drink what you like. Speaking English is apparently what kills you.

A low fat, high carbohydrate diet?

For thirty years or so from the mid 1960's, Western governments and dietary experts talked about a healthy eating pyramid. Do you remember? Lots of foods at the bottom that you can eat once a year, and two or three foods at the top that you are supposed to make meals out of every day. 'High fibre' – so everyone rushed out to buy their Super Bran flakes; 'high carbohydrate' – so everyone started eating rice and pasta; 'low fat' – so everyone bought low fat spreads and low fat yoghurts.

The truth is that adding fibre as an extra to your diet does little for you – the fibre needs to be inherent in the food, wrapped around the sugar stores to ensure their slow release. High carbohydrate diets pushed people (especially women looking to slim) into meals of nutritionally useless, refined wheat pasta. And then there's low fat. Now we are learning that some fats are good for you and even protect your good health!

Frankly, 'Dietary Experts' misled us all for 30 years or more and some Government Health bodies are still doing it today!

The French Paradox

These dietary experts had also to ignore the opening little commentary at the start of this chapter. Joke or not, it is true. For the Western world, the biggest dietary lesson was simply swept under the carpet. The French diet, dubbed a paradox as if it were some paranormal, unexplainable Gallic mystery, sat uneasily with the superficial approval given to the Asian Diet or vegetarian studies.

The French paradox? The French eat more fat than the Americans and British, and consume more alcohol. Yet they have lower rates of cancer and heart diseases, they spend 30 per cent less on health care and enjoy a longer average life expectancy. Several studies have produced this same data. One actually showed that, within France, the area of highest fat consumption was in Gascony – the home of D'Artagnan, broad, beefy rugby playing men and their well built wives. It is also the home of *foie gras*, patés, sausages, many cheeses, cream and of dishes like cassoulet (pork fat, duck breast, bacon and sausages in a bean stew).

And where do the French have the least cancers and heart attacks? In Gascony.

Factors that protect

Ignoring the French Paradox was the biggest mistake dietary 'experts' ever made. Instead they advised us to, *'eat less fat and more carbohydrates'* – a misguided falsehood. The priority should be to cut 'added, empty sugar' and refined carbs and add vegetables and fruits into your diet that can counter inflammation.

One of my best friends lives in Gascony – spend a week or two there. It's a farming community, so plenty of beneficial bacteria in your daily diet, plenty of leeks, onions and garlic, especially chopped and raw. Salads covered in olive oil; red wine with every meal; fruits in abundance throughout the summer and autumn. (They are, like the Thais, always nibbling at a fruit.) They exercise, they play rugby and they move bales of straw. And they eat. Eating is a fundamental pleasure in life – it is a national sport.

Importantly, they believe in 'nourishment' – in real food. I was talking to the local hairdresser about McDonalds. *'Why would we want one here? My children like their food'*, he said. No coincidence then that McDonalds near Ste Maxime is almost only populated by tourists, and had to provide a range of salads (including prawn, and smoked salmon) plus proper potatoes not merely French Fries, to get any French customers into the place. If a French woman wants to diet, she merely eats smaller portions – she wouldn't think of changing what she eats. The British and the Americans seem to have this belief that in some way you can 'eat yourself slim'. Carry on – just switch to low calorie or low fat versions and the pounds will drop off! Who in their right mind would drink a gin and slimline tonic?

Have you seen the film 'Green Card'? There is a wonderful scene that sums this up. The mighty Gaul, Gerard Depardieu, is having breakfast with his American leading lady, Andie McDowell. Incredulous at her breakfast offerings, he goes out and buys a coffee percolator, and his full-butter croissants. When she has her muesli, covered in low fat yoghurt – he looks on in disgust. *'Birdseed'*, he mutters under his breath.

The Mediterranean Diet

One area of France has a diet that does pass muster with the Politically Correct Dietary Brigade and that is the 'Mediterranean Diet'. More correctly it should be called the 'Northern Mediterranean Diet', and I have first-hand experience of this diet too, as I've had a house in France by the Mediterranean for 26 years. The epicentre of this beneficial diet seems to stretch from Barcelona to somewhere near Naples. The diet typically includes:

- A limited amount of meat.
- A limited amount of dairy (from goats).
- Red wine consumption with meals.
- Good consumption of fresh nuts.
- Good consumption of dried fruits.
- High consumption of vegetables, including garlic.
- Low consumption of refined grains and common glucose.
- High consumption of fruits.

- High consumption of olive oils and nut oils (monounsaturated oils).
- High percentage of home-grown, in season, fresh and organic produce.
- High consumption of fish.

The coast line of the Northern Mediterranean is an extended fishing community. The boats still come in every day, and serve their catch at the quayside in France and Italy. Go inland 25 kilometers and you are in farming communities.

Tomatoes, peppers, beetroot, onions, cucumbers and salads. Peaches, oranges, plums, pears, apples. Everything has its season. In May it will be asparagus and strawberries, in June it will be peaches and salad vegetables and so on through apricot season, to the nut festivals when the châtaigne (chestnuts) and walnuts are picked. Fresh, local, in-season produce. And they've never heard of macrobiotics although the similarities are clear!

From my local knowledge I can tell you that the locals shop at the local farms, not the supermarket. 18 per cent of the local produce is organic; they use crop rotation. Our oil is extra virgin organic olive oil or occasionally walnut oil. Olive oil is dribbled on everything. You even dip your bread in it before your meal. Grilled fish is the staple along the coast, inland there is a lot of wild game. Of course you can have the fish stew, or the fish soup. The fishermen of Marseille invented bouillabaisse using the ugly fish in their catch that no one could sell. Salad Nicoise? It's not the one you have in London. It was originally made of lettuce, green beans, onions and tomatoes with the little anchovies the fishermen of Nice couldn't sell, all covered in olive oil and chopped garlic.

The standard cooked vegetable dish is ratatouille – peppers, courgettes, aubergines, onions and garlic stewed with olive oil. Nothing is fried, no salt added.

The fennel, onions and garlic kill any harmful microbes and yeasts consumed. Herbs like oregano and rosemary modulate blood sugar levels and reduce diabetes risk (*University of Illinois*). The local herb, saffron, has been shown to contain three anti-cancer ingredients (crocin, picrocin and safranal).

Coffee is strong and black; it contains diterpines, which have anti-cancer properties. Cheese is almost certain to be from goats as the hinterland is mountainous. And then of course there is the wine – made on the skins and grape seeds. And the sun, which makes vitamin D in our bodies. Simple brick houses with stone floors to keep the heat out in summer and the cold north wind out in winter. At night you sleep in the pitch black, with shutters on the windows, an historical requirement, to protect you from thieves.

Research approves!

Fat? In 2002, a pan-European survey concluded that people on the north shore of the Mediterranean consumed the highest levels of fat, yet had the lowest levels of heart attacks and cancers in Europe. The point is, it is largely 'good' fat.

Bad fat? Two meta studies *(Annals of Internal Medicine,* 18 March 2014; and *Amer. J. Clin. Nutr.* Jan 13 2010) show that people who eat high saturated fat diets have no difference in coronary disease risk over the people who eat little!

Carbohydrate? Research in *JAMA* in 2014 showed that cardiovascular risk is increased through intake of added sugar and refined carbs. There are now major studies on the Mediterranean diet; for example, one in the *Journal of the American Medical Association.* In this, two groups of people were studied comprising over 2000 men and women all aged between 70 and 90 at the start of the eleven-year study. (Importantly, they did not separate food from local lifestyle.)

Here are the conclusions:

- The benefits of diet, alcohol, exercise and non-smoking were described as **dramatic**. People who followed the Mediterranean lifestyle had 65 per cent less risk of death from heart disease and cancer over the control group!!!
- Each of the following areas independently provided benefit:
  *The diet – high in fruit, vegetables, nuts, fish, olive oil, seeds and whole grains, but low in meat and meat products – cut risk of death by 23 per cent.
  * Exercise – defined as 30 minutes per day of moderate activity – cut risk of death by 37 per cent.
  * Alcohol – those people drinking one to four glasses of wine

per day – cut risk of death by 22 per cent. (Indeed non-drinkers were significantly worse off.)

* **Non-smoking** – not one cigarette consumed in the past 15 years – cut risk of death by 34 per cent.

And if you do all four, the total figure is 65 per cent across the eleven-year period.

In the November 2007 edition of *the FASEB Journal,* French researchers have shown that the really beneficial contribution to the French diet is the polyphenol content in FRESH foods. There are several thousand different polyphenols. Many are powerful antioxidants and the scientists showed that they could both prevent and shut down tumours by cutting off the formation of new blood vessels needed for tumour growth. The study also showed dose dependency, with increasing effects as more and different polyphenols were consumed, and showed the benefits for people with heart and circulatory problems. The scientists, in particular, reviewed the 'Mediterranean Diet' and found the polyphenol content of fruits, vegetables, herb teas (infusions), olive oil and red wine was extremely high and very potent – red wine started to have a beneficial effect at the level of just one glass!

Another protective and correct contribution comes from the local consumption of high levels of mushrooms. The local markets are full of different types, local residents will go out on Sunday afternoons for a walk in the forest to pick their dinner, mushroom 'festivals' are joyous occasions.

There is now a huge body of research evidence showing the protective and corrective power of mushrooms. You should consume several types. Some stimulate different elements in the immune system, others help clarify and oxygenate the blood, others kill cancer cells, and some have been shown to reduce tumour size by 70 per cent. That is more than most drugs achieve!

A colourful life

The South of France is a colourful place – its regional hues are blue, orange, yellow and green.

Now imagine that every day in the centre of our big lunch

table we have a one metre long concave piece of tree bark filled with vegetables – fennel, tomatoes, yellow peppers, red peppers, beetroot, cauliflower, radishes, cucumber, sweetcorn, onions, spring onions, garlic cloves. And another for fruit with apricots, peaches, deep red plums, cherries, strawberries, grapes.

The yellows, the reds, the oranges, the greens and the deep purples are all plant pigments that protect. They may be called flavenoids, or polyphenols, or carotenoids or anthocyanins but that doesn't matter to someone living in the South of France or Gascony. They are just part of life's rich tapestry. The vegetables and fruits have all drawn minerals from an ever changing soil. A soil that uses natural manure and organic farming practices. A soil much of which is silted by the rivers coming down from the mountains. Foods for enjoyment; foods that nourish, protect and prevent, as does the wine, the olive oil and the sun.

So let me list for you, just a few of the bioactive natural compounds known by scientists to have definite epigenetic properties – properties that can protect and correct the surrounds of your core DNA code: Vitamin D (sunshine on the skin), resveratrol and grape seed extract (in red grapes), omega-3 (in fish and game), catchetins (in green tea, vinegars, peaches), indole 3 carbinol and sulphoraphanes (both in broccoli and 'greens'), quercitin (in onions and apples), anthocyanins (the dark red of beetroot, cherries, plums), pomegranate, lycopene (in tomatoes), piperine (in black pepper), apigenin (parsley, celery, chamomile tea), polyphenols in olive oil, fisetin (strawberries, grapes, onions), turmeric (curcumin); all these and more have proven epigenetic benefits.

To my mind any diet for health should start with the vibrant South of France Diet as a model. Whether from Gascony, where the fats are counteracted by red wine, olive oil, garlic, onions and plentiful vegetables and fruits and nuts. Or the Mediterranean coast and the benefits of the natural compounds in fish soup, ratatouille, garlic, herbs, vegetables and fruits and nuts. The locals enjoy their outdoor life, and they live longer than we do in the UK, and with their first serious illness coming well after ours.

So, here we have a diet that **protects** AND **corrects** – a diet that both nourishes AND heals. The most telling factor in the research, to my mind, is the finding that this was 'dose dependent' – the more you eat – in terms of volume and width – the lower your risk of illness.

So am I really suggesting a high fat, low carb, high bioactive compound diet?

Too right! Low carb and high fat? It is now clear that eating refined carbs and added sugar gives rise to insulin rushes and leads to chronic inflammation in the body. And chronic inflammation is the precursor to all manner of chronic illnesss, from diabetes to heart disease to cancer. For example, top American cardiologist Dr. Chauncey Crandall, Director of the Palm Beach Cardiovascular Clinic, argues on his Heart Health website, that if the walls of the arteries were not inflamed in the first place, the fat would not 'stick' to them and there would be less risk of artherosclerosis. And inflammation in the body doesn't just aid the development of cancer - it drives metastases.

The traditional Mediterranean diet is low carb and the carbohydrate is provided by legumes, pulses and whole foods. Indeed, research has shown that eating a daily helping of lentils prevents cardiovascular disease and diabetes. On the other hand, added sugar is linked to the development and propagation of cancer.

There is no doubt that some fats like trans fats, the cornerstone of packaged and processed foods, are positively dangerous – they may soon be banned. On the other hand there are 'good' fats like fish, nut, seed and olive oils, which are protective in disease. And it would seem that you can eat 'bad' saturated fats, as long as you eat much higher levels of the good fats and avoid the empty carbs. It's about the balance between the two. Crandall thinks one of the worst foods is ice cream because it contains both sugar and fat.

Finally, you have the fresh and colourful vegetables and fruits – full of bioactive natural compounds that are both protective, and corrective. (You can find more than 130 recipes in our new *Rainbow Recipes* book.)

CHAPTER 9
A DIET FOR PEOPLE WITH CANCER?

According to various expert authorities like the World Health Organisation, a poor diet lies behind up to two thirds of cancer cases while a good diet can prevent cancer. This has been established beyond doubt. So, if you have had treatment and been given the 'All Clear' by your oncologist, logically why shouldn't a good diet prevent your cancer returning?

Understanding the Naysayers

Almost every week people contact CANCERactive with stories that they told their oncologist about how they had changed their diet and were met with a shrug of the shoulders. Some doctors had even ridiculed the patient. Only a very, very few were supportive.

Worse, some UK professors and oncologists will tell you that if you already have a cancer, no diet is going to help you stop the cancer. In fact, one top cancer professor wrote a point of view in the *British Medical Journal* about exactly this, saying he had many studies all showing that changing your diet didn't matter one jot to the outcome. (Interestingly he did not list a single one of the studies so we could not check their validity!) It could be that some were just about the addition of a vitamin, or cutting out meat, or some other such isolated factor. Single and limited action is not what I mean by 'Changing your diet', nor is it what this book is about.

Let us be clear upfront. **The 'Naysayers' are totally wrong.** The opposite is, in fact true. Changing your diet coupled with light daily exercise are two factors that have been shown beyond all doubt to increase survival times.

So why do some oncologists take the opposite view?

Much of the reason is that the UK medical profession wants to control the lives and treatment of their patients one hundred per cent. They may be genuinely scared that the patient might take a supplement that could conflict with one of their drugs, but there is almost nil clinical evidence for this fear. But many 'old-school' doctors and their bosses hark back to the days of 'Doctor knows best, so do as he tells you' and they would like to recreate this dependence and control.

But research shows more than half of all cancer patients want to take back control of their own lives from their oncologist. It is called 'Self Empowerment'. Modern patients often feel there are treatments the doctor has not mentioned and that there are things they can do to help themselves. Patients can join a support group and hear what other patients did, they can search the Internet for potential treatments, or go to American cancer centre websites which are often far more open-minded and positive about diet, and they can go to one of the many complementary cancer centres that have sprung up all over the UK.

There's even CANCERactive. All this must have a significant impact on survival ratings the UK which are known to be improving, despite a paucity of new drugs and the failure of supposedly early diagnostic tests like the PSA test and mammograms.

Patients want to make better-informed, more personal choices and they are more questioning, but their questions expose the doctor or oncologist and his restricted advice. He then becomes defensive and dismissive.

Newly qualified doctors are likely to have spent just a few days studying the subject of 'Diet' during their training. The typical oncology professor has had no formal training in nutrition and is barely informed on up-to-date cancer nutrition, if at all.

Worse, some hospitals now even tell their doctors not to discuss complementary therapies with patients – we had two ladies with breast cancer in one week complaining to us that their oncologist had told them that if he discussed diet and complementary therapies with them he'd be 'struck off'. What rubbish is this?

Worse still, there are people who attack 'complementary therapy' websites like CANCERactive or nutritionists, herbalists, therapists and researchers such as myself, falsely claiming we are quacks and that there is no research to support any complementary therapies. They deliberately encourage media support for their crazy views which, frankly, come between patients and increasing survival times and so are both despicable and dangerous.

The only person who suffers from this mess is the patient who is confused enough anyway! It has to stop. To quote the words of George Bernard Shaw: *"It is easy... terribly easy... to shake a man's faith in himself. To take advantage of that, to break a man's spirit, is the devil's work."*

I actually feel genuinely sorry for doctors. It's not their fault if the British Medical authorities don't train them fully or keep their knowledge up to date. Unfortunately, this lack of knowledge and the subsequent 'cover-up' with the dismissive shrug, damages their credibility.

It is not just unhelpful, it is also against the law. In the UK, your oncologist has a legal duty to fully explain ALL your treatment options. Ignorance is no defence.

Of course, oncologists don't need to talk to you about diet; NHS hospitals have NHS Dieticians. And those dieticians have booklets like the one I was sent by two ladies in a week, both thinking it was some sort of joke. The booklet was entitled 'A Diet for Chemotherapy' and had a drawing of a cheeseburger, a milkshake and a sticky, sugary bun on every page. Meanwhile the booklet and a 2011 article in *The Times* from a top oncologist both encouraged patients undergoing chemotherapy to 'keep their weight up' by consuming calories in the form of fat and sugar (cream, butter, milk, milky sugary tea and so on).

I feel sorry for dieticians. They are worked off their feet. They only get time to see the seven per cent of patients who are suffering from cachexia – a condition where the chemotherapy is causing severe weight loss which will result in the death of the patient. And we cannot possibly have seven per cent of all cancer patients on chemotherapy dying as a direct result of the chemotherapy, can we? So dieticians follow political orders and advise weight-gaining diets. To suggest that this is a good diet for the normal cancer patient is bunkum. A persistent myth that can cause harm.

Interestingly, American cancer centers Memorial Sloan-Kettering and MD Anderson now tell people on chemo to eat healthy diets - low glucose, refined and processed foods, low 'bad' fat diets, just as I have done for 8 years! There is also research that taking fish oils significantly reduces the risk of cachexia.

There are also research studies showing that, for example, breast cancer attacks the bones, the bones then produce growth hormone to defend themselves and the tumour then uses this growth hormone to build blood supplies. Cows' dairy adds growth hormone to your blood stream in the form of Insulin-like Growth Factor 1 (IGF-1).

Why feed the cancer with glucose and growth hormone at the very moment the oncologist is trying to kill it off?

I won't go on. To quote from J F Kennedy, *"The great enemy of the truth is very often not the lie, but the myth; persistent, persuasive and unrealistic"*.

No wonder patients are so confused. It is all a mess, driven by politics and vested interest.

Encouraging patients to employ a good diet is officially part of UK cancer treatment!

Suggesting that positively changing your diet has no effect on cancer outcome and so you shouldn't bother is actually in conflict with the UK's National Cancer Plan (2000), where part of the plan was that patients should be given nutritional advice in order to improve their outcomes! Refusing to give dietary advice, or dismissing your efforts, is thus both illegal and against recommended best practice in the UK!

Correction and Protection

The persistent mantra of "don't eat fat, too much red meat, drink too much alcohol, but do eat five lots of fruit and vegetables a day" is at the heart of UK cancer diet recommendations. But it is slowly changing. I have shown you that there are real lessons to be learned from the French Paradox and the Northern Mediterranean Diet. Put simply, I believe that incorporating a spectrum of bioactive natural compounds from vibrant, colourful foods into your diet, from yellow and red peppers to beetroot, to broccoli, garlic, onions, olive oil, red grapes and organic red wine and herb teas, helps to PROTECT you from cancer and CORRECT the problem if you have it.

As you will see, the benefits of the Rainbow Diet are real and not confined to cancer; for example, research shows it outperforms the current, recommended NHS 'anti-diabetes' diet. Another study, this time of over 10,000 men by the University of Las Palmas, Spain showed that eating a Rainbow Diet could cut depression by 30 per cent.

The Rainbow Diet is full of natural antioxidants. In 2011 an 11 year study on antioxidant supplements was published in the *European Journal of Nutrition*. This concluded that those people with the highest levels of antioxidants in the blood streams had a 48 per cent less risk of dying from cancer.

Australian research published in the *Journal of the American Dietetic Association* showed that different foods from the Rainbow Diet reduced the risk of colorectal cancer in different areas of the colon and rectum. In a randomised, controlled clinical trial, researchers found a reduced rate of proximal colon cancer with high consumption of brassicas (cabbage, Brussels sprouts etc) and a reduced rate of distal colon cancer with dark yellow vegetables and apples.

Research, research, research

Nobel Prizes have been won for showing that natural compounds in your diet can reduce inflammation and for showing how natural compounds can help your immune system better recognise cancer cells. There are American 2011 clinical trials on how stress management techniques increase survival times (counselling, yoga, diet all play a part in reducing cortisol levels or blocking its effects). Suppose your condition merits anti-oestrogen drugs (like Arimidex). Why shouldn't you help your survival chances with a diet that limits oestrogen levels, too?

Cancer Watch (the CANCERactive research centre) has covered more than 150 studies in the last few years on the effects of diet in increasing cancer survival. My views concur totally with the American Cancer Society's conclusions from their 2012 report stating that there had been an 'explosion' in research in the last six years; and 'overwhelming' evidence showing that diet (along with exercise and weight control) can help you **'survive longer'** and that diet can help you **'stay cancer-free'**.

Let's look at just a few of the research studies in Cancer Watch on diet in the last couple of years:

Breast Cancer

Women with the highest levels of carotenoids (the natural compounds that give carrots, yellow and red peppers and sweet potatoes their colour) in their blood have no recurrence of breast cancer; secondly, two cups a day of blueberries reduce triple-negative breast cancer tumours in women by 60 to 70 per cent. (*Journal of Nutrition 2011*)

Prostate Cancer

Professor Robert Thomas of Addenbrook's Hospital, Cambridge has shown that prostate patients can lower their PSA readings with a polyphenol mix of pomegranate, EGCG from green tea, curcumin and broccoli, while broccoli, tomatoes and daily exercise can delay the need for treatment.

Research from the University of Illinois shows that broccoli releases natural compounds called sulphorophanes, but only in the presence of an enzyme called myrosinase, which is destroyed by over-cooking. Researchers at the Institute of Food Technology in Norwich have shown that a gene PTEN blocks tumour growth; but a fault in it encourages tumour growth. Sulphoraphanes could block tumour growth in prostate cancer, even where the PTEN gene was faulty.

Colon Cancer

Leeds University conducted a randomised, double blind, placebo controlled study showing that concentrated omega-3 from fish oils could significantly reduce the size of colon polyps preventing colon cancer or its return. In America similar studies have shown that curcumin can reduce polyp inflammation too. This evidence reduces the need for operations.

All Cancer?

The red grape polyphenols, resveratrol, quercitin and catchetins, have now been used in several research studies. These three natural compounds seem capable of working on their own or in conjunction with the drug gefitinib, which is an anti-EGFR agent (stops blood supplies to tumours). Research concluded the combination 'inhibits breast cancer progression and may increase success of anti-EGFR therapy by inhibition of Akt/mTOR signaling'. (*Universidad Central del Caribe School of Medicine in*

Bayamon, Puerto Rico.)

Oxford University and Radcliffe Hospital scientists reported their studies on aspirin in 2012 concluding that just 75 mgs (take daily with food) could prevent cancer, halt metastases and extend survival times. They felt the results were 'so strong' that they urged NICE to recommend it as part of standard cancer treatment in the UK! Aspirin is the modern equivalent of the natural compound salicylin from willow bark, often chewed as a remedy in previous eras. Other anti-inflammatory agents are available in their natural form and we will talk of those later.

So, do you still think that natural compounds and a good diet cannot make one jot of difference to cancer survival?

Salvestrols

An interesting development has been the work of scientist Gerry Potter, Professor of Medicinal Chemistry at DeMonfort University Leicester School of Pharmacy. In the early 1990s Potter developed a drug (now called abiraterone) as part of a team looking to stop the progression of prostate cancer. The work was a National Cancer Institute project at the Royal Marsden. Potter showed that the drug could shut off a protein, an enzyme CYP17, which caused the male sex hormone, testosterone, to be made throughout the body. The drug stops the cancer 'feeding'.

In 2002 Potter used the same logic to look at foods and cancer cells. Working with another professor, Dan Burke, he identified a cellular **'rescue mechanism'**, which hinged on the metabolic interaction of natural compounds in certain foods with another protein, again an enzyme, found only in cancer cells.

This protein, CYP1B1, is widely regarded by cancer scientists as a cancer marker – that means that if it is present in your body you have cancer, since it does not occur in healthy cells.

Potter noticed that there were a number of natural compounds found in a diversity of foods and that these natural compounds acted as 'pro-drugs' with CYP1B1.

For example, a compound I will talk about later is resveratrol, produced by red grape skins as they come under attack from microbe and fungus predators after the grape's sugars. Potter showed that resveratrol acted as a pro-drug, being attacked by CYP1B1 to produce a toxic drug-like substance, piceatannol, which brings about that cell's death (*Br J Cancer, 2002; 86: 774-778*).

The food list where Potter and colleagues have identified similar pro-drugs is seemingly random:

- Vegetables such as broccoli, cabbages, kales, savoy, brussels sprouts, cauliflower, kohlrabi, chinese leaf, spinach, chard, lettuces, watercress, green beans, broad beans, garden peas.

- Artichokes (globe), red and yellow peppers, beansprouts, celery, salad rocket, avocado, pumpkins, squashes, gourds, marrows, zucchini, cucumbers, melons, gherkins.

- All red fruits such as strawberries, raspberries, grapes:and plums plus blackcurrants, redcurrants, blackberries, blueberries, mulberries, cranberries, bilberries.

- Apples, pears, pineapples.

- And herbs such as parsley, sage, rosemary, thyme, basil and mint.

Interestingly, like me, they argue that these 'salvestrol' natural compounds are in decline – the more you spray to kill the predators, the less the food need to make; GMO foods wouldn't make any. Then there are much changed dietary and lifestyle habits which have seen less of these foods consumed. All this and more leads Potter's group to believe that we consume just ten per cent of the salvestrols we need for proper protection and correction. They argue, again as I do, that newly-diagnosed cancer patients are invariably nutritionally deficient. Their solution is there urgent consumption of corrective salvestrols.

In the *Journal of Orthomolecular Medicine Vol 25, No. 1, 2010* (with authors Brian A. Schaefer, D.Phil.,Catherine Dooner, B.A, M. Danny Burke, Ph.D, Gerard A. Potter, Ph.D) the researchers present case histories involving five cancers: breast, prostate, colon, liver, and Hodgkin's lymphoma. To quote the authors, *"Two of the cases show how rapid and dramatic the improvement can be when nutritional deficits are addressed. In each case of the five studies the patient used Salvestrols to significant effect"*.

You will, as always, have to judge Salvestrols for yourself. But, the foods and the natural compounds are there for anyone to consume.

'Bioactive' food components

The Salvestrols work isn't the only study that turns the theory of the Rainbow Diet into a reality. For example, new research looks at the natural compounds and their ability to control cancer stem cells.

Stem cells have now been clearly shown to be the controlling factor in certain cancers. Stem cells are your normal repair cells in your body. They can divide rapidly and change into any type of healthy cell you need. Sometimes, under the effects of localised oestrogen, they get 'stuck' in this rapidly dividing mode. In 2012, a number of expert scientists showed that chemotherapy may knock a cancer back, but if it didn't kill off these cancer stem cells, the cancer was likely to return.

2012 research from Dr. Young S. Kim of the National Cancer Institute in Bethesda, MD and her team has shown that 'bioactive' food components, which are available in foods or as dietary supplements, may well have a capacity to suppress cancer stem cells and/or prevent them from self-renewal (*Kim et al. Journal of Nutritional Biochemistry; July 2012*).

The researchers say eating inappropriate foods and their ingredients may result in the loss of regulatory molecules and promote the aberrant or uncontrolled self-renewal of cancer stem cells; (epigenetics in action again).

In highly technical terms Kim stated, *'The ability of these bioactive food components to influence the balance between proliferative and quiescent cells by regulating critical feedback molecules in the network including dickkopf 1 (DKK-1), secreted frizzled-related protein 2 (sFRP2), B cell-specific Moloney murine leukemia virus integration site 1 (Bmi-1) and cyclin-dependent kinase 6 (CDK6) may account for their biological response.'*

No. I didn't understand much of it either! What I did understand was that **while some foods encourage the stem cells to re-grow, other 'bioactive' compounds stop this from happening** - the 'bioactive' natural compounds followed by the researchers included sulforaphanes, curcumin, piperine, theanine and choline plus vitamins A and D, genistein, and EGCG from green tea. All of these, according to the researchers, have been demonstrated to be able to modify the self-renewal properties of cancer stem cells. They termed these compounds 'Biotics' and stated that all could be found as supplements.

Eating more than one bioactive compound increases the benefits

There can also be little doubt that many of these bioactive natural compounds in foods have come, over the eons of time, to work synergistically. A bioactive compound in one food may well deliver a benefit, but when consumed with another bioactive compound, that benefit may be enhanced. This has been shown increasingly in research.

For example in a 2012 report in the *American Journal of Clinical Nutrition*, researchers from Spain analysing data taken from dietary questionnaires provided by 40,622 men and women aged 29 to 69 recruited into the European Prospective Investigation into Cancer and Nutrition, have concluded that:

- There is a link between greater (first pressed Virgin) olive oil intake and a lower risk of dying .

- The monounsaturated fats found in olive oil work synergistically with essential fatty acids (for example the omega-3 fat, DHA) to enhance their incorporation into cells and cell membranes.

The scientists found that participants whose olive oil intake ranked in the top quarter had a 26 per cent lower risk of dying of any cause during the 13.4 year follow-up period, a 44 per cent lower risk of dying from heart disease, and a 38 per cent less risk of dying from other causes than non-users.

The researchers noted that olive oil may be protective against certain cancers, against cellular inflammation, and against heart disease. Omega-3 in fish oils is already known to have longevity benefits including the strengthening of telomeres at the ends of the DNA chains. The bioactive compounds in the olive oil were thought to enhance this.

I will give you more examples on how one natural compound seems to enhance the actions of another towards the end of the book.

So - put a little colour into your life

I hope this chapter has gone some way to convincing you to ignore the persistent and negative mythology in UK cancer care by understanding that there is indeed 'overwhelming' research out there which can help you make a real difference to your survival and even prevent a cancer returning.

'Bioactive' natural compounds exist in many colourful foods. They possess the ability to 'protect and correct' your cells. And they help improve each other's action. The more you eat, the better.

The great thing about the Rainbow Diet is that it allows little dietary 'hic-coughs' because it is corrective. It allows you to encompass the maxim 'a little of what you fancy, does you good'. Of course, it is wiser not to overdo the bad things. But the real issue is to ensure you eat the good things – the foods that possess bioactive benefits.

The Rainbow Diet is also very practical. It is not about stewing up special smelly herbs, blending exotic and expensive concoctions or only eating tasteless foods, which the rest of the family can't stand and cause protests.

The Rainbow Diet is actually a short hand summary, an easy to remember descriptor. It tells you to put some vibrancy into your life. Think 'lots of bright, colourful foods, across the week'.

Let us now look at some other diets to see if there is more we can learn.

CHAPTER 10
THE APPLIANCE OF SCIENCE

'The secret of success is consistency of purpose', said Benjamin Disraeli. Nowhere can this be more true than with my late friend Nicholas Gonzalez, a doctor in New York, and with Professor Ben Pfeifer in Switzerland, each with limited clinical trials to support their disciplined and detailed Diet Therapies.

Dr. Nicholas Gonzalez

Dr. Nicholas Gonzalez treated cancer patients for nearly 30 years. His methodology was heavily influenced by the theories of Mancunian embryologist **Dr. John Beard**, later polished and developed by William Kelley.

When studying the foetus in the womb back in 1906, Beard observed that the placenta stopped growing on the precise day the pancreas of the foetus became active and started to secrete its own enzymes (around day 56). He concluded that since there was no logic to the foetus needing pancreatic enzymes to aid digestion (nutrition being provided by the mother via the placenta in a pre-digested form), the enzymes must have another role.

Beard noticed that placental cells (trophoblast cells derived from stem cells) acted rather like cancer cells, and hypothesised that if pancreatic enzymes could stop them growing, maybe they could do the same for cancer. He also noted that around day 56 the first signs of structure started to appear in the foetus – the rapidly growing blob of stem cells was now developing ear, eye and organ cells. Maybe pancreatic enzymes could take rapidly dividing stem cells and turn them into normal, slower growing body cells?

So his theory was simple. A stem cell under the influence of oestrogen, the female hormone, produces a trophoblast cell. This can divide rapidly and is essentially the same as a cancer cell. Pancreatic enzymes can 'convert' this into a normal cell. 102 years ago he even suggested that maybe cancer was like having a baby growing in the wrong place at the wrong time! He wrote a book *'The Enzyme Theory of Cancer'* but after his death in 1923 and, with the emergence of techniques like the radiation work of Marie Curie and then chemotherapy, his work was simply forgotten.

In 1970 a dentist, **Dr William Donald Kelley** was looking for something to help him with his wife's breast cancer. He followed Beard's theories and cured his wife with a dietary programme that included pancreatic enzymes. Kelley believed that cancer progressed because of a lack of cancer digesting enzymes in the body and that the pancreas was the prime cancer fighting organ in the body.

After treating his wife he decided to open a clinic and successfully treated 455 patients with some 26 different cancers over a 20 year period. His treatment programme had 5 parts:

- **Nutritional Therapy** – to break down the cancer cells; megadoses of vitamins (for example, up to 50gms of vitamin C), minerals, bioflavenoids, coenzymes, raw almonds, amino acids and raw beef formula with pancreatic enzymes.
- **Detoxification** – to cleanse the liver and body of dead cells; laxative purges, Epsom Salts, fasts, lemon juice, coffee enemas.
- **Diet** – to rebalance the body and the immune system. (At the outset he felt this needed to be strictly vegetarian but over time changed that view.) He majored on organic foods like nuts (including almonds) and seeds, low protein grains, and raw fruits and vegetables. He avoided processed foods, pesticide residues, refined foods, peanuts and dairy.
- **Neurological Stimulation** – to allow free flow of the body energy to the cancer site, he advocated osteopaths, chiropractors and physiotherapists.
- **Spiritual** – Kelley urged patients to read the Bible, to trust in God and to pray.

Kelley changed his views on a vegetarian diet believing in the end that everybody has his or her own personal 'metabolic code' and that this code determines what foods best nourish that person. He developed his own 'malignancy system' with 10 different 'Metabolic' or Dietary Types, and 95 variations within those. He recorded his Treatment Programme and case histories in a book, *'One Answer to Cancer'*.

Bill Wolcott, who had also followed the work of Dr John Beard and worked with Kelley has developed this Metabolic Typing further still, using nine controls including blood types, endocrine levels, prostaglandin levels, electrolyte levels and more. He claims to have helped over 60,000 people nourish their bodies maximally using his typing programme. You can even go a long way towards the full service he offers on the web: www.healthexcel.com.

Gonzalez became interested in Kelley's work whilst a student at Cornell University Medical School in 1981. As part of his fourth year thesis he reviewed Kelley's work and then turned it into a formal two year project. In his research, Gonzalez tracked 50 of Kelley's patients, all of whom had been originally given a poor prognosis, but all subsequently enjoyed long-term survival after adopting Kelley's regime.

He also reviewed the case histories of 22 patients with pancreatic cancer – a cancer where 5-year survival in America is just 4 per cent. After interviewing the patients themselves, plus families of the deceased and reviewing medical records, his very thorough report showed Kelley's work had clearly out-performed orthodox treatments. In 1986, Kelley decided to retire – and Gonzalez took up the mantle. Gonzalez worked in New York, not just on cancer but on various diseases. He was joined by Dr. Linda Isaacs in 1985.

In 1993 the Associate Director of Cancer Therapy in the NCI invited him to present his work across all cancers.

In preliminary studies comparing pancreatic patients on chemotherapy with an equivalent group on the Gonzalez therapy, patients undertaking the Gonzalez regime lived on average 17.5 months – or three times longer than those taking the orthodox medical approach. The results of this study, supervised by the NCI and funded by Nestle were published in the peer-reviewed 'Nutrition and Cancer' and reported **the best results ever in the treatment of the disease.**

Uniquely the NCI then sponsored a full three phase clinical trial on his work. This was monitored by the FDA and his work paid for ($1.4 million) by the American National Institute of Health's National Centre for Complementary and Alternative

Medicine. Again, it focused on pancreatic cancer in the trials because it is so hard to beat, and results might occur more quickly and noticeably. In the further trials, 126 patients were treated with the FDA approved drug gemcitabine. No-one lived past month 19. In the Gonzalez regime, despite 8 of his 11 patients starting out with grade 4 disease, 5 of the 11 survived 24 months, 2 actually more than 48 months.

From this juncture the whole trial seems to have gone haywire. Gonzalez had already had to suffer no involvement in the selection of the patients on his protocol and they were considerably worse off (at higher stages) than the mean for the drug. There were also far, far fewer of them and clearly the samples were not matched or randomised by the people conducting the trial.

Gonzalez in his book '*What went wrong. The battle for a fair evaluation of the Gonzalez Therapy*' describes it as complete mismanagement. His Protocol was even violated in 'numerous ways' and this was subsequently confirmed by independent regulators. The study report and a misleading article were both produced without his knowledge. The saga was described by Dr Paul Rosch, a professor at New York Medical School as a '*Tragic tale which supports a growing suspicion that the cancer cartel… is devoted more to preserving their enormous profits and reputations than to the prevention and cure of cancer*'.

It always seems odd to me that a drugs company pays for its scientists and pre-selects the patients in a trial very carefully. It receives the report first and some companies have been known to 'massage' the findings. Never does it have to simply hand over the product to a bunch of independent strangers who then conduct the clinical trials and publish a report without its input. Why so for 'alternative therapies'?

Gonzalez didn't just want to cure people though. He wanted his 'Dietary' regime thoroughly tested and incorporated as standard practice within orthodox mainstream medicine. Political Dynamite!

The Gonzalez regime has three basic parts:

1. **Detoxification** – involving a variety of cleanses and two coffee enemas each day.
2. **Diet** – individually designed diets as a result of extensive metabolic typing. Diets avoid refined, processed and prepared foods. Some patients are encouraged to become vegans, others to eat meat, depending upon personal metabolism traits.
3. **Supplementation** – 120 to 175 supplements may be used daily, again, tailored to the individual's requirements. These involve trace minerals, antioxidants and pancreatic enzymes.

Professor Ben Pfeifer

Another person with clinical trials behind their Diet Therapy is Professor Ben Pfeifer, formerly at the Aeskulap Clinic in Switzerland. Although Pfeifer started with prostate cancer patients, he is now moving on to other hormonally driven cancers.

Pfeifer's Protocol was primarily developed for hormone refractory prostate cancer – a state where the patient had little hope of long-term cure. Clinical studies show Pfeifer's treatment programme has a 65 per cent success rate, even though it has been used largely with patients for whom orthodox treatment has failed. His work was covered originally in the *Swiss Journal of Oncology, January 2005.*

Pfeifer uses an individually tailored programme of herbs, glyconutrients, minerals and vitamins. All these are centred on four commercially developed products:

- **Prostasol** – containing herbs such as saw palmetto, pygeum, reishi, ginger, nettles, skullcap, beta-sitosterol, and is licensed in Holland with no tainting from oestrogenic products.
- **Biobran** – is a natural food extract, made from 'pre-digested' rice bran using enzymes from shitake mushrooms. It is a powerful immune system booster which works by stimulating the activity of T- and B-lymphocytes and Natural Killer cells –

the front line in your body's defences. There are over 15 published studies in science journals on this immuno-modulator, highlighting its safety and effectiveness in individuals who have compromised immune systems.

- **Imupros** – is a blend of nutritional supplements including vitamins, trace elements, ginseng, lycopene and green tea extract.
- **Curcumin Complex** – is a mix of **curcumin,** a potent anti-inflammatory and antioxidant compound found in the spice turmeric; and **resveratrol,** a strong antioxidant, plant compound from red grapes; and **black pepper** which enhances absorption.

Interestingly, Pfeifer's protocol doesn't deliver where the patient's cancer is not oestrogen driven, nor when radiotherapy has caused damage.

Although the standard UK orthodox medical line is to ignore the Swiss clinical trials, one hospital – St Bartholomew's Hospital, London – is at least honest enough to say that, in the absence of any worthwhile treatments for this late stage prostate cancer, they may as well give the Pfeifer Protocol a try. It's not an official trial – and certainly not a clinical trial – and only about a dozen patients have been allowed to take up the full Protocol, to see if it provides any benefit. You can read far more on our web site, where we will include updates.

Pfeifer, meanwhile, is now developing his Protocol for other cancer types.

What is common between Gonzalez and Pfeifer, apart from the fact that their programmes are supported by research, is that the exact programme is tailored to you and your cancer, and both involve very detailed testing, and then a very large number of highly active ingredients given with specific purpose to meet specific needs.

The Gerson Therapy

Guaranteed to make certain orthodox medical experts turn puce merely at its mention, you should be clear that the Gerson Therapy has no clinical trial data to support its effectiveness.

Despite the fervoured denial of sceptics, it does have quite a lot of happy customers and anecdotal evidence, more than I first imagined. And I have been to San Diego, met Charlotte Gerson, and met with both Oxford Don Michael Gearin-Tosh and Beata Bishop who used the Therapy and beat their cancers.

The Gerson Therapy was developed by Dr Max Gerson (1881–1959) for migraine but he noted it had an effect with TB, and so started to treat people in the 1920s for an incurable form of TB, where he achieved phenomenal results. The Gerson Therapy is more than just a diet therapy – it is a healing discipline. Although primarily used by people who already have a chronic illness, it is however occasionally used in a preventative context. It may well be hard work but, for some, the effort is truly worthwhile.

"Suffering isn't ennobling, recovery is."
Dr Christiaan Barnard

Let us be quite clear. For a number of people, and many of those for whom orthodox medicine had failed, the Gerson Therapy has been an important part of their 'recovery'. There are many anecdotes, most notably Michael Gearin-Tosh, and Beata Bishop, two of the people who more than beat the odds with the Gerson Therapy. Michael lived 10 full years after being diagnosed with terminal multiple myeloma – sadly he died of something completely unrelated. Beata turned to the therapy 25 years ago with her melanoma when all the orthodox treatments had failed her. You can find much more on our website.

The basic principle behind the therapy is to heal the whole body by returning the body systems, key organs and cells to the state they should be in, if you had a healthy non-toxic body. The aim is twofold: The stimulation of the body's own immune defences to do what they do normally in a healthy body, plus the readjustment in the balance of the molecules and atoms within the cells, returning them to levels normally found in healthy cells. It is a healing, restorative strategy for all diseases, not merely cancer.

Once both parts of this therapy are fully established, the theory is that a diseased body will simply restore itself to full health – just as nature intended. In a few cases patients use the Therapy as an 'alternative treatment', but mostly they start it after orthodox therapies have failed them. This causes a double problem – the patients are usually 'late stage' and their bodies have been well and truly poisoned by chemotherapy. None the less, there are numerous success stories – The San Diego centre is at last keeping records and claim about a 25 to 30 per cent success rate. There is no doubt that this therapy has had notable successes, especially given that patients tend to be in later stages of their cancer, having often tried and failed with all available orthodox treatments beforehand.

However, diseased cancer cells apparently 'liquefy', which in itself creates a further problem. The process of breaking down tumours can be so effective that large amounts of toxins are released into the bloodstream by the diseased cells. (It should be noted that patients frequently experience 'healing reactions' when these large amounts of toxins are released from the cells into the blood system.)

However, as I covered earlier, the largest detoxification organ, the liver, is often seriously toxic itself and simply cannot treat the sudden increases in toxins flooding into the blood stream. So it needs help – it needs to be cleansed itself, and supercharged to help it better eliminate all the extra toxins.

One method of achieving this is to stimulate the liver with up to five coffee enemas per day for a limited period, whilst using castor oil every other day. This causes increases in the levels of bile juices, and a dilation of the bile ducts themselves, making the passage of toxins easier.

Dr Max Gerson was described by Dr Albert Schweitzer as, *one of the most eminent geniuses in medical history."* He originally published *A Cancer Therapy: Results of Fifty Cases,* over fifty years ago. His work is now driven by his eighty-something year old daughter Charlotte, who stresses that the therapy is applicable to a host of diseases, not merely cancer, and that even healthy people should consider a period on the therapy from time to time merely as a precautionary detox.

The total therapy aims to provide optimum nutrition consisting of a deliberate over-abundance of minerals, enzymes and vitamins, whilst avoiding the toxic pesticides and herbicides of normal food by using only organic sources.

The basic principles of the therapy are:

- The use of only organic food to avoid pesticide and herbicide toxins.
- Very limited fat and protein consumption both of which are known to 'feed' cancer cells – no animal fat or protein in the first eight weeks; nor milk and soya.
- No pulses (lentils, beans and, again, soya) to be consumed as they can prevent mineral uptake because of their phytic acid content. (NB. You could just skim this off the surface of the boiled pulses though.)
- All water used for cooking or rinsing must be provided from distilled or reverse osmosis sources.
- Water must not be drunk as it dilutes the power of the juices. A little peppermint tea is allowed.
- Neither plastic nor metal foil may be used as it may contaminate food.
- The diet is limited to
  1) freshly made juices of vegetables, fruits and leaves, consumed within 20 minutes of preparation to avoid losses in enzyme effectiveness, and
  2) large quantities of raw fruit and vegetables, along with some lightly steamed vegetables, stewed fruit, potatoes and oatmeal.
- Organic fresh vegetables and fruit, in season, are the ideal.

The therapy attempts to exclude sodium, whilst dramatically increasing potassium intake as we discussed in Chapter 3. Fresh juices provide more easily absorbed and digested nutrients, whilst not taxing the impaired body systems. The use of hourly juices over the length of the day also avoids calorie and, thus, insulin surges and actually limits the total number of calories consumed per day.

Absolutely **essential** to the diet therapy are:

- Apples – raw.
- Carrots – raw and lightly cooked.
- Potatoes – baked, mashed or in potato salad.
- Sweet potatoes – but only once per week.
- Fresh fruit – grapes, cherries, mangoes, peaches, oranges, apricots, grapefruit, banana, tangerines, pears, plums, melons, papayas (pears and plums may be stewed).
- Dried fruit – apricots, dates, figs, peaches, raisins, prunes.

Absolutely **forbidden** are:

- All things bottled, canned, frozen, preserved, refined, salted, smoked and sulphured.
- Bicarbonate of soda in food, toothpaste and mouthwashes.
- Alcohol.
- Salts.
- Avocado (too much fatty acid).
- Basil, oregano (aromatic oils can cause difficult reactions).
- Berries (except red, black and whole currants).
- Biscuits, cake, chocolate, cocoa, coffee (any sort), tea.
- Cucumbers.
- Fats and oils (except flaxseed),
- Mushrooms, nuts (too much fatty acids/fats), peas (sulphured), lentils, beans, seeds (phytic acid/enzyme inhibitors).
- Pickles.
- Pineapples.
- Refined flour.
- Soft drinks, fizzy and fruit juices (preserved).
- Soya (fat content and phytic acid).
- Spices.
- Sugar (including sweets).
- Tap water.

Forbidden for first eight weeks: all dairy, eggs, meat and fish.

The type of juicer is also crucial. Centrifugal juicers simply do not extract the full volumes of minerals, vitamins and enzymes. Gerson recommended a heavy press juicer that involves two stages and a double press.

The therapy is arduous. A ten-hour day spent juicing plus making and using the coffee enemas is not unusual; and a period of two years to fully cleanse the body is not uncommon. The theory is that it takes a long time for the body to develop the many stages of the cancer process in the first place, and so it takes an equally long time to get rid of them all to restore everything to maximum working order!

So the therapy is hard work. You need time to prepare the fresh juices, as they have to be drunk at their prime. Then there is the preparation and use of the coffee enemas. But as Goethe said, *"The day is of infinite length for him who knows how to appreciate and use it."*

The Gerson Institute has been criticised in the past for not adapting the therapy as new scientific discoveries were made for natural compounds. This has now been addressed and there is now a new book out from Charlotte Gerson that covers the issue: *"Healing – The Gerson Way"*.

Other elements of the therapy:

Gerson used crude **liver extract** to boost his patients liver function, but nowadays this extract is more refined and seems not so potent. While Gerson used his special 'calf liver preparation', most sources now seem to have pesticide residues and campylobacter infection. **Coenzyme Q10** and defatted **colostrum** (the first fluid secreted in a mother's breast) are now used to boost the immune system.

Pancreatic enzymes have always been a part of the therapy, as have **WobeMugos tablets** containing a number of anti-tumour and immune-boosting natural compounds.

Recent additions have included the use of **hyperthermia, B-17** and **ozone therapy**. Supplements like **grapefruit seed extract, Pau d'Arco, selenium** and **chromium picolinate** (which stimulates the pancreas) are used also now. Some critics claim that the loss of the liver extract is major – I have no evidence one way or the other.

What I do observe is that the current therapy is not as random as some critics suggest. Blood tests monitoring all manner of enzyme, toxin and mineral levels are taken on a frequent basis, and adjustments are made as a result.

The Plaskett Therapy

One of the Gerson-needs-to-be-updated critics was Dr. Lawrence Plaskett, formerly vice chair of the UK Nutritional Cancer Therapy Trust. After a degree in biochemistry at Cambridge, a doctorate at London University and a number of years in food companies and Government agencies, Dr. Plaskett turned his extensive knowledge to updating the Gerson Therapy. He now educates new nutritionists to degree level.

His research on natural compounds in food is extremely detailed. Plaskett in the UK and John Boik in the USA really do expose the lack of knowledge inherent in British Orthodox Medicine on this subject.

Plaskett argues that many recent scientific discoveries have proven that Gerson was totally right and considerably 'ahead of his time'. The latest scientific studies have supported, for example, the importance of omega-3 (from fish oils and linseed oil) as an essential element in the good health of cells; the use of coffee enemas to induce raised levels of glutathione S-transferases, the enzymes of liver detoxification; the use of high potassium in the diet and digestive enzymes to help increase absorption.

Where he feels recent studies have added to Gerson is that there is no need for castor oil, iodine and iodide, dried thyroid, liver juices and liver injections. Instead he recommends a very detailed and precise list of supplements, some of which vary according to the cancer.

Plaskett's version of the therapy is vigorously vegan. Dairy products, eggs, fish and meat are excluded, because he argues that cancers thrive on protein and a low protein diet has been shown to be effective against cancer (*Tannenbaum*).

Plaskett is also a firm believer in the eat-to-beat-cancer principle and it is his firmly held view that a nutritional approach to cancer should be nationally available. There are at least 90 trained Plaskett Therapists throughout the UK.

Notable Others

Dr. Contreras at the Oasis of Hope in Mexico (Contreras is Mexican) uses a modified version of the Gerson Therapy, plus

'Metabolic Therapy' consisting of laetrile treatment along with pancreatic enzymes, vitamin C megadoses, spiritual healing and prayer.

Dr. Burzynski who believes from his own research findings that cancer patients lack certain key peptides (chains of amino acids, smaller than proteins). His solution is to analyse which are lacking and then to use diet and supplements to rebuild levels. His work is constantly monitored by the FDA.

The Nori Protocol, is based on research evidence showing cancer needs methionine, an amino acid found in certain foods, or it dies. Foods that are low in methionine are nuts, seeds, vegetables and especially fruits. (Sounds like a Rainbow Diet, doesn't it?). The Protocol directly targets the mitochondria and also uses sodium selenite, which is claimed to be the most effective form of selenium for therapeutic treatment). Genipin from gardenia juice extract and thymoquinone (from black cumin seed) are added active ingredients.

The Hippocrates Health Institute incorporates a colourful, fresh, raw and vegan 'living foods' diet into its comprehensive wellness programme.

There are many others – check out our website.

Summary

> *"Despair is the price one pays for setting oneself an impossible aim."*
> (Graham Greene)

If you have cancer, curing yourself solely through a diet therapy may seem a very tall order. But for a few people with cancer who reject orthodox medicine, it's the place to start. Whichever route you take (diet therapy or the use of diet as a part of your Integrative plan) please remember that your cancer may have taken six years to develop to a point where it could be diagnosed. You are not going to rid yourself of it in six weeks. Please do not despair, whichever route you choose, if 'cure' seems distant. First try to stabilise and calm the situation.

There are a number of similarities between the above therapies. Firstly, patients to date tended to only use these therapies at a late stage of the cancer – often when orthodox medical approaches have failed. Despite this, you may feel the clinical trials and the anecdotes tell a positive story.

Secondly, they are often more disciplined than critics claim, involving detailed blood and biochemical analysis.

Thirdly, the diet therapies are not all vegetarian – they may use metabolic typing to determine whether meat should be consumed or not; or they may be 'fat and protein' free – thus eliminating everything from dairy to soya to meat and fish. It's a moot point but an important one.

Finally, they all have width. They don't rely on a couple of vitamins, or a vegetarian diet or giving up alcohol. They have a total concept – something to tackle the whole cancer process. For example:

- Boosting the immune system with natural compounds.
- Correcting mineral imbalances and deficiencies.
- Trying to return the cells to a healthy normal state.
- Using natural compounds to attack the cancer cells.
- Using natural compounds (like fish oils) to reduce inflammation.
- Using pancreatic enzymes to try to turn off the cancer cells.

As you can see it is totally wrong to suggest changing your diet doesn't make a jot of difference – it can help save your life. Cancer Watch, the research centre in CANCERactive, and the American Cancer Society provide two objective resources and analyses that prove otherwise.

The issue is simple: Rather than taking yourself off to New York, Switzerland, Mexico or California at great expense, are there things you can learn from all this to build into your life right now and so increase your personal chances of beating cancer. And the answer is an overwhelming 'Yes'.

CHAPTER 11
ACID AND ALKALINE BODIES

The human body works best when it is slightly alkaline. In fact an acid body causes the biochemical processes to work poorly and illness ensues. Acid bodies can also lead to cancer. However, you may have read that certain foods cause 'acid ash' in the body, whilst others cause 'alkaline ash'. This is tosh, at best a gross oversimplification of the causes of an acid body.

A neutral, neither acid nor alkaline, solution will have a pH of 7 on a scale where 1 is extremely acid and 14 is extremely alkaline. The body works best at about 7.2 to 7.4. A research team made up of eleven scientists from Arizona Cancer Center, Wayne State and H. Lee Moffitt Cancer Institute, Florida conducted research on cancer tumours in 2009 confirming that the core of a cancer has an acid pH of 6.2 due to the energy production system of glycolysis (burning glucose in the absence of oxygen). They found that an acid body helped the cancer fire off its metastases and also helped them take hold elsewhere. They also discovered that alkalysing the body (they used sodium bicarbonate in solution as a drink) could stop the metastases. And they showed that injecting the same cheap alkalysing compound into the heart of the tumour could stop its chemical reactions, causing shrinkage. Clinical trials are now underway.

So how does your body become acidic in the first place? And how can you make it more consistently alkaline?

1. Consuming good levels of potassium and magnesium but little sodium will help make your cells more alkaline.
As we have told you in a previous chapter. Your immune system and all your organs will become more alkaline, and your body will thrive.

The biggest sources of potassium and magnesium have already been covered but principally they include all fruits and all vegetables (bananas, lemons, plums are excellent potassium sources – as are tomatoes, asparagus, Brussels sprouts and rhubarb, four foods often included erroneously as 'acid forming foods '), herbs, whole grains, whole rice and fresh nuts and seeds.

2. Consuming foods that have high levels of sodium will make your cells more acid.
This list would include:

Mono-sodium glutamate (for example, in Chinese foods)

Common table salt and most sea salt (both refined)

Processed foods

Prepared foods

Smoked foods

Dried meats like ham, chicken breast slices and salamis, patés, sausages, bacon

Mass-market loaves of bread and breakfast cereals

Once sodium displaces potassium inside the cell (because of excesses of sodium, deficiencies in potassium, or deficiencies in magnesium result in the pump that kicks sodium out not working properly) lowered cellular oxygen occurs. When Warburg won his Nobel prize he noted that cellular oxygen was essential to prevent cancer, as were alkaline cells.

3. Other factors can achieve the same damage.
For example, aggressive human oestrogens such as oestradiol can cause havoc inside the cell and the same high sodium, low oxygen combination. Synthetic compounds that are oestrogens or act as oestrogen mimics in the body (like HRT, Bisphenol A, parabens, phthalates, toluene etc) could also cause this situation too. So the list of 'acid cell' formers might include certain pesticides and in-home chemicals, and environmental toxins.

Stress produces the hormone cortisol that can cause negative cellular changes. Steroids and insulin can do this too, whilst a range of natural compounds from fish oils to curcumin, aloe vera, ginger and garlic can counter this.

The Chinese call cows' dairy 'phlegm food'. It contains hormones such as IGF-1 which can make cells divide rapidly and increase oestrogen levels. The high blood calcium levels also affect magnesium absorption and thus reduce the effectiveness of the cellular pump.

4. Certain compounds can counter the oestrogen threat. Weakening or omitting them can cause acid bodies.
Melatonin, a hormone produced during sleep, regulates oestrogen levels. Unsurprisingly, then, IARC has declared lack of sleep to be carcinogenic. But EMFs will also lower melatonin production and cause oestrogen increases in the body.

Being overweight increases body fat levels and this increases oestrogen levels in men and women. Being overweight is not just the product of eating the wrong foods but poor lifestyle habits too (for example eating one large meal a day, large levels of glucose, no exercise etc). Thus reducing excess body fat levels through exercise will make your cells less acidic via lowered oestrogen levels, increased levels of 'happy hormones' called endorphins and lowered insulin levels.

Foods that limit or denature aggressive oestrogens are thus alkaline-forming. These would include foods like 'supergreens', wheatgrass, chlorella, broccoli, lignans, linoleic acid in flaxseed and medicinal mushrooms. There are foods that stop oestradiol attacking the receptor sites on cells and launching the havoc message. Phytoestrogens are highly protective in this way. They can bind to the same receptor sites and stop human ostrogens. Phytoestrogens do not cause havoc inside the cell and occur typically in pulses, vegetables and fruits. Asians have much higher levels of phytoestrogens in their blood streams than their sisters in the West.

Then there are foods that increase cellular oxygen via increasing glutathione levels (all fruits and vegetables, especially green ones). Finally other factors can help alkalise your cells and improve oxygen levels, for example having the correct types and levels of beneficial bacteria in the intestine can help expel oestrogenic compounds from the gut; an excess of yeasts in the body, may cause lowered oxygen levels in a local area, and set up the conditions for ill health. Eliminating excesses of yeasts thus makes for a more oxygenated cellular environment.

Later in the book there is a chapter on controlling oestrogen with food, and one on controlling yeasts. As you can see, producing acid cells and lowered oxygen can be due to a wide variety of factors all capable of being countered quite easily.

So 'alkalise for health'

Some dietary experts recommend taking a teaspoon of sodium bicarbonate in a glass of warm water first thing in the morning or last thing at night to help combat the acidity and return you to an alkaline state. (It can also kill off yeasts). I worry that this is 'missing the point'. It is your cells that need correcting if you are ill. And that means more magnesium, more potassium and less sodium. Also, your gut doesn't need alkalising. Pathogens thrive when acid levels fall. Indeed, good bacteria like acidophilus produce lactic acid and that keeps the pathogens in check. Apple Cider Vinegar has a positive effect here too.

Others recommend incorporating greens (like fresh wheatgrass, chlorella or spirulina) and flaxseed into the diet, or sleeping in a darkened room, avoiding pesticides, and cows' dairy while switching to toxin-free, in-home products.

Then there are those who swear by juicing, perhaps first having undertaken a three or five day fast. Juices usually incorporate a high organic vegetable content. Ginger may be used to add taste (and it will calm inflammation). It is not always advisable to incorporate a high fruit content, especially if you may suffer from yeast imbalances.

This is clearly a very complex issue and there is far more on our website and in the rest of this book, but I hope the above goes some way to understanding just how you can 'alkalise for health', increasing your oxygen levels and decreasing the acid salts in your cells. There is so much you can do.

CHAPTER 12

CLEAN WATER –
THE ONLY SOLUTION

As JB Haldane once exclaimed, *'Even the Archbishop of Canterbury is 85 per cent water!'*

If a plant in your garden is drooping and limp, you may add nutrients to the soil and you will certainly add water. But, if the water is contaminated you know the plant will be affected. Why do you not use this thinking with your own health?

Clean water is essential to our health. It affects all our cells, our enzymatic processes and our ability to detox; treatments such as the Gerson Therapy stress the use of pure water for cancer patients, for cooking and even for washing utensils.

Remember – you drink tap water and you bathe in it. And the skin is not a barrier, as some water companies would ask us to believe. It is a carrier. If it were not, how would a nicotine or oestrogen patch work?

We suspect our tap water is less than perfect but are told that individual pollutants are below government-determined safe levels, so we have no need to worry. And the whole issue on water safety ends up in a dispute between logic and statistics. Governments repeatedly state there is little evidence that individual pollutants are above safety limits and may be causing problems. But surely it is possible that the combined effects may be far worse.

Rain falling brings with it smoke, dust, chemical fumes, germs, lead and strontium-90 to name but a few things. The Swedes blame the UK industrial revolution for clouds of acid rain that wiped out the fish population in some of their lakes.

Water then flows through the soil, in rivers and streams picking up fertilisers, pesticides, herbicides and nitrates.

Some people buy organic food only then to cook it in tap water; or they make their decaffeinated herb tea with boiled tap water. Boiling merely concentrates certain contaminants.

Back to basics – the need for water?

The late Dr Batmanghelidj, formally of St Mary's Hospital Medical School (part of Imperial College, London), provided a strong case for drinking at least two litres of water a day in his book, '*Your Body's Many Cries for Water*'. He argued very convincingly that dehydration can be responsible for a huge range of ailments and degenerative diseases including dyspeptic pain, rheumatoid arthritis pain, stress and depression, high blood pressure, high blood cholesterol, excess body weight, asthma and allergies. He showed how these diseases and ailments originate often from metabolic stress, and one of the biggest contributory factors to this stress is dehydration.

In the author's postscript, he added, '*When will all NHS doctors start looking at dehydration and getting their patients to increase their clean water consumption?*'

Others will argue that two litres of water per day per adult is an absolute minimum for proper cellular hydration, with three litres probably closer to the mark if we exercise or we are ill, having radiotherapy treatment and so on.

But what is the science? When I was in advertising I once asked a famous bottled water company for their support to the need for two litres per day – and they told me that they had none. The European Union scientists have recently decided in their infinite wisdom that you may not claim that 'water rehydrates you' in advertising as there is insufficient evidence! Surely this is nonsense; but how much water is required?

The FSA in the UK achieve a figure of eight glasses a day based on an analysis of how much water you use in an average day, less the water you consume when eating foods such as fruit and vegetables. On average, the body loses 1 to 1.5 litres of water per day, more if you exercise, more if you are in a hot climate.

Too much water can actually reduce levels of salts and important electrolytes in the body. In **icon** we covered the story of a London Theatre artist who sang and danced his way through a two-hour performance every night. He regularly drank 14 bottles of water a night and ended up in hospital with total electrolyte imbalance!

In April 2008 doctors in the Renal Division of the University of Pennsylvania have concluded in the *Journal of American Society of Nephrology* that there is no evidence whatsoever for the claims that 2 litres or more will help you detoxify or help you lose weight or avoid headaches and so on. They do say that drinking more water will help clear the body of salt and urea but conclude that the issue is to drink 'enough', stating that there is no research showing benefit in drinking larger amounts.

So what is enough? And again the answer is as individual as you are. You may be healthy and normal in a cool climate. You may live up a mountain, or in the tropics, you may be ill and having treatments. The simple way to tell if you are drinking enough water is to check the colour of your urine. It should be almost colourless – a very pale yellow. If you are taking B vitamins, or a multivitamin containing B vitamins, or turmeric/curcumin supplements it will be a little darker.

The rule of thumb is that if you have dark yellow or even brown urine you are simply not drinking enough water. The SAS and top sportsmen use this simple system because they know that a 5 per cent drop in body liquids causes tiredness and sluggishness, which can reduce performance by 50 per cent.

The toxins in water

If you have cancer, it is crucial to try to establish what caused the cancer so you can make every attempt to cut it out of your life. What if that toxin were water-borne?

Prime areas of concern in tap water supplies are:

- Chlorine and fluorine
- Heavy metals
- Pesticides, fertilisers and herbicides
- Drugs and oestrogens.

In an Iowa study *(Lynch, Zhang, Olsen)* there were significantly higher levels of female lung cancer and male bladder cancer in towns with surface water supply and shadow wells. Pesticides and other chemicals on the land were implicated.

Chlorine is added to water, for example, to kill germs and bacteria, but it also destroys vitamin E and kills the 'friendly bacteria' in the intestinal tract. Chlorine can damage arteries and can even oxidise other contaminants in the water to produce free-radicals or, worse, combine to produce chloroform, chloramines and other toxic by-products, which are carcinogenic.

The National Research Council in the USA has prepared a 379 page report on trichloroethylene. Always known to be a dangerous pollutant and linked to child leukaemia, kidney cancer and a number of illnesses, the report concludes that TCE is actually 40 times more powerful than originally thought! And levels of TCE have been increasing in tap water as chlorine combines with other increasing levels of pollutants. These two new discoveries mean that in certain regions the water TCE content is now actually above the original safety levels set by the Government.

Another research study published in May 2008 by researchers at Birmingham University analysed birth defects in babies born between 2001 and 2003 in Taiwan, where chlorine levels are almost identical to those in tap water in the UK. They found a doubling in birth defects like hole-in-the-heart, cleft palates, urinary tract defects, brain defects and Down's syndrome. Earlier studies have linked chlorinated water to miscarriage, still birth and bladder cancer. The researchers identified trihalomethanes (THMs) as the cause – and stated that you can increase levels in the womb by drinking the water, or bathing in it.

In a Finnish study on surface water (AMJ August 1999), chlorinated water was linked to increased incidences of bladder, kidney and stomach cancers. The US Environmental Agency has stated that prolonged and frequent swimming in chlorinated pools contributes to skin cancer (*Epidemiology 1992: 3*). Chlorinated water also contributes to miscarriages (*JAWWA 1992: 20*) and gastrointestinal cancer, bladder cancer and rectal cancer (*American Journal of Public Health* 1997: 87).

Some 1000 cities now treat their water with ozone, which has had a significant effect on purity.

Fluoride: Fluoride is an acknowledged 'equivocal carcinogen'. It was downgraded (for reasons beyond my comprehension) a few years back from 'clear evidence of carcinogenicity'.

All the original tests used by governments worldwide to encourage fluoridation of water purported to show that fluorine was a tooth and bone protecting agent. Calcium fluoride was the proposed additive. Approval was given on that basis. But life moves on and now in the UK we use sodium fluoride, formerly used as a rat poison and a by-product of the aluminium industry, which causes it to be contaminated by metals such as aluminium and even arsenic. This water treatment is illegal in Sweden, Denmark and Holland, since apparently sodium fluoride contains too many heavy metal contaminants, and in addition fluoride can inhibit thyroid function and damage the immune system. Hypothyroidism is a known consequence of too much fluoride.

While governments and water companies add chlorine to water to treat water, they add fluoride to water to treat people. Without our consent.

It is medically contra-indicated – for pregnant mothers (US Government, 1966), formula-fed infants, diabetics and people with kidney impairment. What are they supposed to do; move home?

It's not as if we don't get enough fluoride in this modern world. Sulphuryl fluoride, for example, is used as a fumigant on nuts, wheat and over 150 US foodstuffs many of which are sold in Britain. Residues on these foods can be 130 times higher than the level in our water. It's a psychotropic drug and the cousin of Prozac.

Worse, toothpastes commonly contain sodium fluoride. In the USA there are on-pack warnings which read, '*As with all fluoride toothpastes, keep out of the reach of children under 6 years of age. If you do accidentally swallow more than used for brushing, seek professional assistance or contact a poison control officer immediately*'.

There is virtually no hard evidence that fluoridation improves children's teeth, indeed, quite the opposite. Teotia and Teotia conducted the largest dental study in the world in India. Over 30 years, they examined 400,000 children and found that tooth decay <u>increased</u> with fluoride concentrations in the water and decreased with calcium concentration.

In the USA, The National Institute of Environmental Health Sciences investigated a Harvard professor who was sponsored to the tune of $13 million to look into child bone cancer and fluoridation. He actually reported to Federal Officials on his study that no link between child bone cancer and fluoridation was found. However, when the full report arrived, the detail showed there was clearly a risk, especially to boys of a young age! His links to the toothpaste companies are also being investigated.

Some states are now moving away from fluoridation of water.

Aluminium: is present in significant quantities in tap water, as it can be added to clarify the water during treatment. A detailed review paper published in March 2002 discussed the powerful evidence showing that aluminium from drinking water and other sources is a major contributory factor to Alzheimer's disease, which is becoming increasingly common amongst older people.

Adding insult to injury, research shows that aluminium can react with low-doses of fluoride in water, causing more aluminium to cross the blood-brain barrier and become deposited in the brain. Julie Varner and her colleagues showed this definitively in a detailed 52-week study of rats, published in the prestigious peer-reviewed journal *Brain Research*. Aluminium is a potent neurotoxin and has even been implicated as a co-factor in the initiation of cancer.

Other metals: Old pipes in the water system and chemicals deposited in streams can lead to **lead**, **mercury** and **copper** contamination. Mercury's negatives are well chronicled; both lead and copper inhibit zinc uptake in the body and zinc is important in a variety of ways from enhancing vitamin C effectiveness to protecting against prostate cancers. One theory of prostate cancer is that the lower levels of zinc found in prostate patients are due to heavy metals like mercury and cadmium displacing the zinc.

The National Academy of Sciences (September 2001) showed that even very low levels of **arsenic** in the water were linked to cancer (the United States EPA set standards in 1975 and may well have set them wrong, was the conclusion). Studies have been made from China to Chile and arsenic is increasingly found to seep into the soil from natural sources, agriculture and industrial waste.

Parasites are now common in 20 per cent of the British population. In Carolina 82 per cent of the population were getting theirs from the water system as the microscopic parasites had become immune to chlorine.

Nitrate and nitrite: A study of 22,000 women in Iowa showed that **nitrate**, common in rural areas was associated with bladder cancer. 20 per cent of ingested nitrate was shown to be transformed in the body to nitrite and N-nitroso compounds causing cancers such as colon and bladder (May 2001 study).

Scientists from 19 countries at IARC in Lyon (2007) have concluded that high **nitrite** levels, especially in conjunction with low vitamin C levels are linked to various cancers especially stomach, oesophageal and brain. Of special concern was the run-off of water from pesticides in the fields, with nitrates and nitrites either directly promoting cancer through the water supplies, or indirectly via the by-products of their effect on stimulating cyanobacteria in the soil which go on to poison crops and then us all.

Radon: The National Association of Scientists in America in 1998 showed that radon in the water supply was linked to lung cancers. Radon can leach into water supplies where the underlying rock contains even small uranium deposits. This is a potential risk in some areas of South West and North West England.

Drugs: Another debate concerns **oestrogen** levels in the recycled drinking water of major cities, originating from ladies who take HRT and contraceptive pills. This has been blamed for reduced fertility, and for increases in testicular cancer. Sperm count is down 20 per cent in the UK in 25 years, whilst testicular cancer is up 80 per cent. It has also been blamed for male fish showing female organ development and young human male offspring developing testicle problems and even reducing penis size. Hormones are very powerful substances – they can work in concentrations of less than one part per billion, the sort of levels it is almost impossible to selectively remove from water.

The counter claim is that in Denmark and Scotland, where there is no use of recycled water, oestrogen levels in the populations are also rising. The blame is put on a variety of chemicals in the environment, particularly endocrine (hormone) disrupters like chemical oestrogen mimics (xenoestrogens), for example from white lined cans, plastic bottles, even plastic children's toys, and plastic wrapped food and plastics in general. Certain plasticisers are worse than others and one really has no idea whether the plastic bottle or cup in front of you is harmless or dangerous. Recent US research showed that where a hot liquid was used in a plastic container made of certain plasticisers, harmful chemicals were released at a 40-fold increased level, and continued to be so even on subsequent use with cold liquids.

Then there are xenoestrogens from petrol fumes, cleaning agents, toiletries and detergents, as we covered previously.

Whatever the reason, the issue is: 'Do these harmful chemicals get into your drinking water?' Roger Lilley of Friends of the Earth blames a lack of monitoring by water companies, particularly of local rivers. Both the river Aire in Scotland and the river Lee (from where London gets drinking water) are, in varying degrees, already toxic to wildlife, according to Friends of the Earth.

Nowadays with our increased use of **drugs** (like steroids and antibiotics; or Tamoxifen and statins both of which have recently been shown to remain active in the body for more than 5 years) combined with the increasing numbers of old people who already consume over 60 per cent of all drugs in the UK, synthetic oestrogen is not the only drug that potentially could make it into a big city's water supply. There is even German research that detected six different 'sweeteners' in tap water! Is it enough to hope that all these drugs are removed in your recycled drinking water?

Action?

What are we to do? What is increasingly clear is that there is no such thing as 'generic' tap water, only 'local' tap water. The concentrations of different potential carcinogens vary greatly by region and many are not totally removed under normal conditions. The issue isn't just about drinking, of course. You wash your vegetables in it, and your cups and plates. You cook in it. You bathe the baby in it.

Plastic bottled water is increasingly felt to be less than perfect because of the plasticisers I talked about above, potentially leaching from the plastic into the water. These can be carcinogenic even in minute quantities and as Dr Anna Soto of Tufts showed, they can be cumulative.

Boiling the water merely increases the concentration of the toxins dissolved.

Distillation, if you had the time, money and the apparatus, can work but it is hard to provide enough volume for all your rinsing and cooking needs on top of water levels for drinking.

The most convenient way of removing contaminants is through **filtration.** A double carbon filter can be installed under the sink. It is relatively cheap, but seems to be rather limited in its filtration abilities.

Then there is a **reverse osmosis water filter.**

The great advantage of this system is that it eliminates nearly all of the fluoride, parasites and bacteria, oestrogen, chlorine and aluminium in your drinking water, as well as a host of other potentially toxic chemicals, hormone disrupters and drugs, as long as the filters are changed regularly. Measuring the more common impurities (in parts per million), a recent test I witnessed showed scores of:

Tap water	400–700
Jug filtered tap water	275
Plastic bottled mineral water	175
Reverse osmosis filtered	6

And therein lies the problem. Reverse osmosis removes virtually everything – including the minerals that are important for good health. These minerals are normally dissolved in water and as a result it has a pH of about 7.2. So you see natural water is slightly alkaline, reflected in the ideal body pH which is also slightly alkaline. However, remove all the minerals and you don't just remove potential 'nourishment', you make the water much more acidic. One man in Ireland I know measured his water's pH after reverse osmosis at 5.2.

There has been a lot of press comment and concern about this 'dead' water issue. You could 'compensate' a little by doubling your daily intake of minerals. But you might still miss certain trace elements.

The counter argument is that reverse osmosis water has been consumed throughout South East Asia for the last 25 years without any apparent ill effects. There are mass market machines outside apartment blocks – you simply put a coin in a slot and you fill up your very large container! The big beer companies like Singha, and also Nestlé and Coca Cola have launched brands of this 'Clean, drinking water.'

A new development is that of re-mineralisation. After the first two chambers take everything out of the water, a third chamber runs the water over rock salts to put the important minerals back. And this, in turn, alkalises the water again.

Another idea is a **water ioniser,** with claims that it filters the water effectively, keeps it alkaline and keeps it 'alive'. The good news is that prices of these have declined from the early models at £1000.

For now the most cost effective solution is probably glass bottled spring water from the original source to drink, if you can get it (restaurants can), and use a reverse osmosis filter to provide the inert water for washing and cooking the vegetables and washing the dishes.

Whether you already have cancer or are keen to prevent it, you should take a realistic view of the above facts and plan your action. Water is vital to your body and good health; you simply don't need the impurities that come with it.

CHAPTER 13
CUTTING OUT THE BAD GUYS

Yes, I'm sorry. I did say that other diet books told you what to avoid and cut out; and I implied this book was going to be different.

My personal view is that you don't have to deprive yourself of all your favourite foods – and I do believe a little of what you fancy does you good. But nonetheless, if there is top quality evidence against certain foods, it is my duty to tell you and your right to know.

Cows' Dairy

The *White Lies* report handed to the UK Government by a team of experts in 2007, in the words of the UK press, 'hammered' dairy. I have been warning readers for 15 years now.

In 2002, the Karolinska Institute produced an epidemiology study: On the links between dairy consumption and prostate cancer risk, they found a straight-line correlation; the more dairy you consume, the greater your risk.

Other studies have shown a less exact, but similar correlation between increased cows' dairy consumption and increased breast cancer risk.

In fact, the evidence against dairy is almost unarguable – there have been quite a lot of studies on several different cancers – we have covered them all in **icon**.

For example: 61,000 women were tracked for 13 years in a US study *(American Journal of Clinical Nutrition)* – a glass of milk a day (or equivalent) doubles ovarian cancer risk.

For example: 5000 people were followed for 65 years – those children who grew up in families consuming the highest amounts of cows' dairy (two cups per day each) had three times the colorectal cancer risk later in life *(Jolieke, Queensland)*

And bad news for the British – adding milk to tea ruins the health benefits of tea according to the Charité University Hospital, Berlin. The casein (milk protein) content of the milk, sticks to the beneficial polyphenols of the tea and negates them.

People come to me after speeches and ask if consuming low-fat or skimmed milk or organic milk would be all right?

The average dairy cow in the USA now produces 50 (yes, 50) times the volume of milk over its predecessors 20 years ago. How? Through hormones, drugs, genetic changes and 'super' feeds, which are often derived from animal protein even though cows are herbivores. The fat in milk is a solvent likely to bring with it all manner of hormones (natural and injected), antibiotics, pesticides and herbicides from the fields. Organic milk might have less of these toxins in it and low fat might also be better for you.

But the real problem does not go away with low fat or organic milk. The issue is bigger than drugs or pesticides. It is a hormone, Insulin-like Growth Factor 1 or IGF-1, which helps a baby calf grow to full size in about 10 months. IGF-1 causes cells to grow rapidly, and we humans don't need this turbo-charged growth, in fact it is dangerous. IGF-1 has been shown to cause cancer cell proliferation.

Monsanto, the giant American food company, and the FDA in the USA claim IGF-1 does not cross in any volume from the gut into the bloodstream. Specific Japanese research with mice clearly indicates otherwise.

As I told you earlier, the high levels of fat and protein in milk prevent absorption of elements like zinc, crucial to vitamin C absorption and action, and also important in the prevention of prostate cancer. Both cows' dairy protein and high blood levels of calcium actually depress circulating magnesium, potassium and vitamin D levels, and prevent the absorption of calcium into tissues and bones. There is increasing evidence that too much blood calcium may even cause cysts or ductal disturbances in women's breasts, and even cancer, while it is increasingly clear that vitamin D can help with both the prevention and treatment of a great many cancers.

But. Raw cows' dairy from grass fed, outdoor, organic cattle actually has two benefits. Firstly, the raw milk contains a wealth of helpful bacteria and immune-boosting compounds. Secondly, cows have rumens and in these the bacteria use the grass to make isomers of linoleic acid. Although linoleic acid is of questionable benefit, the isomers are not. Collectively, they are called Conjugated Linoleic Acid, (CLA), which has been shown, for example, to build up in breast tissue and be highly preventative of cancer. It can stop cancer appearing in the other breast, it has been shown (in rats) capable of correcting cancer, and it is proven to have epigenetic benefits!

Patients fighting cancer do not need high levels of protein and fat in their diets, and nor do they need IGF-1. You should try to cut down on cows' dairy as much as possible. You can get more than enough calcium from a daily helping of 'greens'. A little goat's cheese would be a good replacement for cows' cheese as we have been eating this for historically longer and it is more easily digested in the gut. You can try rice, almond or soya milk if you need to. But do not switch your large volume of milk consumption directly for a large volume of soya. Soya has a high fat and protein content too, and for this reason was cut from the Gerson Therapy. Personally, I am increasingly concerned about the possible dangers linked to GM soya which are covered in detail later.

Fat myths

In the Western world, we have two problems with **fats and oils:** We consume too much of them, and we consume largely the wrong sort!

Firstly, fats and oils are basically the same types of chemicals. Fat is the solid state, oil is the liquid state.

Next, understand that fat is very high in **calories:**

1 gram protein	=	4 calories
1 gram of carbohydrate	=	4 calories
1 gram fat	=	9 calories.

In the USA people regularly consume 50 per cent of their calories as fat, whereas in rural China this figure can be below 10 per cent. We noted earlier that several research studies show that high calorie consumption can produce more free-radicals and lead to more cancer, whereas calorie restriction is an important anti-cancer weapon.

Over the last two years it has become increasingly clear that calorie restriction and fasting can restrict cancer cell growth, halt progression and metastases and induce cancer cell death *(for example: De Lorenzo et al Caloric restriction reduces growth of mammary tumors and metastases.* Carcinogenesis. *2011 Sep; and Champa CE et al. Oncologist. 2013;18:97-103)* and increase or potentiate the effects of chemotherapy and radiotherapy. Good weight control is also one factor reported by the American Cancer Society to aid survival and even prevent a cancer returning.

Consuming fat is important as we will see. Consuming excess is dangerous, especially if the wrong sort.

Hydrogenated, or Trans Fats

For too many people in the West most fats and oils consumed are 'hydrogenated'. These are found in junk food, fast food, chicken nuggets, battered cod, onion rings, bagged snacks, crisps, salted roasted peanuts, processed foods, supermarket bread, biscuits, soup, chips, rice mixes, pasta mixes, pizzas and even some breakfast cereals, health bars and healthy bran-rich products; the list is endless.

Possibly the worst offenders are the modern 'vegetable oils'. Seemingly beneficial in name, these oils are often well known and have been used for centuries all over the world.

However, the food companies now refine these so that they do not spoil, using hydrogenation to extend the 'shelf-life' of supermarket and fast food products.

Firstly, the natural oils, corn, sunflower, and so on, are taken to very high temperatures in the refining porcess and virtually all nutrition that was originally present in the seed or vegetable is lost. Worse, the refining process can use gasoline, ethylene, methylchloride and chlorination leaving behind chemical traces. Finally, in many cases the resulting liquid is fully or partially hydrogenated – they add hydrogen to make it more solid at room temperatures. This may be reheated and then pressed to make what you or I may think are healthy 'vegetable oil' margarines because the label talks of 'sunflower oil' or similar. A wolf in sheep's clothing.

When oils are hydrogenated they are termed **trans fats**. For a number of years, people thought that the refining process just took out all the goodness and you were left with some sort of inert, nutritionally worthless oil. Not so. The Mayo Clinic comments, **"A recent study of 80,000 nurses showed that women whose diets were high in both saturated and trans fats had an increased risk of heart attack. But of greater interest was the finding that nurses who consumed considerable amounts of trans fat faced an ever higher heart attack risk than nurses who ate a lot of saturated fat."**

Ooooops!!

The Mayo Report continued, **"The research adds to previous evidence that trans fat may be as bad for your heart as saturated fat. In fact, trans fat may even be more damaging because in addition to raising your 'bad' (LDL) cholesterol level, it also appears to lower your 'good' (HDL) cholesterol level."**

We'll come to good and bad cholesterol later – let's not get confused!!

The end product of the digestion of trans fats, just as with smoking, is free-radicals. Lots of free-radicals. As we said earlier, these molecules are incomplete; they have a missing piece and are quite happy to rip the replacement from any molecule they come across, in turn making this molecule incomplete. This in turn, rips pieces off other molecules until it is the surrounding 'soup' of the genetic code that is being attacked, thus affecting the messages it directs. And that increases your risk of cancer – enormously.

Trans fats have been linked to higher levels of colon cancer *(University of North Carolina)* and to pancreatic cancer *(NCI)*.

Several research studies have shown that trans fats increase tissue inflammation in the body, through their stimulus of prostaglandins. Such inflammation increases risks of many chronic diseases from heart disease to cancer.

The FDA have at long last decided to act on these dangerous fats. In 2013, Commissioner Dr Margaret Hamburg has announced that *'trans fats are not generally recognized as safe for use in food'*. Walter Willet of The Harvard School of Public Health backed this announcement saying it was, *'strongly supported by massive scientific evidence that trans fat has many adverse effects on health'*. Already, many products in the USA state on the pack that they are 'Trans Fat Free'. Do yours?

Saturated fats

Good or bad? That's the new question. In the French paradox, the locals consume quite high levels of saturated fats; but these fats are known to increase inflammation in the body and to stimulate the production of oestrogen. Saturated fats have spent almost 40 years on the 'bad fat' list. But that is changing. In October 2013 The British Medical Journal ran a piece concluding that saturated fat was NOT the cause of heart disease and supporting the French Paradox. *'The mantra that saturated fat must be removed to reduce the risk of cardiovascular disease has dominated dietary advice and guidelines for almost four decades. Yet scientific evidence shows that this advice has, paradoxically, INCREASED our cardiovascular risks'.* The article then talks of government obsession with cholesterol and the 'overmedication of millions of people with statins'.

Cardiologist Dr Crandall demystifies the fat issue in his Heart Health series. Cholesterol is far from a bad guy – you need it for your brain, to produce important hormones, to make vitamin D, for your cell membranes and the transport system in and out of the cell and for good food digestion. As we will see 'HDL' is good cholesterol and found in seeds, nuts, olive oil and walnut oil. It is an important part of the Mediterranean diet and French Paradox. Typically Saturated fat is linked with 'LDL', often called bad cholesterol. But Chandler says that it's not all bad, just a subsection called 'Pattern B type', which is mainly derived from trans fats.

Unsaturated fats

Finally, we have **'unsaturated'** fats – although even this category is not 'straightforward' to understand. Again, let me try to simplify it.

There are two main types of unsaturated fats:

- *Polyunsaturated fats*
  Polyunsaturated 'fats' are liquid at room temperature and are essential because the body cannot make them. Many margarines were launched on a healthier-for-you platform because they originated from these polyunsaturated oils. The list includes soybean, sunflower and safflower oils.

  But again, you must be very sure they haven't been through the processing and refining mill. Furthermore, cooking with them obviously raises their temperature and starts to damage them.

  Polyunsaturated oils should provide around 2 per cent of your calories. In excess they can inhibit HDL levels (good cholesterol – see later) and also render vitamins like beta-carotene inert.

- *Monounsaturated fats*

  The 'healthiest' oils are monounsaturated oils found in, for example, **olive and walnut oils.** Bottles of pressed oils like these are easy to find around the Mediterranean and olive oil, in particular, has a high unsaturated, good fat content plus added benefits like polyphenols; a number of research studies have linked its consumption with a decreased cancer risk.

  Ideally, you should choose bottles of these oils from a respected supplier and in an untreated state. Oils high in monounsaturates are better for cooking as they have a high oxidation threshold and they remain stable on heating – so they do not become hydrogenated or saturated easily. Figures for the percentage of monounsaturated fat in nuts and seeds and oil are:

Olive oil	73%
Rapeseed oil	60%
Hazelnut	50%
Almonds	35%
Cashews	28%
Brazils	26%
Sesame seeds	20%
Pumpkin seeds	16%

But you still need to be careful of misleading claims for margarines containing them. The content could be minimal, and the margarine could be heavily refined and even hydrogenated.

The nuts themselves have huge benefits. For example, consumption of walnuts has been shown to reduce prostate cancer risk, and people eating fresh nuts daily have lowered cancer and heart disease risk.

Fish oils, flaxseed, linseed and other 'friendly' oils

There is another group of oils – a group I am going to call 'friendly oils'. Fish oils give you long-chain omega-3; whilst flaxseed, linseed and evening primrose give you predominantly short chain omega-3, omega-6 and a little omega-9. They are all essential oils, needed by our bodies.

I will cover this in more detail later, but suffice it to say here that you need as much long-chain omega-3 as you can get in this modern world, to balance the bad fats and to correct the over provision of omega-6 and -9 available in modern diets.

Omega-3 actually calms inflammation by switching off the enzymes that make prostaglandins.

You should observe some simple rules on your 'eat-to-beat cancer' diet.

- Ideally reduce total fat consumption to 10–20 per cent of total daily calorie intake.
- Eliminate all trans fats from your diet.
- Reduce consumption of saturated fats.
- Never eat fried food; especially away from home.
- Eat fresh food whenever possible.
- Focus your oil and fat consumption on pure oils (e.g. olive, walnut), ideally from a source you can trust.
- Consume more oily fish, seeds and fresh nuts.

Cholesterol

There is a mania in the Western world against cholesterol at the moment; a mania constantly stimulated by statin manufacturers who would like the entire population to take their very profitable pills. (In the USA they are even now giving them to children!) However, all cholesterol was not created equal. There are two main forms: High Density Lipoprotein (HDL) and Low Density Lipoprotein (LDL). LDL has several types and Pattern B type seems to be the dangerous one that blocks arteries if they are inflamed.

High 'bad' LDL cholesterol causes stagnation of the whole metabolic system and inhibits the ability of the liver to detoxify the blood and therefore the tissues. High LDL cholesterol leads to more negative hormone production, especially oestrogen and eicosanoids, and an increased risk of cancer.

However, medical authorities and the media don't simply confuse the various types, they also don't understand how you come to have high levels in your body. The traditional medical view is simply that you eat too much of it.

Most people with 'high cholesterol' will be told to reduce their cholesterol intake (eggs, butter, lobster, shellfish, liver, cheese etc.) and that this will reduce their cholesterol levels in the body. This is tosh. The cholesterol molecule is far too large to cross the intestinal wall. In other words, cholesterol is formed in the body from smaller molecules. And these smaller molecules could have even originated from carbohydrates! Research has shown that certain beneficial bacteria in the gut, when fed whole foods containing soluble fibres like pectins and lignans, produce short-chain esters, which actually block the formation of bad cholesterol in the blood stream.

Failure to expel cholesterol via the liver and hereditary factors also play a role in your cholesterol levels and cholesterol balance.

Certain nutritional factors can help reduce your liver cholesterol levels, for example magnesium, vitamins C, B-12 and B-6, and lecithin (choline, inositol, linoleic acid). As discussed earlier, people with high cholesterol levels may well have bile duct blockages and gallstones and should look seriously at undertaking a liver flush.

Chandler says it is the BALANCE of fats that is important. You need high HDL, and low Pattern B. You can change the balance in your favour by consuming fish oils, extra virgin olive oil, the fibre in whole porridge oats, garlic and policosanols (natural statins found in cane sugar, yams and beeswax), especially when combined with flaxseed. Several studies on olive oil, policosanols, plant fibres like lignans and omega-3 show they each lower LDL, whilst leaving HDL levels unaffected.

But, to return to one of our main themes, *"fat isn't so bad. It's refined carbs and added sugars that cause the problems'*. Chronic illness finds its origins in chronic inflammation in the body. And the Rainbow Diet overcomes this because its good fat content is high and its bad carb content is low.

Common Sugar

Common sugar, or glucose, causes and drives cancers. It weakens the immune system and, via insulin, it causes chronic inflammation. It also causes epigenetic blocking effects on genes. Furthermore, it is linked to epilepsy, dementia, diabetes, arthritis and heart disease.

The Rainbow Diet, the Mediterranean Diet, the Gascony Diet contain no added sugar, no fluffy, refined biscuits, cakes and ice cream. No fizzy soft drinks, no puddings, no supermarket fruit juices, no sugar in tea or coffee.

In *JAMA* on Feb 15th 2014 there was a research study about the dangers of common sugar to your health. Daily 'added sugar' calories should be no more than 8 per cent of total calories consumed. 70 per cent of Americans consume over 10 per cent. Over 21 per cent, and your risk of dying from heart disease more than doubles. 37 per cent of these added calories come from fizzy soft drinks alone. Ice cream and dairy deserts are 6.1 per cent; grain deserts 13.7 per cent; biscuits, cakes and chocolate bars are 5.8 per cent and supermarket fruit juices and smoothies 8.9 per cent.

But glucose is the food of fermentation, the energy system of the cancer cell. Earlier I told you of Professor Thomas Seyfried and his belief that cancer is a metabolic disease which can be reversed by a high good fat, low carbohydrate and lowish protein diet. He calls it the Ketogenic Diet. I call it the Rainbow Diet.

Since 2012 there has been research covered in Cancer Watch on the benefits of Calorie Restriction (eating 15 per cent less calories than you need – in practice it was less carbs) on improved results from chemotherapy and radiotherapy. Another showed fasting for just three days significantly improved the quality of the immune system.

Starve your body, and glucose supplies in the blood run out after about 12 hours (quicker if you exercise). But 70 per cent of people with cancer don't like the idea of a three to five day fast even if it lowers insulin, oestrogen and IGF-1 levels, halts cancer progression and metastases, and improves the success of chemo- and radiotherapy! There's no pleasing some people

So, in America they have started clinical trials with a calorie restricted, 'good' fat rich, low carbohydrate, low protein 'food' called *KetoCal*. French Paradox? Moi?

There is mounting evidence that common glucose drives and even causes cancers – consume it at your peril.

Refined foods, processed foods and preserved foods

The food industry has a lot to answer for. Nowhere more so than in its use of refining. Above we covered what they do when they refine oils.

Grains: laughably, the food industry makes a virtue out of foods being 'vitamin enriched' or having 'added fibre'. They caused the problem in the first place. When they refine wheat, the grain loses at least 75 per cent of its B vitamins, at least 90 per cent of its mineral content, at least 98 per cent of its vitamin E and at least 99 per cent of its fibre.

You are eating pap. No wonder recent research in **icon** showed we are all becoming deficient in folate and several other B vitamins. This is costing lives and money: The NHS is even working with the drugs companies to perfect a 'Heart disease lowering pill' – one of its five ingredients is folic acid.

B vitamins like folic acid/folate are essential to the proper division and copying of our DNA.

Refined grains are used in processed foods and, along with chemicals, sugar and salt, E numbers and other additives; the consumer is getting little other than moderately toxic, nutritionally empty calories.

Ladies who lunch and go for their slimming plate of pasta and their glass of chardonnay are eating a food devoid of almost all its nutrition, where the refining process has actually increased the calorie level by about 7 per cent. Without a doubt, the glass of chardonnay provides more nourishment.

I have a simple rule – only put whole foods in your mouth.

Sadly, that won't solve all the problems with grains. The overproduction and storage of grains in the EU has meant moulds are increasingly common, resulting in the presence of aflatoxin in the grains – and this is carcinogenic.

Meats and Meat Products: There is no requirement to label meats or meat products so the hormones, food additives, the drugs, antibiotics and chemicals used to fatten and treat the animal go unmentioned.

Nitrates are frequently added to brighten the meat. In fact sodium nitrite and nitrate are widely used in dried meats, bacon, pepperoni, sausages, hams and hot dogs. Children who consume more than a dozen hot dogs a month have a considerably higher (9.5 times) risk of leukaemia. Women eating these foods during pregnancy produce offspring with a higher incidence of brain cancer.

Pickling is linked to stomach and throat cancers (the Japanese eat a lot of pickled foods). Smoked meats and fish are also linked to stomach cancer.

But preservatives abound. In 1995 Americans each consumed on average ten pounds of preservatives. Britain is not far behind. Many different chemicals are used as preservatives, and yet no-one knows what effect this mix has on our bodies, and many of these chemicals may well have the ability to stay in our tissues for long periods of time.

A French police friend telling me about road accidents in France said that exhumed bodies were hardly decomposed two years after death, such was our exposure to chemical preservatives!

Caffeine

Caffeine depletes the body of vitamins, especially B vitamins, essential for the correct division of cells. It is a poison and has a negative effect on the immune system and on potassium and magnesium levels. Recent research showed that taking paracetamol with coffee could cause liver damage.

Sweeteners

Aspartame is often linked with possible increased risk of brain tumours. There was one research study with rats but there has never been any evidence with humans. However research in 2005 and again in 2012 has linked a daily diet soda drink containing aspartame to greater risk of leukaemia, lymphoma and multiple myeloma in humans *(Cancer Watch 2012)*.

Aspartame is in more than 5,000 food and drink items – from diet drinks to low fat yoghurts. It was originally developed as an ulcer medication but the FDA refused it a licence, deeming it unsafe for human consumption *(FDA Public Board of Inquiry, Sept 30, 1980)*. Now permitted as a food additive, aspartame is a mix of six chemicals such as methanol, a cumulative poison known to affect sight. Methanol can also be converted under certain conditions to formaldehyde, a known carcinogen. Other ingredients include phenylalanine (linked to problems of the nervous system), and diketopiperazine, which has been demonstrated to cause brain tumours in animals.

Monosodium Glutamate (MSG)

MSG is a totally unnecessary chemical food additive and flavour enhancer. It was developed by a food chemist in Japan. Early studies showed that it was addictive and could put weight on rats. John E. Erb wrote in his book *'The Slow Poisoning of America'*, that the whole purpose of adding MSG to food is to encourage people to eat more by enhancing taste. No legal limits have been set for the additive although it can cause a 'morning after' hangover, nausea, chest pains and numbness. Yummy.

Acrylamides

Panic set in early in 2002 when a Swedish scientist looking at whether toxins might be passing from plastic packaging into foods instead discovered highly toxic acrylamides present in chips (especially overly cooked ones), crisps and potato-bagged snacks, branded breakfast cereals, biscuits, crispbreads and crackers. Seemingly any oven-baked processed food where the temperature was taken over 120°c was liable to be contaminated.

The World Health Organisation says that the safe limit for acrylamides is zero, such is their concern. They immediately called together 26 of the world's top scientists to develop a viewpoint and some 'solutions'. Despite the severity of the findings no hard action has yet been taken – six years later! A study announced in January 2003 by Cancer Research UK attempted to say that the levels found in these foods were not found to cause 'long term' problems. Readers are nevertheless encouraged to exert caution as the findings came from a study lasting barely three months!

Indeed, in 2008 research from the University of Maastricht scientists analysing the eating habits of 120,000 people showed those who ate chips or crisps regularly were significantly more at risk of cancer.

For those concerned about acrylamides, three eat-to-beat cancer tips are:

• If you like to **snack**, make your own – put out a bowl of organic sunflower, pumpkin and sesame seeds, with a few chopped nuts.
• If you want a genuinely healthy **breakfast cereal** make your own with oats (unrefined), millet, chopped nuts, dried fruits, seeds, a little soya milk, rice milk or even water. Or eat organic whole oats – porridge made with water – and sprinkle some linseeds on top.
• Never roast quickly at high temperatures, only slowly at lower ones.

Eating 'out of home'

This may seem an odd inclusion, but not after you have given it some thought.

Some fast food chains only fry their food; some chains only microwave all their meals. Many restaurants will keep certain meats and fish in the freezer and microwave it to defrost it and avoid wastage.

Microwaved food is genetically modified food. When a microwave heats food it does it by exciting the electrons in the atoms of molecules. When the microwave is turned off do you think the electrons will all be in their original orbits? Kirlian photographs show microwaved food denuded of its natural energy and William Kopp has gathered together extensive German and Russian research. This shows that microwaved food is nutritionally deficient, and the number of cancer and pre-cancer cells circulating in the bloodstream rises after a microwaved meal.

Far Eastern food is little better. The Chinese food in the UK is often greasy and oily, with monosodium glutamate and sugar widely used. You can get 6–12 gms of salt from one meal! Much of the dish Pad Thai is carbohydrate and oil in the UK, complete with added sugar and nothing like the meal in Thailand.

The majority of restaurants use mass produced ingredients, and only those 'freshly' supplied by the supermarket down the road! Refined pasta, sugar and salt and dairy-laden sauces abound. It's a minefield for someone concerned about the quality of what they put into their body.

Summary

Above I have detailed some of the factors that could cut out perhaps 80 per cent of potential problems. But in all cases, I have tried to avoid the negative – providing simple ideas and alternatives you can use, from putting out bowls of nuts and seeds, to only using olive oil, to taking probiotics, to eating whole grains, and whole oats – all of which can help you reduce the levels of free-radicals and cancer-feeding and cancer-producing agents in your body.

It's really not that hard, is it?

CHAPTER 14
ORGANIC FOOD – LIVING FOOD

Organic food really is better for you

There has been all too much mythology, false claim and counter claim about organic food. The debate is now over. Organic food really is better for you.

Various small studies have been trumpeted by the UK Soil Association over recent years. But now the arguments must surely cease. The EU has commissioned the definitive, £12 million study, growing organic crops and comparing them with mass-produced ones in several locations. (Quality Low Input Food, or the QLIF study). With the first results in, Professor Carlo Leifert (a patron of **CANCERactive**) and his team leading the study are quite clear: Organically produced crops and dairy milk usually contain far more 'beneficial compounds', like bioactive compounds, omega-3 and antioxidants. More detailed results are expected over the next few years as the study continues.

We did know already. Over the last seven or eight years there have been some very serious and detailed studies conducted using matched research samples. What has become increasingly clear is that there are small increased levels of minerals in organic food, bigger increases in vitamins, while the biggest differences come in levels of certain important natural compounds like phenols, anthocyanins and so on. The production of these is not just inhibited by pesticides and herbicides, but often the nitrogen-rich fertilisers limit the plant's ability to manufacture these key, health providing factors. Here are just a few examples:

- Organic practices increase vitamin C levels in potatoes *(Hajslova 2005)*.
- And strawberries *(Asami 2003)*.
- Beta carotene levels are higher in organic crops *(Lombardi-Boccia 2004)*.
- And high nitrogen fertilisers depress levels *(Leclerc et al 1991)*.
- Plums grown organically with a ground cover of clover have

127

more polyphenols and quercitin *(Lombardi-Boccia 2004)*.

- Organic potatoes and apples have higher levels of polyphenols and flavenols *(Harmouz 1999)*.
- Organic strawberries have significantly higher levels of glutathione *(Wang and Lin 2003)*.
- Resveratrol is 26 per cent higher in organic grapes.
- Phenolics are 33 per cent higher in organic peaches.
- Antioxidants are 220 per cent higher in organic spinach *(Ren et al 2001)*.
- Organic Chinese cabbage and Welsh onions have 1.3 to 10.4 times the anti-mutagenic flavenoid concentrations *(Ren 2001)*.

Is your food organic?

What really is organic food? My definition would be that it is a natural food, grown in its fully natural state, in balance with its natural environment. Crop rotation plays an important part in my definition. For example, it allows nitrogen fixing bacteria to play their role and different crops to recharge the soil to the benefit of the next crop.

Our bodies and our DNA have evolved to be in balance with the world around us over hundreds of thousands of years. It was a slow steady process of development. Most of us are wise enough to realise that pouring chemicals into our modern environment leaves our bodies unprepared to meet the sudden changes. So too with food.

But, since the days of the ancient Egyptians, we have always strived to create bigger chickens, potatoes that avoided the blight or new crops that grew even with low rainfall. When we cross-bred two potatoes in the eighteenth century, was the resultant potato natural? When we cross-bred wild turkeys to create the domestic version, or two breeds of chicken to make a better egg-layers, are our bodies ready? Or seedless grapes and oranges, are they truly natural?

But now 'cross-breeding' has reached new levels. Led by American food company scientists we now 'play' with the natural DNA freely producing 'genetically modified seeds'. Approximately 99 per cent of the GM seeds now used are of two types – about 79 per cent is herbicide-resistant, and 20 per cent is pesticide-producing. The claimed benefit is that the volumes of crops produced per acre will grow, and that ultimately we will need less herbicides and pesticides in our fields. The reality is that the levels of these chemical toxins required do not seem to have declined by the fifth year and herbicide-resistant weeds are now on the increase. And every year farmers, however poor, need to buy new seed instead of gathering their own because these special GM seeds, uniquely, have been allowed to be patented by the US Government. The farmer even has to contract to buy the herbicide solely from the seed company too.

Critics claim that the process of genetic modification can generate other potentially dangerous genetic fragments within the seed. They are concerned that the seed companies have been allowed to write their own rules, the FDA granting them virtual self regulation. There also seems to be insufficient testing, especially for potential side-effects.

The French, for example, have resisted American companies' suggestions to grow genetically modified crops. And the decision seems to be supported by the facts. There are already studies showing increased cancer risks from GM potatoes *(Institute of Nutrition of the Russian Academy, 1998)* and several others using potatoes, corn, soy and canola have shown liver damage in animals, while others have shown that GM fed animals had impaired gene expression, greater mortality and more organ damage overall. Smaller babies are also observed. In other cases (for example with GM Soy) higher incidence of allergies is noted.

Perhaps most alarming is an observation by Judy Carman an epidemiologist and GM expert, when reviewing Food Standards Australia New Zealand conclusions about the safety of GM foods, that they overlooked potential problems including birth defects, cancer and long-term nutritional deficiencies. '*A review of 12 feeding trials includes none with people, and one where the seed was not even tested with animals*'. Tests usually only monitored effects after 7 to 14 days and then only looked for any effects from the planned genetic change and not for any side-effects or unplanned effects. Some experiments tested the foods with only five or six animals!

More concerns are emerging over crops with genetic

mutations designed to resist bacteria; could they have a detrimental effect on the beneficial bacteria in your intestine? The FDA has actually prepared a report on the fear that Antibiotic Resistant Marker genes (ARM) could transfer into the beneficial bacteria of the intestine. One FDA report actually wrote in capital letters that ARM could be a SERIOUS HEALTH HAZARD as they could create a new breed of bacteria immune to antibiotics.

The French are, however, looking seriously at allowing one crop to 'go' GM: Grapes! Between 1999 and 2005 there have been 25 tests on GM grapes in America. And the French have been working on GM grapes with the Italians, Germans and Australians. GM strains for herbicide resistance and mould resistance have been developed; one even helps the grapes to resist mould by producing hydrogen cyanide! As you will understand later, the development of mould on the skins of organic grapes actually causes the grape to produce resveratrol, which we are only just learning is a highly important natural compound in the fight against cancer and a number of other diseases such as Alzheimer's. And it is the very compound that gives the grape, and red wine its image of health.

Seven out of every ten supermarket foods in the USA now contain GM strains.

And how can a judge decide that it is 'safe' to have a GM crop 60 yards or 80 yards from a natural one? Birds eat seeds, they fly, they deposit the seeds miles away and the next year the pollen interacts with a natural crop. Is our evolution really to be left to ageing judges with no knowledge of science and Darwinian principles?

One estimate I read stated that there could be no natural crops in the USA in five years time. Is that what we want in Europe?

Even Organic food is not beyond political influence: The demand for organic food has grown dramatically in both the US and the UK. The two countries have had rather different solutions. In the US the solution was merely to change the rules and regulations, bringing with it concerns that the food could not be trusted to be truly organic. By contrast the Brits kept the stringent rules in place and import foods to make up the shortfall.

Let us hope that the Soil Association has world-wide policing of Kenyan green bean crops and Vietnamese mangoes. Why am I so concerned?

Mass production

The sad truth is that when it comes to food we continually confuse quantity with quality, volume with value, eating with nourishment.

One example of this is the emergence of 'Hydroponic farming'. There is now a complex in Kent the size of ten soccer pitches growing 1.3 million tomato, pepper and cucumber plants all year round, using no soil but a liquid food supply instead. Current estimates are that this one 'factory' will produce 15 per cent of the UK's salad crop production – reducing reliance on imports. While natural predators not pesticides will control pests enhancing the 'organic' image of the end product, the 'food' is grown on rock wool – rock that has had air blown through it and resembles candy floss – in a water-based solution of nitrogen, phosphate, potassium and magnesium. If the tomatoes are receiving no trace minerals, how will you? The debate has started in the press, but it is one of overcoming food shortages versus loss of food taste. Does anyone think about nourishing your cells anymore? Has anyone conducted any proper research on vitamin, mineral and natural compound content of these all-year-round crops compared to the natural, organic varieties of our forefathers?

But producing more lettuces unnaturally is really the tip of the iceberg. There are a number of basic reasons to be concerned about mass-market, supermarket crops. Firstly, fields are repeatedly sown with the same crop. the idea of crop rotation seems to have died in the Middle Ages. Of course there was a reason for it. Crop rotation was used to recharge depleted soils with certain bacteria and nutrients across the 4 year cycle. Now chemical fertilisers are expected to do the job just as well. Unfortunately they don't and they can't. Take the loss of minerals for example. One study using the UK Government's own figures over a 50 year period to 1990 showed losses of minerals like calcium in green vegetables reaching 70 per cent, and another showed vitamin E declines to merely one sixth of the levels 100 years ago. How could synthetic fertilisers be expected to make up these shortfalls in fields planted with the same crops each year?

Furthermore, in the attempt to sell more higher-priced products, or simply to keep their shelves fully stocked, supermarkets seek more produce from abroad. But vitamin levels are all about the ripening process of the vegetable or fruit. And they are lost quite quickly in stored fruit and vegetables. Within four or five days of picking, most green vegetables have lost 50 per cent of their vitamins and a potato has lost three quarters of its vitamin C (and potatoes are the UK's best natural home-grown source of the vitamin). By the time the produce has reached the UK, been unloaded, shipped to a central storage location and then out to the supermarkets, what nourishment can we expect to have left?

Frozen vegetables fare little better with 25 to 50 per cent of the vitamins disappearing upon freezing.

Minerals are absorbed from the soil throughout the full development of the fruit. Pick the food after only 60 or 70 per cent of its full growth span and expect the consequences.

How could we ever expect the same vitamin and mineral content in supermarket produce as in 'Locally grown fruits and vegetables, in season and picked ripe and eaten fresh'? Macrobiotic principles don't seem that absurd at all.

But it is not simply a question of vitamins and minerals. Kirlian was a Russian who, about 50 years ago, invented a photographic system able to show the energy emitted around life forms. I have Kirlian photographs of mass market foods and their organic equivalents, and they show clearly that organic food has more 'energy' in it than non-organic. To repeat: Food is supposed to nourish my body and provide it with vitality. How will eating lifeless, energy-less, vitamin and mineral reduced foods do this?

Pesticides and herbicides

Another benefit of organic foods is that they should contain no pesticides or herbicides; no toxins to weaken our immune systems or damage the balance of hormones inside our bodies. With 'normal' vegetables and fruit there is little legislation restricting what pesticides and insecticides are used, nor how often. Over 400 fertilisers, herbicides and pesticides are available for use on our farms. Is it any wonder that farmers have a higher incidence of multiple myeloma and leukaemia?

Pesticides and insecticides have also been linked with brain tumours, connective tissue tumours (especially with children), and liver cancer and are thought to be behind the recent rapid growth of kidney cancer. Whilst individual pesticides might be found in any food at a level lower than UK Government-designated safe levels, the Government has done little research on the interaction of all the chemicals, or indeed the cumulative and interactive build up over a number of years within the tissues of the human body.

In the USA, the lifetime maximum safe limit set for these chemicals is exceeded when a baby reaches the age of 18 months!

Fruit orchards can be sprayed a dozen times, then the fruit is waxed, locking the pesticide in. Long gone are the days when chickens populated orchards to eat the bugs before the bugs could climb the trees!

Worse, when Western governments banned DDT, they only banned its use. Some unscrupulous companies are still free to sell these chemicals to third world buyers. And do you know where your green beans and lettuce were actually grown? The Food Standards Agency in the UK stated in 2006 that certain imported foods increasingly contain higher levels of pesticides than is deemed legally safe. But do we actually ban their sale?

Worry about bees

Albert Einstein said that if all the bees died out man would only live another four years. This could be prophetic. The issue facing world leaders is not the price of oil and food, but the loss of bees. They are dying out. Various theories have suggested causes such as GM crops, EMFs, mites (cuckoo-like bugs that get inside the hive and lay their eggs inside the bee brood cells) while German research has 'proven' the cause is pesticides.

Flowers, most vegetables, virtually all fruit (except bananas), clover and wild herbs would all die out. That also means great reductions for cotton, feed for cattle and even precursors for herbal medicines and drugs. Olive oil, nuts, grains like corn and oats, and rice would still be with us – they don't need pollination. The

Armageddon scenario has actually started. In some regions farmers are pollinating orchards by hand. Whatever the cause, someone in power needs to come up with some answers soon. Meanwhile, since there is not a lot you and I can do about this, let's keep going with our current plans to improve our nourishment:

Saving money while going organic

'Going organic' is not an option for everybody because of the increased expense. The good news is that not all contaminated foods were created equal! According to the Environmental Working Group of Washington DC, people can lower their pesticide exposure by 90 per cent by choosing their fruits and vegetables wisely. Eating the 12 most contaminated fruits and vegetables will expose a person to nearly 20 pesticides each day, says the EWG. So these are the ones to buy in 'organic' versions. At the other end of the spectrum there are foods which are sprayed little and/or absorb little. If you just want to avoid the chemicals you might as well buy the supermarket versions. For your information, three studies have now been completed and the findings have been consistent, with fruits worse than vegetables.

12 most contaminated		12 least contaminated	
Apples	Peaches	Asparagus	Mangoes
Red bell peppers	Pears	Avocados	Onions
Celery	Potatoes	Bananas	Papaya
Cherries	Red Raspberries	Broccoli	Pineapples
Grapes	Spinach	Cauliflower	Peas
Nectarines	Strawberries	Kiwi	Sweetcorn

A 2000 Study by the Consumer Union reflected the same pollution. Apples, peaches, pears, grapes, green beans, spinach, strawberries and watermelon were the foods with the highest levels of pesticide residues.

However, it may not be hard to put matters right. Another group of scientists, this time at the Centre for Disease Control and Prevention at the University of Washington, funded by the US Government, tested the urine samples of school children in

Seattle for 'organophosphate pesticides'. During a 15-day trial, those consuming organic foods saw their levels drop to zero.

Meat and fish

Nearly 60 per cent of the calories we consume from processed animal products (for example meats, dairy, cheese, etc.) come from fat. As we said earlier, fat is a wonderful solvent and contains toxic chemicals and antibiotics from the upbringing and diet of the animal. Over one hundred such substances have been identified and 40 per cent of them are carcinogenic.

In the USA 82 drugs, hormones and chemicals are legally allowed to be given to dairy herds. Growth hormone and oestrogen are two of these and one has to accept that any meat consumption comes with these chemicals contained in the flesh and especially the fat. Dairy consumption brings a similar chemical concoction.

Then there are the antibiotics, colourings and, depending upon the previous crops in the fields where herds graze, possibly high levels of pesticides and insecticides. The foodstuffs may not even be natural. BSE in cattle was brought about by feeding animal food products to herbivores. Whatever happened to the concept of animal husbandry?

Farmed fish often do not consume the sorts of food they would have eaten in their natural habitat. Natural plankton is essential for their omega-3 levels, but will hardly be found in the waters of farms. Farmed fish also have 20 per cent more 'fat' than their wild ancestors due to their own 'sedentary' existence!

The mass market animals have weakened immune systems and are more prone to parasites, bacteria and viruses. The incidence of liver fluke in British livestock has increased four-fold since 1997. Recently, Asian prawns and chickens, which had been banned for consumption by humans because of toxins, were found to have been shipped for use by EU farmers as animal food! The toxins entered the food chain nevertheless! Volume and profit margins have become the Holy Grails of food production. Nourishment is an old-fashioned concept.

Action?

- Eat-to-beat cancer means that you should take more trouble over selecting the products that go into your mouth. Know a few reliable suppliers. And buy locally-grown, fresh, in season and organic where possible. Shop more often if necessary.
- Why not start your own vegetable garden and plant a few fruit trees? You will be surprised how easy they are to grow along the fence instead of those fir trees.

CHAPTER 15
DERIVING THE MAXIMUM NOURISHMENT FROM YOUR DIET

Say 'beneficial bacteria' to most doctors and they just might mention something about little milky drinks with more than an added hint of marketing.

But the truth is very different. **Without large volumes of the right types of beneficial bacteria in your gut you greatly reduce your personal odds of preventing or beating cancer or any chronic illness.**

In the last 10 years we have seen a huge scientific breakthrough in our understanding of the role and crucial importance of beneficial bacteria to the body's health systems. My new book *'The Secret Source of your Good Health'* covers that research in detail. Over 4000 research studies, 80 clinical trials and major reports in magazines like *Science or Nature* demand new thinking from the medical profession. No longer are we to be considered 'organisms' of 25,000 genes and 7 trillion cells. We are 'super- organisms' living in a community of 100,000 genes and 100 trillion cells, all working together in one giant ecosystem.

The secret source of your good health

In the nooks and crannies of each of us lie microbes and bacteria. What used to be considered parasites are now understood to be contributors; fully paid-up members of a larger community, each providing something towards the health and wellbeing of the whole, the super-organism. Nowhere is this more true than in the gut where bacteria and microbes are essential contributors to your good health. The intestinal flora, or microbiome, performs at least six general functions, which you cannot do without:

1. They are the first line of your immune defences. At night when you sleep, they attack and digest most of the microbes and yeasts you ingested during the day – ones you would rather

not have in your body at all.

2. They are not just the front line foot soldiers, they actually direct the formation of about 80 per cent of all your immune defences throughout your body! They also control your 'immune memory'.

3. They don't just work with your digestive system to extract certain natural compounds from your foods, they actually MAKE some of them, like vitamin K, B-12, folic acid, biotin and niacin and more. Without them you just cannot derive full nourishment from your foods.

4. They also make short-chain esters, which, for example, reduce levels of 'bad' cholesterol forming in the blood stream.

5. One of these esters in sodium butyrate. It is strongly anti-inflammatory and has epigenetic effects. Sodium butyrate has even been shown in a number of separate studies to kill cancer cells. (You could take sodium butyrate but it tastes foul – an alternative might be the B vitamin niacin.)

6. They can chelate to (bind with) toxins (like oestrogen, nitrosamines and heavy metals) using certain natural compounds in fibrous foods and help to expel them from your body.

With the exception of a few complementary therapists and an occasional professor waving warning flags, the orthodox medical community and the drugs companies have been damaging and/or killing them off willy-nilly with little regard for their importance.

Diversity and absolute numbers are essential

Over 800 different types of bacteria live in your gut. About 400 have been identified. Hardly an illness remains that has not been linked to bacteria in the gut, whether it be *Clostridium C. perfringens* type B in people suffering from MS, or *Ruminococcus* and *Collinsella* linking to inflammation of the arteries.

By 'infecting' us, bacteria stimulate an immune response. It's an example of 'action and reaction'. They increase the numbers of T- and B- lymphocytes, immunoglobulins, cytokines and Natural Killer cells in our bodies. Rather like certain vaccines, they help 'immunise' us against a worse attack that might come in the future. Without them your immune system withers, and is less prepared to face a major threat if and when one occurs. Obviously over thousands of years many 'beneficial bacteria' have developed with us and now just provoke an immune response through their mild, harmless presence. Pathogens (the 'bad guys') may provoke a much stronger response, and even death. The continued presence on beneficial bacteria produces a continued response and now experts believe that beneficial bacteria are the ongoing stimulus for our immune memory.

Research (and this includes a major American study 'The Human Microbiome project', involving 200 scientists, 5 years and $173 million) has shown that almost all illness is predated by a loss in volume and diversity of your gut bacteria. They get ill first – then you get ill.

This is not merely caused by a weakened immune system, but more by a loss of the good guys in the microbiome keeping the bad guys in check. When the bad guys dominate, they produce toxins, inflammation and even immune response and any or all of these may contribute to physical diseases like cancer, diabetes, arthritis and IBS, or mental issues like dementia, Parkinson's, Autism, or mood swings, depression and aggression. Gut bacteria don't just cause tummy upsets on holiday; they can cause illnesses from constipation to colon cancer.

Breaking the relationship that protects us

Three hundred years ago when we lived on farms, we all ate a bit of dirt daily. Hands that touched chickens, horses and dogs then fed the babies. We constantly ingested bacteria from a variety of sources. Importantly these could have included some not-so-common strains. For example, when young children 'pick up colds' it may just be that they are reacting to a new bacterial strain that has entered their system. Research studies show that children brought up on farms, and children brought up in homes that have animals have much stronger immune systems. For life!

Babies in the womb are sterile, so the outside world is very dangerous. Natural birth babies have much stronger immune systems; they pick up bifidobacteria when passing through the birth canal. Mother's breast milk contains specific polysaccharides called glycans, which human enzymes cannot digest, but bifidobacterial enzymes can. Thus the number of these bifidobacteria increases, creating an early immune system and affording protection. Caesarian babies are disadvantaged. And bottled milk has no such effect.

Now our sanitised world that is no longer rural but sees 72 per cent of us living in towns and cities, offers surgical not natural birth, and pasteurises, sterilises, irradiates and cleans fastidiously results in far lower levels of beneficial being ingested.

Worse, in our new world we continually kill them! With prescribed antibiotics and drugs, chemotherapy and mercury-based vaccines, but also with everyday factors like chlorinated water, or antibiotics in our food, or too much salt which changes the acidity of our digestive juices to a point where the bacteria don't like swimming in it. Our friendly bugs can be wiped out in unfriendly conditions in just three days.

And when we kill them off, some of them are not so easy to replace – the bacterium you ingested from the cat when you were four years old may be found only occasionally. All that immune response and protection may be lost forever.

Also, research shows that they don't die off equally. Many bad guys are more resistant to drugs and antibiotics. When your oncologist tells you that he doesn't want you supplementing, but would rather you ate 5 lots of fruit and vegetables a day, he is condemning you to poor nourishment. His drugs killed off your good guys and without them you just cannot make certain essential natural compounds like biotin, B-12 and folic acid. These microbes are now understood to uniquely produce molecules capable of regulating the human biochemistry and potentially the genome! They are the ultimate epigenetics.

But humans do not understand their needs - we no longer give them the foods they enjoy, like whole foods, vegetables and importantly fibre and so we break our 'deal' with them. And it's a deal that has built up over several million years. 'You look after me – and I'll look after you!' It is called symbiosis.

Your health depends on their health

Your microbiome gets ill first – and you cannot get better until it gets better. For example, in American hospitals *Clostridium difficile* is an infection that can follow antibiotics. The disrupted microbiome leads to severe IBS and 14,000 deaths a year. But now doctors have found a way of calming the gut. They use enemas of the stools of healthy people and the majority of infected people recover! American clinical trials showed that if you have problems with your gut microbiome, you should only tackle them naturally. Drugs and antibiotics actually amplify imbalances and make matters worse. The important question for someone who is ill becomes 'Am I really ill, or is it really my microbiome?'

An example: Colon cancer

Various research studies on colon cancer show that it is linked to low B-12 and folic acid levels, localised cellular inflammation in the intestine and localised oestrogen. Risk doubles if you double your salt intake and if you smoke. Washington University and Tokyo Medical School have shown that the potential metastatic secondary, liver cancer, can be halted by vitamin K supplementation.

I have long held that the cause of colon cancer with its frequent spread to the liver, was driven by microbial or parasitic infection that produced the above symptoms. In 2007 American research showed exactly that. A weak microbiome (thanks to antibiotics, poor diet, or smoking for example) can allow microbes, pathogens and parasites to dominate. Many of the factors research has shown to be associated with colon cancer are in fact factors associated with a disruption of the microbiome allowing 'bad guys' to take over.

Eat-to-beat cancer

Clearly the starting point is to avoid chlorinated tap water, and mass-market meats with added antibiotics. You might also decide you should avoid drugs, salt, and especially antibiotics. Common sugar will feed their foes – the yeasts.

If you can't live on a farm, you might 'top up' every day, especially if you are over 50 years of age when bacterial levels start to fall. We used to eat foods like fermented vegetables (sauerkraut would be an example) and raw milk. In fact, thanks to the French who ignored European bans on raw milk, you can buy raw cheese in British supermarkets and find UK farmers selling raw cows' milk on the Internet. As I said earlier, the benefits of drinking a little 'top up' raw cows' dairy may even outweigh the negatives of milk, especially if the cows are grass fed and thus make Conjugated Linoleic Acid (CLA).

If you are ill and have been treated with drugs, especially PPIs or antibiotcs – you should follow the HUG (Heal Ur Gut) Protocol on my health website. The short version is:

Start by taking probiotics containing Lactic Acid Bacteria *(L. acidophilus* and *L. rhamnosus)* and *Bifidobacteria.* These 'Hold'; they keep pathogens in check. Then food supplements like caprylic acid and oregano can be used to 'Kill' yeast overgrowth, while artemesinin (sweet wormwood), pau d'arco and black walnut can be used against pathogens. The third step is to 'Replenish' – adding lost bacteria with sauerkraut, kefir and kombucha. Finally, you should 'Heal' the lining of your gut.

A **Probiotic** cannot be called a probiotic unless it has been shown in clinical trials that the beneficial bacteria in the bottle can reach their desired destination (the way through the stomach is paved with acidic danger) and, once there, they can deliver a clear, proven health benefit. There is also research that shows it is pointless taking a few pills (of 3 -10 billion bacteria) if you don't feed them properly. Their foods are termed **Prebiotics.** Eat apples and carrots with the acidophilus – they love pectins. Eat endives and onions (for inulin) or polysaccharides with bifidobacteria. The next day there will be trillions of them in your gut. Personally, I take Protozymes from Modere. Always take the pills with cold water.

This is a very serious subject. You can read far more about it in my book *'The Secret Source of your Good Health'*.

Ignore this chapter at your peril!

CHAPTER 16
VITAMINS AND MINERALS IN THE FIGHT AGAINST CANCER

If you ever need an example of people being seriously confused, you need look no further that the Medical Community and their understanding of 'Vitamin Supplements'. Increasingly they class these as part of 'CAM' – Complementary and Alternative Medicine. Note the word 'medicine'. It means that someone somewhere wants to regulate vitamin supplements just as they think they do with drugs!

Before we get into the detail of this section I want to make my views clear up front – they are all based on scientific research.

1. **Nothing is better for you than eating the actual food with its natural compounds.** For example, research scientists gave identical matched samples of people, identical doses of vitamin C from synthetic tablet, or from fresh orange juice. At intervals between three and 24 hours later, blood samples from each group were stressed with hydrogen peroxide, and oxidative damage measured. The blood samples that had come from the orange juice takers, resisted the damage quite significantly. The samples from the synthetic pill takers had no effect. Researchers felt that the reason for the difference was that natural orange juice had a combination of advantageous factors over and above vitamin C, like flavones, carotenoids and cyanidin-3-glucoside plus the natural sugars to enhance the effect. *(Guarnieri; British Journal of Nutrition 2007; 97).*

2. **Chemically synthesised supplements may offer little health benefit and may even cause harm.** There have been several mega-studies from the USA, the Nordic Cochrane Institute and others, all claiming that antioxidants like beta-carotene and vitamin E did little good and could even reduce life expectancy. Importantly, while researchers laid themselves open to criticism by actively selecting less

than 10 per cent of possible studies available (causing bodies like Cancer Research UK to question the objectivity), the research studies chosen featured synthetic compounds and not natural vitamins, a fact which few people have picked up on!

3. **Antioxidants are just a few of the supplements that might help cancer patients.** There is an on-going problem in the media and amongst doctors and oncologists. Namely, a complete confusion between 'antioxidants' and other supplements. Antioxidants neutralise free-radicals and include vitamins A, C, E, lycopene and others my doctor had neither heard of or could spell. But there are many, many more supplements that are not 'antioxidants' but play a variety of roles in countering stages of the cancer process; for example vitamins D and K.

4. **Natural compounds are the next best thing to whole foods. In fact, in some cases they are better because they are concentrated.** While the majority of high street vitamins seems to have been 'dumbed down' to synthetic and limited copies of the real thing, natural compounds like fish oils, curcumin, ellagic acid, quercitin, indole-3-carbinol and resveratrol have very clear benefits in research and are a totally different matter. These are being shown increasingly to offer significant anti-cancer benefits and are capable of being used at concentrations way above those found in even a 'healthy' diet. Many of these compounds from natural sources with their associated co-factors are proving much better at fighting cancer than synthetic antioxidants.

5. **Mineral supplementation is becoming increasingly essential.** While minerals such as selenium and zinc are commonly quoted as essential to the anti-cancer process, other minerals, especially trace minerals like boron, are now being found to play important roles too. But, whether due to mass production farming, soil depletion, lack of crop rotation, or hydroponic growing methods, mineral levels are in serious decline in our everyday foods.

Toxicity and nutritional deficiency

Earlier in the book I explained that when I talk to, or correspond with, newly diagnosed cancer patients it takes but a very short while to find proof that they are both toxic and nutritionally deficient – leading to a weakening of their immune systems and the development of disease. **Toxicity** can be divided into two parts:

* **Toxicity from external third party sources** – like chemicals, drugs, pesticides, EMFs, etc. I believe I have shown that in many of these cases, there are effective ways of detoxing the body. By this I do not mean running off to the health food shop for a herbal drink. It is known that selenium will help displace heavy metals like mercury from the body; chlorella has a similar ability to bind to such poisons; so do plant lignans and, as we will see, indole-3-carbinol in broccoli and greens is being developed and patented by pharmaceutical companies, such is its excellent abilities. All this is aided by the action of the correct beneficial bacteria in the gut. There is much research on this and even many clinical trials.
* **Toxicity due to mineral imbalance** – again I believe I have covered the need to ensure you are a potassium- and magnesium-rich machine, not a sodium- and dairy calcium-rich one.

Nutritional deficiency is a product of our modern lifestyles, and the rubbish purporting to be food that surrounds us these days.

The Food Standards Agency in the UK has told us that, *'People do not need supplementation if they are eating a balanced diet.'* When we asked what a balanced diet was they told us that it was, *'Eating a bit of everything, with emphasis on starchy foods and 5 portions of fruit and vegetables a day'* (we have the letter).

Firstly, people like doctors and the FSA forget that the NHS actually recommends supplementation themselves – for example folic acid in certain cases like pregnancy and heart disease. There is even talk of adding vitamin D to milk.

Secondly, define 'supplements' please. Doctors regularly hand out supplements, for example synthetic hormones like HRT and Thyroxin, which are many, many times more powerful than vitamin supplements. And they have well-researched, negative side-effects. I've never seen studies on vitamin C that show it can cause more cancers, heart problems and even kill people.

Next, our modern lifestyles are not totally of our making but they can control our diets. For example, a businessman flying to Frankfurt for a day's meeting at 6.30 in the morning has little choice but to supplement. Modern no-frills airlines have only crisps, bagged snacks, and refined flour sandwiches to eat. A hastily taken sandwich often substitutes for lunch. Where is the nourishment in this? Surely a multi-vitamin and mineral supplement would be a good, if not essential, idea?

Finally, we have covered the poor diets of our children and their pizzas and crisps and chocolate. But if they turned to the staple foods in our supermarkets to *'eat a bit of everything including starchy foods'*, what would they find? Nutritionally worthless foods like refined rice and pasta, and white bread, and sugar. In some supermarkets you cannot find wholewheat pasta, or whole brown rice. The vegetables and fruit are not a lot better. Often picked unripe and shipped half way round the world – not exotic ones but potatoes, green beans and broccoli, raspberries and pears. Red peppers, tomatoes and lettuces grown in 'nourishing' liquids, not soil, to shorten the growing time!

Vitamin and mineral depletion

Our soils are increasingly depleted. Crops are grown for volume and frequency; crop rotation is rarely used, natural seasons have been shortened; some fields barely rested as one crop of wheat follows another.

In February 2004 David Thomas, a mineralogist, published a paper reporting the decline of mineral levels in our fruits and vegetables from 1940 to 1990, using the Government's own figures. The report showed major declines of up to 70 per cent in potassium, magnesium, iron and calcium. A second, separate study, by Anne-Marie Mayer of Cornell University was published in the *Bristol Food Journal* and came to similar conclusions.

The US Senate minutes in 1936 stated that laboratory tests had proven that US farm soils were becoming minerally depleted, as was the produce, and that people were developing deficiencies. This was repeated in the Senate hearing in 2002. The fact is that the FSA recommendation that you don't need supplementation is in complete contrast to US recommendations – there have been three Senate hearings on the subject and the recommendation was that people should supplement, especially with minerals as the soils growing the crops were increasingly depleted.

But our weakened soils are only the start. Other factors reduce vitamin and mineral intake and nourishment:

- Much of the produce we eat has travelled a long distance. It may be a week between picking and eating, or more.
- Much of the produce we eat, especially fruit, has been picked unripe anyway so that it does not go off during the week of travel nor when on shelf in store.
- Fruits gain the majority of their vitamins as they ripen. Unripe fruit may be 50 to 60 per cent deficient.
- Broccoli, brassicas, spinach, asparagus lose 50 per cent of their vitamins within five days of picking. A potato will lose 75 per cent of its vitamin C within 5 days. Fruits can lose 50 per cent of their vitamin C within 1 day.
- Frozen vegetables lose about a third of their vitamins during the freezing process.

Also, the FSA tell us that there is no need to supplement – but they don't seem to have studied the latest scientific research. For example, vitamin E depletion in vegetables like cabbage and lettuce has resulted in levels around one sixth of those found in 1900. If you look at the research being done on vitamin E and cancer, the scientists show that levels of 200 mgs (about 300 International Units or IUs) for vitamin E give results. If I started to eat vitamin E rich food when I woke up and carried on all day, I would be lucky to get past 100 IUs. Without supplementation how am I going to get to the levels scientists show are effective?

Then there are important compounds like Coenzyme Q10. As we age we make less of it, but it is vital to the perfect workings of our cellular power stations, the mitochondria, and is used by Gonzalez and Gerson to fight cancer. The good news is that you can supplement. US research showed that supplementation of 30-50 mgs per day (any more is wasted) produces results after about 3 months and restores levels to those found in people in their mid-twenties. If we take the FSA route of eating a bit of everything to increase our levels, then you will need about 3 meals a day of brains, liver, kidney and other offal. Delicious – I think I'll take the supplements.

Do antioxidants work with cancer?

Let's start with simple antioxidants and multivitamins. Four very large real life studies show they do. These were not done in a laboratory, in a test tube or with mice. These were all real time studies with humans and matched samples.

- The US conducted a five-year study of 38,000 people in China, finishing in 1993. It showed that the group of people supplied daily with three antioxidants (beta-carotene, vitamin E and selenium) had a 13 per cent reduction in cancers, and a 21 per cent decline in death from cancer despite their already supposed healthy diets.
- The French completed the seven year Su. Vi. Max study in Autumn 2003. 17,000 people took a single pill containing 5 antioxidants (zinc, selenium, beta-carotene and vitamins E and C) in a random, blind test. During the research period there were 31 per cent fewer men's cancers and 37 per cent fewer cancer deaths overall.
- A 30-year diary study on eating habits in the USA on colon cancer showed that those people who took a multivitamin and mineral supplement at least 4 times per week went on to develop 40 per cent less colon cancers. This study finished in 1994; the question is 'Would the dumbed down multivitamins of today deliver these results?'
- An 11 year study *(European Journal of Nutrition 2010)*, designed to sort the debate out once and for all, showed that people taking antioxidant supplements had a 48 per cent reduction in the risk of cancer mortality. In addition, the risk

of dying from all causes (all-cause mortality) was 42 per cent lower among antioxidant supplement users. Interestingly, taking only a basic multivitamin and mineral supplement - the sort repeatedly 'dumbed down' by Health Authorities in Europe - offered no protection against cancer or all-cause mortality.

Antioxidants do appear to deliver; while my fears on synthetic mass-market supplements seem to be supported. I think it is safe to conclude you should always use specialist, naturally-sourced supplements.

'New' vitamins

But, it is too easy to focus on 'the famous 5 antioxidants' as if they were the panacea for everything. Part of the reason is that doctors and press alike have just about understood that free-radicals rush around in our bodies 'oxidising' things and so antioxidants are there to stop them. And so vitamin C, beta-carotene and vitamin E are pulled out of the cupboard again and again to be extolled or attacked, depending upon which day of the week this is.

This belittles the important scientific evidence being produced by researchers all over the world.

You will also find doctors and other health professionals – I even heard it from the CEO of a UK cancer charity – saying, *'There's just no evidence to support the use of supplements'*. If they believe that they are clearly very ignorant. Apart from the four studies above, go to any US cancer web site – try Harvard Medical School, the Mayo Clinic, UCLA, MD Anderson; and in the UK, go to www.canceractive.com and you will see just how ignorant! There you will find that:

- The EU approved form of vitamin E – synthetic alpha tocopherol – is the form of least ability. In contrast, the four tocotrienol forms have considerable new research behind them (from the USA and Japan especially) on their cancer preventing effects. Indeed alpha-tocopherol may even block the action of tocotrienols.

149

- Vitamin D is seen by Harvard Medical School as essential in the fight against cancer – cancer cells actually have more vitamin D receptor sites than healthy cells and vitamin D kills them. Recommended Daily Allowances (RDAs) were set for the prevention of Rickets – the new research shows them woefully low in relation to anti-cancer needs.
- Vitamin K is now being shown by the Universities of Washington and Tokyo to be able to stop some cases of liver cancer and leukaemia. RDAs were originally set for blood clotting issues – again they are woefully low for cancer prevention.

Vitamin supplementation with orthodox therapies

Many patients go to their doctors asking if it is safe to carry on taking their supplements when he is giving them his orthodox concoctions of radio or chemotherapy. Since he doesn't actually know anything about supplements, but worries that his medicine anyway may fail, he will tell patients that they should stop taking the supplements as they can interfere with his clever stuff. He may say they are contra-indicated with the drugs or use other similar terms of *'doctorspeak'*. He will then probably add that they should just eat a healthy diet including five lots of fruit and vegetables a day. Clearly then he believes that a healthy diet is devoid of all vitamins and minerals that could possibly interfere in any way at all.

We have even had **icon** kicked out of hospitals because we dared to say that there is research showing certain vitamins and natural compounds can **improve** the success of radiotherapy. The oncologist in charge said we were irresponsible and said that our suggested supplements were contra-indicated. When we asked for his evidence to pass on to our readers, we received none at all. It simply doesn't exist. In fact, the opposite is true.

In 2001, John Boik of MD Anderson stated that Natural Compounds could actually enhance the effects of radio-and chemotherapy. This was after he had reviewed over 4,000 scientific research studies for his book *'Natural Compounds in Cancer Therapy'*. This was also the conclusion of UCLA in 2004 who stated that whilst healthy cells controlled their uptake of antioxidants and 'stopped' when they'd enough, cancer cells had lost this control and antioxidants could move into a cancer cell in excess and help the radio or chemotherapy destroy it.

Ralph Moss has reviewed the evidence for and against. Originally the debate used to mention only 'antioxidants' as some were felt to limit the way a chemotherapy drug attacked (oxidised) the cancer cell. Now doctors and nurses regularly confuse the terms 'antioxidants' and 'supplements'. Moss showed that even with antioxidants, no supporting research existed that suggested you cut them out.

Moreover, the truth is that **there are clinical trials that support the benefit of supplements with chemotherapy.** Here are just a few little examples:

* Tocotrienol vitamin E actually enhances the effects of Tamoxifen, so much so that you need 25 per cent less of the drug if you take the right dose of vitamin E in the right form. You won't hear too much about this research as far less Tamoxifen would be sold if women decided that they'd rather take some vitamin E and cut their risks of side-effects and womb cancer. There are also clinical studies on indole-3-carbinol, a natural compound, which also reduces the volume of Tamoxifen required.
* MD Anderson in 2007 showed that both vitamin K3 and vitamin C improved the success rates of chemotherapy drugs in clinical trials in bladder cancer.
* Canadian researchers *(British Journal of Cancer)* showed that using fumaric acid, a natural compound, helped activate an enzyme which enhances the activity of a drug called mitomycin C, used against solid tumours in the bowel and bladder. The combination allowed the drug to be used at lower doses with less side-effects.
* MD Anderson have also proven that resveratrol has a huge potential for fighting cancer and it can also improve the success rates of chemotherapy, appearing safe even in high doses.
* Other US cancer centres use vitamin D especially with breast cancer patients.
* The herb Uno de Gato (cat's claw) has been shown to protect healthy cells during chemotherapy, whilst having no

interference with its action on cancer cells. It also boosts the immune system simultaneously.

And with radiotherapy:

- St Thomas' Hospital has some research (but no clinical trials as yet) to show that both isoflavones and selenium can improve the success of radiotherapy.
- MD Anderson repeated German research using astragalus to deliver enhanced radiotherapy results. They have found that it can double survival times.
- Harvard and others have used vitamin D with radiotherapy and shown improved outcomes.
- Two 2011 studies showed that both flaxseed and probiotics could reduce damage to healthy cells during radiotherapy.

Protection to nearby healthy cells, while minimising side-effects like hair loss, can be helped by eating foods such as organic eggs, whole grains and greens for the organic iron and B vitamin (especially folic acid) content. Or you can supplement with B complex containing 400 mgs of folic acid. This has been proven to help reduce damage to the healthy cells.

Fish oils and aloe vera will reduce inflammation during the therapies. Medicinal mushroom extracts can boost the immune system, enhance chemo and radiotherapy, and reduce side-effects like hair loss and nausea.

An amino acid supplement of N-acetyl cysteine containing glutamine (which stimulates the liver to produce glutathione, a natural compound that repairs damaged cells) and L-cysteine (which is particularly important in DNA repair) may help you keep your healthy cells stable. Or you can eat lots of raw carrots, asparagus, avocado, cruciferous vegetables – broccoli, Brussels sprouts, cabbage etc – which are especially strong in glutathione; and kelp, eggs and garlic for L-cysteine. And go out in the sunshine for your vitamin D. Remember magnesium-rich foods, or supplements, soya lecithin, bold tea, dandelion and milk thistle will help de-fat and strengthen your liver during this time. And later you can rebuild your immune system with supplements like echinacea, cat's claw, total vitamin E, chlorella. And MGN-

3 (Biobran) on top of the astragalus you are already taking.

Don't forget, that many drugs are no longer traditional chemotherapy agents but clever 'biologics' that target a damaged gene and try to replace lost proteins. Why would supplements interfere with those?

KEY VITAMINS IN THE FIGHT AGAINST CANCER

More detailed information with references can be found at www.canceractive.com under nutritionals.

VITAMIN A

Information: Vitamin A cannot be synthesised in the body. Must be ingested directly or made from precursor carotenoids like beta-carotene. Fat soluble. Too much is highly toxic to the liver, so it is best to supplement with only a little natural vitamin A, and top up with beta-carotene allowing the body to make more if it needs it.

Sources: Deep sea, not farmed, oily fish is the best source. Cod liver oil supplements.

Daily anti-cancer 'dose': Female 700 micrograms; male 900 micrograms

Known benefits: Many studies show its cancer-fighting abilities. For example, it protects in breast cancer *(Iowa study)* and can cause remission in leukaemia *(Sloan-Kettering)*. Researchers at Chicago University have shown how a derivative of vitamin A (retinoic acid) blocks the damaging action of oestrogen in breast, prostate and colon cancers, by genome mapping.

BETA-CAROTENE

Information: Carotenoids and, within this group of natural compounds, beta-carotene are readily available in foods, but are water soluble. So if supplements are taken, they should be with food and spread out across the day. Importantly natural beta-carotene comes in two forms (all trans, and 9-cis) – synthetic supplements tend to have just the former which may account for the poor reviews the supplement receives occasionally.

Sources: Carotenoids are typically orange/red in colour (see also lycopene). The orange pigment in carrots, peppers, apricots and pumpkins. Tomatoes, kale, cherries, sweet potato, chicory and chlorella also have good levels.

Daily anti-cancer 'dose': Normal levels are 6 mgs – but anti-cancer dosage can go to 60 mgs per day. Smokers should not take synthetic beta-carotene; there are two studies suggesting it increases risk.

Known benefits: Several prevention studies show a reduction in cancer risk by 40 per cent, using beta-carotene supplementation. Studies with colon cancer show an immune boosting effect; it increases NK cells and cancer cell inhibition.

B VITAMINS

Information: Wide range of benefits from this range of vitamins, some of which have quite individual characteristics

Sources: Primarily whole grains, but also 'greens' and nuts

Most notable components in the fight against cancer are:

Folic Acid

Information: Folate levels have declined by as much as 16 per cent on average in just the last five years according to research in MMWR. But it is essential for making perfect copies of our genetic code when cells divide or send out messages.

Sources: Leafy vegetables, avocados, pulses, carrots, melons, apricots, whole grains. Its release from foods is controlled by beneficial bacteria in the colon. It is destroyed by oestrogen and oestrogen mimics.

Daily anti-cancer 'dose': 400 mgs

Known benefits: Essential for accurate copying of cellular genetic code and helps in the development of key messengers, enzymes and proteins. (It even has an anti-ageing role in the brain and also a role in heart disease.) A lack of it is noted in some cancers especially colorectal cancers.

Niacin

Information: A water soluble B vitamin also called nicotinic acid or vitamin B-3. Important in the formation of key enzymes and in the energy development process.

Sources: Good sources include yeast, meat, poultry, tuna, salmon, cereals, seeds and vegetables. Can be made from tryptophan.
Daily anti-cancer 'dose': 20 mgs per day.
Known benefits:
* Incorporated into niacin co-enzyme NAD and NADP, NAD level influence the cellular response to DNA damage.
* Involved in DNA repair.
* Involved in cell-signalling pathway and cancer prevention.
* Depletion of NAD shown to decrease levels of *p53* repair gene protein in breast, skin and lung cancer.
* Niacin deficiency linked with increased risk of leukaemia.
* Niacin deficiency also linked to deficiency in lymphocyte (white immune cell) production.
* Sodium butyrate (produced by beneficial bacteria) and niacin both shown to cause apoptosis (cancer cell death).
* Increased intake of niacin linked to decreased risk (circa 40 per cent) of throat, mouth and oesophageal cancers.
* Niacin has benefits with insulin control, diabetes, cholesterol levels, heart diseases and AIDS.

Vitamin B-12

Information: Essential vitamin – a lack of which is known in breast cancer, colon cancer and stomach cancers. Vegetarians also show deficiencies. A deficiency is linked with a deficiency of folic acid.
Sources: Liver, kidney, lean meat, oysters, seafood, chlorella, although beneficial bacteria are crucially involved in its release from foods.
Daily anti-cancer 'dose': Take Chlorella, if you don't want to eat meat.
Known benefits: Involved in over 300 chemical reactions in the body. The natural and active version is methylcobalmin; the common synthetic and injected form is cyanocobalmin, which converts to methylcobalmin in the body.

B-17

Information: Not a vitamin; amygdalin, the natural compound, has some similarities with B-12 (cyano-cobalmin) and 2014 in vitro studies showed in stopped cancer cell progression. B-17 can be broken down by enzymes unique to a cancer cell (but not in healthy cells) to release cyanide, which kills the cell. Pharma companies currently working on drugs to do exactly the same job!

Sources: Apricot kernels, pips of apples, grape seeds, certain nuts like cashews, pecans, macadamia and almonds, gooseberries, blackberries and other berries, barley, millet and brown rice, water cress, bamboo shoots, sweet potato, papaya.

Daily anti-cancer 'dose': Prevention experts say six apricot kernels a day. For people with cancer: Never take more than six in 90 minutes; never more than 35 in a day; and ensure you have a healthy liver to detox the by-products.

Known benefits: Fans claim that B-17 can selectively kill cancer cells, but there are no clinical trials to support this view just five small studies, three with animals, two with humans.

Biotin (B-7)

Information: Involved in carbohydrate and lipid metabolism. Crucial to DNA repair and stability. Deficiency where beneficial bacteria activity is impaired in intestine.

Sources: Nuts, whole grains, brown rice. Beneficial bacteria are essential for the release of biotin – it is often erroneously claimed that they 'make it'.

Daily anti-cancer 'dose': In B complex or 0.3 mgs supplement

Known benefits: Actual anti-cancer action uncertain, but seems to work as a co-factor to vitamins A, C, B-2, B-6 and niacin and has a boosting effect on the immune system.

Choline

Information: A phospholipid and vital component in membranes, cell signaling and neurotransmission throughout the body; important in the brain where it essential for cognitive function, IQ and development. Clearly, it crosses the blood-brain barrier. The US National Health and Nutrition survey concluded that only two per cent of post-menopausal American women consume the recommended daily intake! Staggeringly low. Vegetarians may be especially low in choline.

Sources: The reason for the low consumption is poor dietary advice (again). Choline is found in soya beans, soya lecithin, steak, chicken, cod, whole brown rice, egg yolk, spinach, cruciferous vegetables, cauliflower, wheatgerm, almonds. Destroyed by alcohol.

Known benefits: Anti-cancer activity not clear. Research shows anti-inflammatory role, and to be a bioactive compound in cancer stem cell growth prevention. It works in conjunction with other B vitamins and without it fat becomes trapped in the liver. It is a major source of the 'methyl' chemical which converts dangerous homocysteine to methionine. There are indications that low choline levels are linked to increased risk of liver cancer, higher homocysteine levels, decreased methylation of DNA and increased oxidative stress.

VITAMIN C

Information: Readily available; always better to eat the natural fruits and vegetables as it is in such plentiful supply and comes with co-factors, like enzymes and bioflavenoids, that help its action. It is water soluble so a little should be ingested at various times throughout the day. You won't store excess. Humans are one of the few animals that don't make it in the body.

Sources: Best are red peppers, broccoli, papaya, berries, cauliflowers, citrus fruits, potatoes and tomatoes

Daily anti-cancer 'dose': Linus Pauling suggested 4 gms daily – but up to 10 gms if you have cancer. The problem is that only about 7 per cent of standard oral supplement doses reach the blood stream and tissues. The new (but more expensive) liposomal products wrap the vitamin in small balloons of fat as happens under normal digestion. This delivers far higher blood levels. Injections of vitamin C give far higher delivered doses than oral consumption.

Known benefits: Vitamin C boosts the immune system, protects cells and cell walls from attack and, in large doses of 20-50 grams (mega-doses), helps oxygenate cancer cells by increasing glutathione levels (since cancer cells can't use oxygen, this kills them). It can also neutralise the toxins from parasites.

COENZYME Q10

Information: CoQ10 has an important role in the energy production system of the cellular power stations. It is found in larger quantities in highly active tissue like muscle, brain, heart and kidneys. Unfortunately, levels decline as we age, but research has shown that supplementation of 50 mgs can restore cellular levels to those of normal 28 year olds. 90 per cent circulates in the blood stream as Uniquinol. The ubiquinone version is the precursor and cheaper! Has proven epigenetic benefits.

Sources: Offal.

Daily anti-cancer 'dose': 30-50 mgs per day. Doses above this seem wasted.

Known benefits: The US National Cancer Institute has stated that CoQ10 can help the body resist infections, including cancer. It has stated that CoQ10 can both prevent cancer cells growing and cause cancer cell death. Researchers in the National Cancer Centre in Tokyo showed it cut cancer rates in half, in rats induced with colon cancer. There are also studies on its benefits with brain tumours and prostate cancer. Statins deplete levels of CoQ10.

VITAMIN D

Information: Essential vitamin to have in your prevention and treatment repertoire, tthere is research on its effects with all types of cancer from colon to breast and prostate. Great amounts of new research from the USA, particularly Harvard Medical School. Acts like a hormone with strong epigenetic effects. Prevents AND corrects: 2009 research showed it helps fight cancer too – cancer cells have large numbers of vitamin D receptors and the vitamin can kill cancer cells and *'can adjust almost everything in the cell from its genetic messaging to its cytoskeleton'*. *'It can even switch genes on and off'*. Other studies show it is essential in activating the T-cells in your immune system, or they cannot attack rogue cells. Pharmaceutical companies have tried to synthesise it and failed to get a concentrate through clinical trials. Everybody should spend 40 minutes every day in the sun, or supplement. Recommendations are 1000 IUs to 5000 IUs. There is extensive coverage of vitamin D on the website, with all references, and in the fourth edition of '*Everything you need to know to help you beat cancer*'.

Sources: Made by the action of sunlight on the cholesterol layers below your skin. No other source comes even near this. A little is found in oily fish, and far less still in dairy.

Daily anti-cancer 'dose': Scaremongering about the negative effects of sunshine, coupled with office jobs, indoor lifestyles and gloomy weather seem to be causing a crisis. Research shows deficiencies now appearing in urban populations. Supplement with vitamin D3 which your liver will convert to the active ingredient. RDA is currently 5-6 micrograms or less than 1000 IUs but research now shows levels of 20-30 times this are perfectly safe – you will get 40,000 IUs from a day on the beach. Two mega-studies from Moores Cancer Centre in San Diego have shown huge potential cancer reductions. One concludes spending 15-20 minutes and taking 2000 IUs per day would result in a 50 per cent reduction in breast cancer, while the other concludes colorectal cancers would be reduced by two-thirds if people took enough sunshine or supplements. Black people living in poor sun environments should definitely supplement. All recent reports suggest 4000 to 5000 IUs per day is the correct level for cancer patients.

Known benefits: Harvard say it is protective for more than 15 cancers from breast, to prostate, to colon and pancreatic cancer. Their professor (Hollick) says 25 per cent less women would die from breast cancer if they took adequate amounts. In another study which followed 1.1 million men and women for 30 years, those with higher blood levels of vitamin D had significantly less deaths from cancer. The sun belt in the USA has long been associated with lower cancer rates. It seems the sun, supported by plenty of green vegetables, really is a strong factor. It prevents – and it seems to help you beat cancer too. Research from Kings College says sunshine actually keeps you younger inside as well! Research also shows it may improve success in radiotherapy.

VITAMIN E

Information: Recent research is throwing official recommendations to the wind. There are eight forms of vitamin E: four forms of tocopherols, and four forms of tocotrienols. (alpha, beta, gamma, and delta of each). The EU only officially permits the sale of synthetic alpha tocopherol, a form that may increase risk of death, reduce longevity and even block the action of beneficial tocotrienols!!

Sources: Give up crisps and bag snacks and put out bowls of seeds and nuts instead. Sunflower, pumpkin, sesame and linseeds, plus almonds and other nuts. Also found in whole grains, spinach, cabbage, lettuce, eggs.

Daily anti-cancer 'dose': Levels of this vitamin have been declining in natural foods. To get an all round benefit you should think natural and 'total' – a totally natural vitamin E, with all the 8 forms. 400 IUs per day

Known benefits: Over 800 studies suggest benefit from this vitamin. It stops fats turning 'rancid' and damaging the immune system, low levels are linked to many cancers and it is a proven immune booster. A review of 12 studies in 2005 alone showed the importance of tocotrienols in beating breast cancer. Recent Japanese research shows that two forms of natural tocotrienols (alpha and delta) directly inhibit a cancer promoting enzyme (DNA polymerase), disrupt the formation of blood vessels by tumours, and can reduce metastasis. MD Anderson, in 2009 research, showed that a higher intake of NATURAL vitamin E cut the risk of lung cancer by 55 per cent.

GLUTATHIONE

Information: A very powerful antioxidant that is produced in all cells in the body – an important part of the power production, it keeps the cell's oxygen levels up and 'knocks out' free-radicals.

Sources: Widely available in fruits and vegetables; top providers are avocados, asparagus, watermelons, grapefruit, strawberries, raw tomatoes, oranges and lightly boiled or steamed cabbage, Brussels sprouts, cauliflower and broccoli.

Daily anti-cancer 'dose': Little need for supplements if you eat the above foods. Its action is enhanced by selenium.

Known benefits: Older people with the highest levels of glutathione in their bloodstream, overcome illness quickest. This highlights the science behind why eating real foods is good and junk food is no good for you. It neutralises free-radicals and harmful fats. Glutathione levels have now been shown to be inversely proportional to homocysteine levels, and high homocysteine seems to indicative of increased risks of diseases such as cancer and Alzheimer's. Keeping vegetable and fruit intake high, possibly supplementing with glutamine, selenium and B complex (especially B-12) may help increase glutathione and decrease homocysteine levels. A healthy gut flora is essential especially as you age so multi-strain probiotics may help.

VITAMIN K

Information: Used traditionally to aid blood clotting, the RDA level set is miniscule and only three groups of researchers study it in the world. That may change.

Sources: Green leafy vegetables, broccoli. But the vitamin K cannot be released without the involvement of beneficial bacteria.

Daily anti-cancer 'dose': The RDA was set at 50 micrograms to aid blood clotting. No official recommendations on dosage – but levels of up to 500 times have been shown to be safe. Take vitamin K2 supplements or sort out your beneficial bacteria and diet. Or both!

Known benefits: First researchers in Washington and Tokyo showed that it could stop some liver cancers completely. Then a benefit was shown with leukaemia and pancreatic cancers. This is hardly surprising; 200 years ago we ate a lot of greens and we had healthy intestinal flora. Research is not totally clear but in some way vitamin K helps vitamin D 'activate' your T-cells before they can attack rogue cells in the body.

LYCOPENE

Information: An epigenetic antioxidant and carotenoid, but not commonly mentioned. It binds to, and breaks up certain fats in the blood stream and tissues.

Sources: Tomatoes, tomatoes and especially cooked tomatoes which release the vitamin more readily

Daily anti-cancer 'dose': 10-15 mgs.

Known benefits: Harvard Medical School showed that eating ten helpings of tomatoes per week could reduce prostate cancer risk by 40 per cent. And if you had the cancer already, it could reduce the symptoms by 40 per cent as well. It is known also to displace certain heavy metals bound in fatty tissue.

KEY MINERALS IN THE FIGHT AGAINST CANCER

CALCIUM

Information: It helps regulate the power-producing activities in healthy cells; and low calcium causes a hormone calcitriol to be produced, which increases fat stores in the body. However, Gerson believe that too much calcium can increase cancer risk. Some cancer experts also believe this too. Calcium may cause problems directly, or excess calcium can reduce magnesium and vitamin D levels both of which protect.

Sources: Increasingly depleted in our soils, calcium is in a wide range of green vegetables, grains and nuts. It is easily absorbed,

Daily anti-cancer 'dose': The issue with calcium is not intake – a helping of spinach or cabbage is enough for a day. The issue is storage and depletion. Calcium is easily absorbed, stored and re-usable as long as vitamin D and magnesium are present. Smoking, oestrogen and alcohol deplete the stores. Coral calcium and other similar organic supplements are excellent providers. A maximum intake of 1 gram per day is plenty.

Known benefits: Several studies have shown that low blood calcium levels are linked to breast and colon cancers. However, Rudolf Keller and Dr Max Gerson believed that calcium stimulated tumour growth. The Karolinska Institute has warned on dairy consumption and the Fox Chase Cancer Centre in Philadelphia has warned on its high calcium levels (May 2005). Men with the highest intakes of dairy calcium are 2.2 times more likely to develop prostate cancer. Personally, I feel that if your intestinal flora are fine and you are eating enough 'greens', there should never be the need to touch a supplement or cows' dairy.

MAGNESIUM

Information: Essential mineral for the transportation of other minerals into and out of the cell. 40 per cent of adults are deficient in it.

Sources: Pulses, whole grains, 'greens', apples, pears, jacket potato, nuts.

Daily anti-cancer dose: Just eat the fresh food listed. Magnesium is available in organic supplement form.

Known benefits: Without enough magnesium, the calcium and potassium transport system into your tissues cannot function correctly, and a build up of sodium will occur, leaving the cells acid and with lower oxygen. The Karolinska Institute has shown that the higher the intake of magnesium, the lower the risk of colorectal cancer.

POTASSIUM

Information: We really should be potassium people – and we are not. We should have an intake of potassium five times greater than our intake of sodium.

Sources: Lentils, jacket potato, broad beans and peas, whole grains, nuts bananas, fresh fish, green vegetables, brown rice, carrots, apples, pears, oranges.

Daily anti-cancer 'dose': No real need to supplement unless correcting an imbalance with sodium, in which case there are organic salts available.

Known Benefits: Ensures the power stations, or mitochondria, produce their energy in a normal cell way. Without potassium they will adopt an anaerobic method and may become cancer cells.

SELENIUM

Information: The FDA in America has clearly stated that selenium 'can reduce the risk of cancer', but it is deficient in European diets. One of the most important anti-cancer minerals. Selenium deficiency is common in cancer patients. Selenium is known to destabilise the AK15 protein causing cell division in prostate patients, and the AK13 protein in melanoma. A deficiency has also been linked directly with stomach and breast cancers. It is known to increase cellular oxygen and glutathione peroxidase activity.

Sources: You will hear about Brazil nuts as the best source, but you need to crack these fresh yourself. Shelf lighting with see-through bags depletes the nuts of selenium and can turn them rancid. Best sources are some types of garlic, tuna and oily fish, lobster, onions, sunflower seeds, tomatoes, wheatgerm, bran, eggs and chicken breast.

Daily anti-cancer 'dose': 100-200 micrograms, (never exceed 200 micrograms) Smoking and 'bad' fats deplete its levels.

Known benefits: It works to enhance the action of vitamin E as an antioxidant. It also can displace mercury, lead and cadmium from cells, and it can even help eliminate some chemicals and oestrogen mimics from the body. There is a large body of research from Germany showing its benefits in both the prevention and treatment of prostate cancer, a cancer that has links to heavy metals and to chemicals.

ZINC

Information: It is arguable that zinc is not itself an antioxidant but it does help others like vitamins A and C do their daily jobs. It is known to accelerate healing time.

Sources: Meat, eggs. pumpkin seeds, sunflower seeds, sesame seeds, wheatgerm, brewers' yeast, shellfish and oysters. Alcohol and vitamin B-6 can deplete it. Dairy blocks its absorption.

Daily anti-cancer 'dose': Recommended levels are 15-20 mgs (there is some indication that levels above 100 mgs can cause cancer).

Known benefits: Particularly important in the fight against prostate cancer. There is some evidence that prostate cancer is linked with heavy metals and chemical toxins. The prostate is the store of zinc in men, and zinc (like selenium) can displace these toxins – or be displaced by them. White flecks on your finger nails are a sign of deficiency. Supplementation of 15 mgs a day has been found to reduce prostate cancer risk by 40 per cent.

Summary

As the science of epigenetics progresses, some of these vitamins (like the tocotrienols of vitamin E), Co Q10, and B vitamins, and particularly minerals like selenium and iodine (kelp), are being shown to have extremely important anti - DNA message blockage benefits. Our knowledge can only increase.

CHAPTER 17
HERBS IN THE FIGHT AGAINST CANCER

Surrounding Hampton Court 500 years ago were not rose gardens, but herb gardens. Herbs were just a natural part of our environmental nourishment. Eating herbs helped prevent – and treat – illness. Just as poorer Asians eat all manner of green plants nowadays, so did we 500 years ago.

We used herbs not merely as 'treatments' but as protection. Stuffing the chicken with sage (an astringent) and onion (an anti-viral) kept the germs away.

In the 'Handbook of Organic Food Safety and Quality', various professors and scientists studying cattle have noted that the animals chose to graze in certain parts of fields where different types of herbs grow. The milk contains higher levels of natural compounds, like omega-3, as a result. I can imagine the same situation for humans 500 years ago. We ate those foods that surrounded us and were in season – and herbs would have been a part of our diets. Sadly this is no longer true, and our health may be paying the price.

For example, Professor Dr. Thomas Efferth from Deutsches Krebsforschungszentrum in Heidelberg has analysed 76 medicinal plants that are believed to treat malignant tumors and other such growths. Extracts from 18 of the plants were found to significantly suppress the growth of cancer cells. He describes the results as '*way above*' the results you could expect from drugs.

In Europe, Herbal Medicine is legally recognised as a legitimate healthcare system under the banner of 'Traditional Medicine'. This means that where natural herbs have traditionally-defined medicinal value and/or have documented scientific research studies on them, claims can be legally made about their specific scientific effectiveness, and their safety.

Unfortunately, this is not the case in the USA, where they are simply dietary supplements. There, scientific research is always required and, even then, claims of medical efficacy are not allowed. In my opinion, this is nonsense as it greatly compromises the worldwide acceptance of, and belief in, herbs as healing agents. As in many things, the view of Americans dominates – and here it is palpably wrong.

Not least, herbs are less likely to feature in everyday conversations on illness if they are dubbed chemicals. And if no effects can be claimed, there is no point in prescribing them and so, they must be deemed worthless. As Europeans with 4000 years of history in treating illnesses, we know that is simply not true.

A further, but minor, complication is that when discussing health matters with European Medical Herbalists, they rarely differentiate between what you and I might call a herb (thyme) and other active ingredients from plants (e.g. Quercitin, from apples and onions). In this chapter I will try to stick to 'Herbs'!

Hoxsey

In 1988 the Office of Technology Assessment (OTA) of the United States Congress commissioned a report on the Hoxsey Therapy. It was the first federal agency to review the therapy and did it as part of a study into alternative cancer treatments. Patricia Spain Ward PhD, a medical historian from the University of Illinois, completed a background paper for Congress; this paper details the full story. You can read a full summary on our website – here is the shortened version!

Harry M Hoxsey (1901–1974) developed and practised a cancer treatment. Since his death, Mildred Nelson, his long-time nurse and assistant, has continued his work. In 1963 Hoxsey chose a site in Tijuana, where today stands the thriving Bio-Medical Centre, home of the therapy.

Hoxsey became a healer in the 1920s. He believed that cancer was systemic – a disease of the whole body – and developed a herbal mixture to kill it off.

His first 'therapy' was in fact an external paste, made of antimony sulphide, zinc chloride, bloodroot and other occasional ingredients like arsenic sulphide, herbs and talc. With the help of Dr Frederick Mohs, a surgeon and the Dean of Wisconsin Medical School and several of its staff, he treated surface cancers that were then surgically removed with success. Hoxsey's 'red paste' and the experiments were written up extensively in the 1940s. Dr Mohs published in 1941 in the *Archives of Surgery* and in 1948 in the *Journal of the American Medical Association*.

However the AMA attacked and attacked, even claiming that Hoxsey and Mohs had used different pastes. One report claimed that Hoxsey's active ingredient in the 1950s was arsenic, but it turned out the AMA was using an early 1920s paste! Hoxsey had developed a caustic treatment and was an ex-mining quack. Mohs was a doctor and a surgeon, and his treatment by contrast was acceptable. In fact both men were using sanguinarine, an alkaloid in bloodroot which has potent anti-tumour effects *(Young 1967)*.

Worse, Hoxsey had an 'elixir' for internal cancers. And he refused to tell people, especially the AMA, what was in it although he identified alfalfa, buckthorn, red clover and prickly ash, he did not name the others.

Unfortunately, Harry Hoxsey's success as a healer, the wealth it created, and his refusal to divulge the exact ingredients of his elixir made him enemies in high places.

By 1950 the FDA used the courts to demand ingredient labeling and block interstate shipments. This forced Hoxsey to reveal all, and he detailed a core set of ingredients, with variant extras depending upon the individual and their type of cancer.

The basic solution was:

Cascar *(Rhamnus Purshiana)* and potassium iodide

The additions might include any of the following:
Poke root *(Phytolaeca americana)*
Burdock root *(Arctium lappa)*
Berberis root *(Berberis vulgaris)*
Buckthorn bark *(Rhamnus frangula)*
Stillingia root *(Stillingia sylvatica)*
Prickly ash bark *(Zanthoxylum americanum)*

Both the AMA and FDA dismissed the potion as *"worthless, without any therapeutic merit in the treatment of cancer"*, and did not even analyse it.

In the *JAMA* 1954 the AMA insisted that *"Any intelligent physician could testify that all these substances were worthless."* All Hoxsey's case histories at the subsequent FDA trial were dismissed as lacking in evidence and neither the FDA nor the NCI provided any detail counter evidence or laboratory trials on cancer efficacy or otherwise. Commissioner Larrick warned Hoxsey publicly in 1956.

However scientific research now does support the ingredients. For example:

- **Pokeweed** – Triggers the immune systems, increases lymphocytes and increases levels of immunoglobulin *(Farnes 1964, Downing 1968)*.
- **Burdock** – 'Considerable anti-tumour activity' *(Szeged University 1966)*. 'uniquely capable of reducing mutagenicity' *(Morita et al 1984)*.
- **Burberry** – Anti-tumour activity *(Hoshi et al 1976)*; contains lycbetaine, an anti-tumour substance *(Owen 1976)*.
- **Buckthorn** – Anti-leukaemia substances; anthraquinone works against tumours *(Kupchan 1976)*.

Even the least studied herbs, stillingia and prickly ash, have anti-inflammatory or anaesthetic properties and are used in European folk remedies.

An eminent US botanist, James Duke PhD of the United States Department of Agriculture, has confirmed that all of the Hoxsey herbs have known anti-cancer properties and have long been used by Native American healers to treat cancers. Even as long ago as the 1850s Dr J W Fell of the Middlesex Hospital was using bloodroot and zinc oxide directly onto malignant growths with great effect.

Hoxsey also had his 'converts'. The Assistant District Attorney of Dallas, Al Templeton, arrested Hoxsey almost 100 times until in 1939 his brother developed a cancer and was cured by Hoxsey. Templeton became Hoxsey's lawyer.

Esquire magazine sent journalist James Burke to Texas in 1939 to write a story *'on the quack'*. He stayed six weeks, wrote **'The Quack Who Cures Cancer'** and became his publicist!

In 1954 an independent team of ten US physicians made a two-day inspection of Hoxsey's clinic, then in Dallas, and concluded that he was 'successfully treating pathologically proven cases of cancer, both internal and external, without the use of surgery, radium or x-ray'.

But the fact is that still the FDA and AMA have not tested the therapy! Even in 1965 Morris Fishbein, former long term editor of *JAMA* and voice of American Medicine for 40 years referred to Hoxsey as a charlatan and talked of *'ghouls and cancer quacks'*. Patricia Ward in her report to Congress quotes this sort of attitude as setting the *'low level of discourse and the emotional rather than analytical tone.'* Hoxsey sued Fishbein – and won.

By 1976 the Cancer Chemotherapy National Services Center researching plants used in folklore, noted that they often had anti-cancer activity.

Hoxsey's clinics were shut down in the 1950s, when even a 1953 Federal Report to the Senate stated that the FDA, AMA and NCI had organised "a conspiracy" to suppress a fair and unbiased assessment of Hoxsey's methods *(The Fitzgerald Report)*. At the time the Dallas clinic had 12,000 patients.

Today the Bio-Medical Center combines the flexible Hoxsey formula with diet, vitamin and mineral supplements. Liquorice and red clover (also used in Essiac and examined in tests with breast cancer at Royal Marsden) are frequent herbal additions. The Centre is outpatient only. You arrive, ideally with all your reports and tests, and they see you for a day or two. You leave with enough potions and medication to last three or more months.

Dietary advice is usually to avoid foods that conflict with the herbs; like pork, carbonated drinks, alcohol, vinegar and tomatoes. Supplements include immune stimulants, yeast tablets, vitamin C, calcium and laxatives. However the Centre does offer treatments like homeopathy and even chemotherapy.

External cancers like melanoma are frequently treated, as are cancers of the blood system. There are many case histories for all cancers from breast to colon. According to director Mildred Nelson, about 80 per cent of patients seen at the Centre 'benefit substantially'.

Essiac

Another 'herbal' therapy that has run the gauntlet in the USA is Essiac, an eight ingredient herbal tea. Currently Essiac is 'unapproved for marketing' in the USA. However the Resperin Corporation, the current owners of the full formula, has a special agreement with the Canadian Health and Welfare Dept. and this allows 'emergency releases of Essiac on compassionate grounds'.

So what's the fuss all about?

The original formula was given to Nurse Rene Caisse by a hospital patient who claimed her cancer had been healed some 20 years before by an Ontario Indian medicine man.

Caisse used the blend of herbs to treat patients for a number of years, setting up her own clinic in 1935 in Braceridge, Canada. Caisse's view was that it alleviated pain, and at the same time broke down nodular masses to form a more normal tissue. (Eventually the tumour would start to soften after an earlier hardening. Patients frequently reported a discharge of large amounts of pus and fleshy material as the tumour broke down.)

Her clinic was free, and by 1938 supporters tried to win Government approval for her work, failing in parliament by three votes. Nine doctors had petitioned the Canadian federal health department as early as 1926 asking that Caisse be allowed to test her cancer remedy on a broad scale. In their signed petition they testified that the herbal treatment reduced tumour size and increased life expectancy.

Caisse's own view was that, if it doesn't actually cure cancer, it does afford significant relief. Whilst in Canada, Caisse treated her own 72 year old mother with the tea under the supervision of Dr Roscoe Graham, consultant and specialist. The tea was administered 12 times a day for 10 days, and her mother lived to 90 years of age.

By 1942, without official approval and fearing arrest, Caisse shut her clinic, although she continued to treat patients at home. In 1959 at the age of seventy she went to the Brusch Medical Centre in Massachusetts, where she treated cancer patients under the watchful eye of 18 doctors. Dr Charles Brush, who treated President Kennedy amongst other members of New England's elite, reported in 1991 that he had been taking Caisse's formula since 1984 when he himself had cancer operations.

The original herbal ingredients were:

- **Burdock root** – A well-known blood purifier which has been reported by Hungarian and Japanese scientists to decrease cell mutation and inhibit tumours. It has reasonably high selenium content.
- **Sheep Sorrel** – A traditional Indian remedy for everything from eczema to ringworm; it does have an effect in herpes, ulcers and cancer seemingly by stimulating the endocrine system.
- **Slippery Elm** – Calcium, magnesium and vitamin-rich, it has a healing effect on the lungs and internal organs. It also helps reduce acidity in the body.
- **Indian Rhubarb** – Very cleansing to the liver and intestinal system. It also helps transport oxygen throughout the body and has an antibiotic and anti-yeast action and reduces inflammation. In 1980 studies showed that it also had a clear anti-tumour effect.

Whilst working with Dr Brusch between 1959 and 1978, Nurse Caisse added four other herbs to the original formula. The new formula became **Essiac**, her name spelled backwards.

The four additions are:

- **Watercress** – Strong antioxidant effects, contains bioflavenoids; it is a good source of vitamin C.
- **Blessed Thistle** – A blood purifier and immune booster.
- **Red clover** – The herb of Hippocrates, the flowers are currently undergoing tests for breast cancer control.
- **Kelp** – Like chlorophyll, chlorella and spirulina, kelp is a strong provider of natural minerals especially iron and calcium in an organic and easily assimilated form. Kelp is anti-bacterial; sea vegetables, in general, help reduce acidity in the body thus improving immune function.

Nurse Caisse recommended 12 – 13 cups of the infusion per day, although there are several reports of it being administered by injection. Shortly before she died she sold the 'secret' formula to the company Resperin.

Without proper clinical trials it is impossible to come to any definitive conclusion about Essiac and a degree of mythology has clouded some of the story.

What is apparent though is that the ingredients of Essiac, if nothing else, make it an excellent all-round immune system booster although some ingredients do have scientific research on their anti-cancer roles.

Black Salve

Of interest, although not for actual consumption, is the poultice Black Salve, which contains Graviola *(Annona muricata)*, Bloodroot and Chapparal along with zinc chloride and galangal root. It seems a modern day alternative to Fell's treatment mentioned a few pages back. We have anecdotes, with photographs, on our website of this poultice impressively dealing with small breast tumours.

The role of herbs in the 'eat-to-beat-cancer' diet

The fact is that our bodies have co-evolved with the plants around us for hundreds of thousands of years, and this cannot be said of drugs.

Some orthodox medical practitioners will say, 'But we do not ignore herbs' pointing, for example, to the development of the drug Taxol from the periwinkle. But this is a synthetic and toxic cellular killer, using but one active ingredient of the herb. It has little to do with Herbal Medicine, for it is not the use of the whole herb by the 'animal' in its natural local environment. It reflects neither synergistic evolution nor a balance with the world around us.

Others will correctly say that no single herb can cure cancer. As we at **CANCERactive** continually point out, no single anything (drug, herb, vitamin) will cure cancer and it is a fool and quack who says otherwise. The whole point of this book is to try and help people cover all the bases and build an effective anti-cancer programme. It would be a foolish person who said herbs had no role to play. Let us look at herbs in a little more depth.

Immune response

A common misconception is that merely stimulating the immune system to generate more foot soldiers will be enough to kick out cancer. Maybe, in a few cases it will. But, by and large, the problem with cancer is two-fold: The immune system is overwhelmed, and, the immune system doesn't fully recognize the cancer cells. It is a quantity and quality issue. The issue is to make lots of different foot soldiers AND stimulate the system in such a way that the cancer cells appear on the radar screens.

So, in Herbal Medicine two therapeutic requirements are essential when treating cancer – **Immuno-modulating** herbs, and **Adaptogenic** herbs. BOTH are required and work synergistically.

Immune system components (T-cells, B-cells, Natural Killer cells, cytokines, immunoglobulins etc.) may be increased in numbers, for example, by the use of grape seed extract, pine bark extract, vitamin E, turmeric, echinacea and cat's claw to name but a few of the best. The second step may be helped by herbs such as Korean ginseng, Pau d'Arco and astragalus, which has been shown to aid rogue cell recognition. There is a lot of research on the role of polysaccharides in helping cells communicate too.

But even this might not be enough as vitamin D (possibly aided by vitamin K) has been shown to 'activate' the attack process.

No wonder drugs like interferon and interleukin don't work too well on their own.

Attacking the cancer process

Herbal Medicines have a wide variety of potent properties and certain herbs with certain properties are known to attack different steps of the cancer process. In my personal view, a trip to a qualified medical herbalist should be an essential part of building an anti-cancer programme.

Here is an indication of the phenomenal strength of herbs, using just a few. There is much more information on our website. On a personal note I found that cat's claw, astragalus, turmeric (curcumin) and echinacea can be an excellent immune system re-boosting combination after treatment with radiotherapy or chemotherapy when we gave this mixture to Catherine, after the chemotherapy

173

drugs had reduced her white cells to desperately low levels and the standard immune-stimulating drugs on offer simply wouldn't work. Her white cell levels recovered in less than two weeks.

NATURAL HERBS THAT MAY HELP

1. ASTRAGALUS

Astragalus membranaceous is a truly all-round anti-cancer agent. It has been used in Chinese medicine for two thousand years. It is known as 'haung qi', or chi, because qi is the word for energy and the herb boosted natural body energy levels. It is taken from the root of a plant needing four to seven years to mature. This herb is also known to boost the immune system and specifically to treat burns, abscesses and hepatitis. In Chinese hospitals it is now used to help people recover from the negative effects of radiotherapy and chemotherapy.

FDA to approve role in cancer?

Its wide usage in China as an immune system booster brought interest from Europe, Japan and America. A considerable amount of detailed German and American research has confirmed its powers and potential role in cancer therapy. The FDA did once say it was looking at granting astragalus approval to be used as an anti-cancer agent. Don't hold your breath. They have never yet approved a herb!

An excellent immune system booster

Astragalus has phenomenal and positive immune system modulating effects. In tests at the Hiroshima School of Medicine in Japan, it was shown to directly increase B-lymphocyte and T-lymphocyte levels, interleukin and antibody production. Astragalus contains bioflavenoids, cholines, and a polysaccharide, astragalan B, amongst other active ingredients.

Astragalan B controls bacterial infection and viruses by binding to their outer membranes and weakening their internal systems. Its use as an adjunct to fight AIDS is increasingly important. But this membrane-binding ability seems to make astragalus an important adaptogenic herb too, 'offering up' viruses, bacteria and even cancer cells to be seen by the immune system. In cancer therapy, where so many cancers 'hide' from the immune system this makes astragalus a natural compound of huge value.

Improves the effectiveness of radio- and chemotherapy

One extremely important conclusion from several US and German studies is that astragalus seems to help the immune system differentiate between healthy cells and rogue cells, thereby boosting the body's total 'cancer-fighting system'. A consequence of this is the added benefit of improving the effectiveness of radiotherapy and chemotherapy treatments.

MD Anderson Cancer Center (Texas) researchers reported that cancer patients undergoing radiotherapy had twice the survival rates if they took astragalus and this prestigious cancer centre has conducted a considerable amount of research on the herb.

It should be taken with meals at a total intake of 2000 to 3000 mgs per day.

2. ECHINACEA and CAT's CLAW

Two more immune system boosters: **Echinacea:** Generally known as an immune system enhancer against colds, the polysaccharide, arabinogalactan, in echinacea is effective in activating macrophages, interleukin and interferon with an increase in T-cell activity. Research also shows that it can stimulate the immune system to kill microbes and directly cause cancer cell death. Separate studies show that it has had positive effects with brain tumours and more work is currently being carried out in this area.

I have read reports that it should not be taken for more than eight weeks at a time as it thins the blood, so special care should be exercised if you are taking blood thinning drugs. There is an EU health warning not to give it to children under 12 years of age because of rare allergic reactions!
Cat's Claw: Alkaloids are very powerful natural plant

compounds and there are six oxindole (or oxyindole) alkaloids in Uno de Gato bark. This natural ingredient is found in the Peruvian rain forest and China. It is known to be anti-viral, anti-inflammatory, an antioxidant and an immune-stimulator and it is known to increase various white cell levels stimulating the production of NK cells. Four alkaloids in particular boost phagocytosis where the white cells attack, wrap up and carry off the rogue cells to be neutralised and excreted from the body – be they microbes, viruses, antigens and even cancer cells.

Research studies have shown the herb to be very powerful in its use with AIDS and cancer therapies. Research shows an action in decreasing the size of some tumours.

It can reduce the damaging side-effects from radiotherapy and chemotherapy as it seems to offer protection to healthy cells and enhances the attack on, and removal of, cancer cells.

As an anti-cancer aid it can also be combined with wild yam and aloe vera forming a very strong anti-viral, anti-bacterial immune boosting force.

It has also been shown to boost the body's natural energy levels.

One gram per day seems to be the dosage for cancer patients.

3. THOROWAX

Also called Hares ear or *Bupleurum scorzonerifolium*, research shows its ability to enhance natural interferon production and according to medical herbalist it seems especially useful in bone cancer/multiple myeloma.

4. ALOE VERA

Used by the Ancient Egyptians and Greeks for bites, burns, lesions and skin 'cancers', research has shown its potency in internal usage as well.

Aloe has two principal actions.

Firstly, it contains very active polysaccharides and one in particular, acetyl mannose, boosts cytokine levels and enhances the immune response to cancer. It is known to increase levels of T-lymphocytes, and interferon. Research has shown also that it stimulates tumour necrosis factor shutting off the blood supply to tumours and also preventing tumour formation.

Secondly, aloe vera contains six or more anti-inflammatory agents. Natural compounds such as salicylate, gamme-linoleic, gibberlin, sterols and amino acids, tryptophan and phenylalanine all have significant anti-inflammatory benefits.

It is also anti-viral and anti-bacterial in its action.

5. WORMWOOD

In 2007 the five malaria aid charities all agreed that the Chinese herb, *Wormwood artemisia*, did a more effective job than the anti-malarial drugs. It is strongly anti-parasitical and anti-fungal – indeed so powerful that it need only be taken for a few days to 'clean up' your blood system. It can be used to kill parasites, yeasts and microbes while leaving beneficial bacteria unharmed.

Recent research suggests that it also has an oxidative effect on the cell, and may even play a small anti-cancer role, particularly in controlling iron levels.

6. GOLDENSEAL

Has an action against pathogens (rogue invaders, like *Helicobacter pylori*) and has been shown to be stronger and more selective than antibiotics. It improves blood supply to the spleen and produces a higher immune response. It has been shown also to inhibit tumour formation.

7. SUMA ROOT

Contains 19 different amino acids and a number of trace minerals. The high germanium content boosts oxygenation at a cellular level. Suma root contains saponins, which help regulate blood sugar, and inhibit melanoma in research. It is immuno-stimulating and research suggests it inhibits cancer cell and tumour formation. Two of its ingredients have now been patented for cancer treatment by pharmaceutical companies.

8. FEVERFEW

For centuries feverfew – which has small daisy-like flowers – has been used as a tea for treating ailments like arthritis and migraine. In 2005 researchers from Rochester University in New York showed that in higher concentrations parthenolide, the active ingredient, kills leukaemia stem cells whilst leaving healthy cells intact. When the researchers compared it to the chemotherapy drug cytarabine they found in turn that the drug showed only 'modest toxicity' to the leukaemia stem cells, but 'relatively high toxicity' to the healthy cells.

The FDA has put parthenolide onto its 'Rapid Access Programme', which is a fast track designed to take experimental drugs quickly into clinical trials. Meanwhile the scientists are saying that leukaemia patients should not take feverfew (or any other herbal supplement) without consulting a doctor first. Lead scientist Dr Craig Jordan says that, anyway, a patient would not be able to take enough of it to produce an effect.

This really sums up the whole issue with herbs. Here clearly is a herb that 'works'. Naturally toxic to a rogue cell but, as we have lived with it for thousands of years, it clearly doesn't harm healthy cells. Next, the researchers 'pan' the current drug – but has it be withdrawn four years on? Then they suggest that leukaemia patients could only get enough of the herb active ingredient in a new, and as yet unmade, drug – haven't they heard of tinctures? And finally you shouldn't take a herb without consulting your doctor. Considering in the USA he knows less than nothing about nutrition (according to the US Government themselves) or supplements, and thinks herbs have no medicinal value at all as that is the medical stance in the USA, how is he going to advise you on feverfew?

So ignore the natural compound that works – while you wait for a drug that might not, and meantime use something that is not very good anyway. Brilliant.

9. BLOOD ROOT

Blood root or *Sanguinaria canadensis* has research which shows consitent anti-neoplastic activity. It seems effective against certain cancer tumours and, according to medical herbalists, can shrink them; it has proven very useful with sarcomas.

10. BUTCHERS BROOM

(Ruscus aculeatus): The active ingredients of this herb has been found to be the ruscogenins which have tumour-shrinking and anti-oestrogenic abilities. It may be used in the treatment of breast cancer.

11. NEEM

A native of Burma, and widely found throughout India, where it is called the 'Village Pharmacy'. An immune system booster, anti-fungal, anti-viral, anti-bacterial; The National Research Council in Washington said, *'It could benefit everyone living on this planet'*.

12. CARCTOL

Is a combination of 8 herbs, each with active anti-cancer ingredients. It is used as part of a strongly body-alkalising diet and must be prescribed by a qualified medical practitioner.

With the new European Laws, medicinal herbs must be prescribed after a face to face consultation with a medicinal herbalist in the UK. The EU has decided, correctly, that medicinal herbs are powerful; surely this is all the more reason to visit a qualified medical herbalist if you want an effective anti-cancer programme.

Sadly, the mythology continues

Of course, many oncologists will throw their arms up in horror if you tell them that you are taking herbs to boost your immune response, while they are treating you with radiotherapy or chemotherapy. But the truth is that there is an enormous amount of research on herbs *per se*, and there are a number of studies showing herbs can help in protecting healthy cells, boosting the immune system, helping cancer cells be identified, and limiting side-effects during such orthodox treatments. Berberine has recently been shown to help the drug temozolomide with brain cancer. In other words, all the evidence points to herbs helping orthodox medical approaches deliver results.

Recently, there have been moves in the UK to ban herb mixtures on the grounds that, although the individual herbs may have effects that are scientifically accepted, there is little research on the effectiveness or safety of mixtures.

Experienced herbalists find these attacks laughable since people have been taking combinations of herbs for centuries and, where there are conflicts, they are already well understood and documented. It also seems rather odd that medical authorities can suddenly make pronouncements like this without having spoken to the leading experts in Herbal Medicine first to find out what research exists. Indeed, qualified Herbalists would have more credibility and evidence attacking the Orthodox Medical Profession – as I said earlier, the medical profession making the attacks has properly tested only 15 per cent of their drugs in clinical trials, and increasingly prescribes cocktails of four drugs or more, when the combinations have never been near a test of any sort. And these cocktails are actually causing 28 per cent of hospital admissions in the USA – and rising. '*Let he who is without blame cast the first stone*'.

Herbs can be taken in a variety of forms. Personally I believe they should be consumed as freshly prepared tinctures as this ensures maximum potency.

Anyone wishing to learn more about herbs and what they might do for a particular aspect of a cancer diet programme should consider contacting either the National Institute of Medical Herbalists in Great Britain or the more traditional Faculty of Herbal Medicine, under the International Regulatory Cooporation for Herbal Medicines (IRCH). Remember you want a fully qualified medical herbalist with expertise in cancer. These people will almost certainly be better qualified than the average GP in the minefield of oncology.

CHAPTER 18
HELPING HORMONES

Hormones are chemical substances that deliver messages in the body. They are so powerful that they can be effective at the level of a few parts per billion. (This is why some chemicals in everyday products are so worrying – they can act like hormones in the body, and yet Government safe limits are set in parts per million – a thousand times more concentrated!!)

Three hormones have been especially indicated in cancer prevention activities: Melatonin, Human Growth Hormone and DHEA.

All three peak in production terms in our bodies around the age of sixteen. Their volumes then decrease dramatically as we reach our fifties. Albert Einstein was being philosophical when he opined *"The tragedy of life is what dies inside a man when he lives."* But he could have been talking about these three essential hormones.

Melatonin

Poor sleep – a carcinogen

Melatonin is produced by your pineal gland, which sits underneath your brain, about 90 minutes after you go to sleep in a darkened room. It helps to push you into a deeper sleep.

This is a vitally important hormone in the fight against cancer. Changes in blood melatonin levels are reflected in changes in the levels of two cancer-stimulating hormones, IGF-1 and oestrogen, each of which rise as melatonin levels fall.

A number of studies has shown that people who have sleep deprivation or irregular sleep patterns have a much higher risk of cancer. For example, night shift nurses and long-haul airline hostesses have a much higher incidence of breast cancer than the norm. Male night shift workers have a higher risk of prostate cancer. So much so that the International Agency for Research on Cancer (IARC), the foremost international body on the disease, is considering officially labelling night-shift work as a "probable" human carcinogen.

The Royal Commission on Environmental Pollution has also made a clear link between exposure to light at night and cancer. Never sleep with a light on and try to have thick dark curtains if light from outside is coming into your bedroom. IARC have confirmed that cancer in general has been shown to be 60 per cent more common amongst night-shift workers and that there is even a similar risk increase among women who stay up late more than two or three times a week. Conversely, totally blind women are only half as likely to contract cancer.

Most interesting was research from the National Cancer Institute and the National Institute of Environmental Health in the United States where human breast cancer tumours were grafted on to rats. In the early hours of the morning, the rats were then given blood which had been previously taken, either from women during normal darkened-room, full sleep, or from women sleeping in artificial light conditions. The blood taken in darkness slowed the growth of the tumours by 80 per cent, whilst that taken after exposure to light accelerated it.

EMFs – the same effect?

While important cancer bodies rush to dub 'night shift working' carcinogenic, officialdom still ignores the issue of Electromagnetic Fields, or EMFs for short. Although the UK Government does urge caution on living within 200 yards of power cables or on the use of mobile phones by children, little is said about telephone masts and WiFi and other such sources. Yet, if you read the Government's own review board booklet, which resulted from a study of all the research to date (some 400 studies were chosen) you would quickly conclude that EMFs deplete melatonin levels in just the same way as a lack of sleep, with an identical knock-on effect to higher IGF-1 and higher oestrogen levels in the body. Clusters of cancer cases around phone and other masts are increasingly observed and in South Korea the Government ordered the dismantling of 1500 such masts because of their concerns over 'health risks including cancer'.

Melatonin – three powerful benefits

Melatonin 'works' in a number of ways, three of which are vital to beating cancer:

- It is a hormone and stimulates the thymus gland to produce immune cells which seek and destroy rogue cells.
- It is also a known antioxidant and free-radical neutraliser.
- It regulates levels of oestrogen, and IGF-1.

Indeed, melatonin is proven to have preventative and corrective epigenetic benefits. In a 2009 research review 'The role of melatonin in epigenetic regulation of breast cancer' scientists *Ahmet Kormaz, Sanchez-Barcelo, Tan and Reiter of the School of Medicine, Ankara, Turkey,* summarised five different avenues of research evidence where melatonin was shown to correct blockages in DNA messages in breast cancer patients.

You can incorporate certain foods within your diet to stimulate the precursors of melatonin (I will tell you more later) but frankly the simplest thing is to supplement. Levels of 3–6 mgs are the doses usually taken, while levels of 10 mgs and above have been known to cause hallucinations.

Such supplements are easily obtained in the USA where synthetic melatonin can be purchased in most supermarkets. However in the UK and Europe the open sale of these hormone supplements is banned, although like HRT they can be prescribed. However, I doubt that your doctor fully understands the importance of melatonin, probably merely thinking that it helps you sleep better.

There is also some concern that synthetic melatonin loses its potency before most people finish the bottle. And anyway, as readers know, I am quite against synthetic supplements and especially synthetic hormones.

Better might be to try a plant melatonin – there is a very good source, called Asphalia, grown with Government grants in Wales.

Meanwhile, steer clear of EMFs (don't live near masts, turn the WiFi off when not using it etc.) and get a good night's sleep in a darkened room away from all artificial lights, power points, electric appliances, electric blankets, computers and TVs.

Human growth hormone (Hgh)

Hgh is also produced about ninety minutes after falling asleep. Its production peaks at puberty and declines to almost zero in your fifties. The good news is you can generate more by going to the gym. Hgh production can be stimulated at almost any age by resistance training when the muscles are overworked and 'tear' slightly.

Hgh helps mobilise and burn fats and stimulates the conversion of protein into lean muscle. Most importantly it also stimulates the production of the seek-and-destroy immune cells.

Even after fifty years of age, diet can also restimulate Hgh production but you will need to take a number of amino acids, vitamins and minerals for best results (argenine, tyrosine, ornithine, tryptophan and glycine work synergistically with vitamins like the B vitamins, vitamin C and minerals zinc, calcium, magnesium and potassium).

Argenine is found in nuts, brown rice, oatmeal, raisins, seeds, meats and wholemeal bread. It is interchangeable in the body with ornithine. Argenine production (from the pituitary gland) ceases in adults around the age of thirty. Trauma will also stop its production.

It is very interesting to note that calorie restriction limits insulin production but also stimulates Hgh production, having the double benefit of controlling negative hormones whilst aiding the levels of this significant cancer fighter.

DHEA (dehydroepiandrosterone)

This is a natural hormone produced by the adrenal glands. Again its production declines with age. It is protective against free-radicals and some people use DHEA supplements although results are very mixed and some increased cancer risks have been noted. It seems to be weakened by oestrogen and stimulated by progesterone. Wild yam acts as a precursor and natural stimulator of DHEA (as for progesterone), and has also been shown to be an excellent booster of the immune system.

Based on the very mixed results from the research I have read, I'm not too sure that people should be supplementing with this hormone at all. However, it has its fans in the USA.

Thyroxin – poorly understood

Finally, I want to mention **thyroxin**, the hormone of the thyroid gland. Again, it's one of the hormones that declines with age. Importantly, it controls your general metabolic rate. High thyroxin levels increase your metabolism. With low levels you put on weight and become easily tired and listless.

Thyroxin came to my attention because we received Personal Prescription application forms from three very different women, of different backgrounds, age and physical appearance. All had breast cancer and all were taking synthetic thyroxin prescribed by their doctor because of poor thyroid function.

Co-incidentally, I received research from the USA which said that women with poor thyroid function had <u>less</u> cancer risk. So I did my homework. Sure enough, if you have an impaired thyroid, and therefore lowered natural thyroxin production, the research indicates you develop less cancer. It's not surprising really, is it? With high thyroxin you'd expect higher metabolic rates and more free-radicals, waste products and toxins.

Thyroxin shares similar pathways with oestrogen. What surprised me was that the fat, short patient was taking the same levels of daily thyroxin supplement as the thin, short one and the thin, tall one. Exactly the same daily dose?! Can this be right? And then I found research in America dating back over 30 years which warned that people should be careful taking synthetic doses of thyroxin as it increased metabolism and increased cancer rates. I published a paper on my monthly e-newsletter. It brought protests from two doctors. Apparently different levels of thyroxin are supposedly prescribed depending upon age, weight, sex and even weather conditions, they claimed. All I could reply was that in the case of my three ladies that simply was not true.

A further complication, quoted in the American research, was that too few doctors investigate why someone has low thyroxin production. One possible explanation is a low intake of iodine. Levels of iodine are important to thyroxin production and some diets are deficient in iodine.

If that was the underlying but undiagnosed cause, and you have been encouraged to take a standard dose of synthetic thyroxin supplement, but then have an iodine-rich dinner (oysters, shellfish), you can easily end up with too much thyroxin in your blood stream and a heightened metabolism. And you wouldn't want that at all. It would increase your risk of cancer.

If you have a problem with your thyroid, please make your first port of call a nutritionist or naturopath or other diet expert.

Summary

I am not a fan of synthetic supplements, especially synthetic hormone supplements. I've read the research on HRT!

So, I suggest that you would be wise to steer clear of EMFs as much as possible and, if over 50 years of age, to supplement with asphalia. And you should always sleep in complete darkness (and so should your children).

A regular visit to the gym is an option, where you might try lifting a few weights under supervision.

I think an annual visit to a specialist nutritionist would be no bad thing either. You service your car once per year – why not yourself?

SECTION 2

RE-BUILDING A LIFE

"Life is something that happens when you can't get to sleep."
(Fran Lebowitz)

And this is a fair summation of the problem. Too many people seem to think of life as passive – it's something that happens. Getting cancer is just bad luck.

This attitude, by and large, is rubbish.

You get out of life what you put in, and nowhere is this more true than with your health. Of course, genetics plays some part; and even your wealth, or lack of it. But by now you will have seen that even the poorest people can be happy, healthy and avoid cancer. The problem is that life in the West is 'broken', with toxicity everywhere, stresses, sedentary jobs and nutritionally deficient, non-nourishing foods.

And so you have to build your own micro-climate; your own little protective cocoon. You need to maximise your immune system, cut out the dangers and nourish your body – we've already seen what the issues are.

Now it's time to start to prepare some plans.

CHAPTER 19
EAT-TO-BEAT OESTROGEN?

Fuelling the fire of cancer

A large number of cancers, both male and female, are hormonally responsive and the prime culprit is often oestrogen. Oestrogen fuels the fire of many cancers and it seems to act in a number of ways.

Earlier in the book we saw two principle theories of cancer formation:

* Where oestrogen can cause stem cells to stay in their rapidly dividing trophoblast state.
* Where an aggressive member of the oestrogen family, oestradiol, can sit on cellular membrane receptor sites directing havoc inside the cell – increasing cellular sodium levels, lowering oxygen levels, creating an acid environment and reducing the cells energy and repair systems.

Oestrogen may act in many other ways to propagate human cancers. For example:

* Oestrogen is known to help cancer messages bind to receptor sites on cells, thus spreading the cancer. Indeed, it has been known to cause and spread cancers since the mid 1990's *(NCI)*. When oestrogen is added to cancer cells *in-vitro*, those cells proliferate *(Dr Anna Soto, Tufts Cancer Center)*.
* In excess, it reduces zinc levels in the body (the prostate, for example, is a store of zinc and low zinc levels are associated with increased risk of cancer).
* It destroys folate and biotin, both vitamins essential in DNA replication and the immune system.
* It weakens the insulin control of blood glucose – the food of the cancer cell.
* Research studies in 2009 show it actually can cause epigenetic mutation directly.

Excess oestrogen is linked to cancers in both males and females from melanomas to ovarian, from prostate to colon.

Oestrogen is linked to all manner of cancers in both males and females. Non-small cell lung cancer is up from 12 to 40 per cent of cases in 20 years. You don't have to have smoked. It is driven by oestrogen.

Oestrogen excess has been linked to other illness: water retention, osteoporosis, fatigue, memory loss, increased blood clotting and histamine levels, along with allergies, depression, dry skin and even diseases like Alzheimer's!

What is oestrogen (estrogen)?

Oestrogen is a family of chemicals, each of which have a similar ability to bind to specific receptor sites in cellular membranes. Often defined mistakenly as the 'female sex hormone', oestrogens come in several shapes and sizes. Actually, oestrone is the female sex hormone and is made in the ovaries. Levels of oestrone increase during the first two weeks of the female 'cycle', decreasing in the second two weeks as the balancing hormone, progesterone, increases its levels. Guy's Hospital in London showed that premenopausal women who had their operations in the second half of their cycle when oestrone was lower, had better survival rates.

Oestradiol is made principally in the fat stores of the body, by aromatase enzymes; in men and women.

Oestradiol is the 'aggressive sister'; about 40 times more 'potent' than oestrone it causes havoc inside cells. Far weaker still are the plant oestrogens, called phytoestrogens.

In fact experts now believe that the high levels of phytoestrogens in the blood streams of South East Asian people actually protect the individuals by binding to the receptor sites, and blocking the ability of oestradiol to take up the same position. This blocking action is also the theory behind Tamoxifen, the breast cancer drug.

The fact is that the 'oestrogen pool' is far larger in our bodies than ever before and it's killing us. (We have a book specifically on the subject detailing the best ways of cutting your oestrogen levels – *'Oestrogen: The Killer in Our Midst'*.) Cancer Research

UK estimated that blood oestrogen levels were growing by seven per cent per year in women! And breast cancer is growing by two to three per cent.

Which takes us to a fourth group of oestrogens, that the drug-sponsored charities seem to deny exists: Dr Soto showed there was a large number of chemicals found in everyday toiletries, cosmetics, perfumes and household cleaners, disinfectants, plastic bottles and packaging and also in fertilisers and pesticides that, once inside our bodies, can mimic the action of oestrogen. These are often termed 'oestrogen mimics' or xeno-oestrogens. She has also proven, worryingly, that their effects can be cumulative.

Oestrogen levels are rising in our bodies, whether from our own natural hormones, ingested animal versions, synthetic copies like HRT, or from those chemicals that 'mimic' its action.

Each week people ring our magazine **icon** to ask about breast cancers, prostate cancers, colon cancers, melanoma and even rare cancers like Hurtle's cells, all of which have been linked with high oestrogen levels. Many more cancers are linked to this same hormone, even some lung and brain cancers.

Although it is relatively easy for a woman to understand that oestrogen might be involved in her cancer, men find it hard to believe that this 'female' hormone could have anything to do with theirs. However it is clearly implicated in, for example, both prostate and testicular cancers.

Let us start with the most obvious link.

Oestrogen and breast cancers

The Bush people of the Kalahari Desert in Africa have a diet largely from vegetable sources with the odd, lean and usually small animal as a treat. Of course, they also have no stress, pollution and electro-magnetic radiation to worry about. Seven per cent of their population is over 65 years of age. They have worn but not bad teeth, whilst in some parts of Europe a third of the population has no teeth at all. They eat little or no animal fat and never dairy from cows. And they have no breast cancer.

Breastfeeding is the norm and continues until the child is four to five years old. In the West some mothers do not breastfeed their children at all, whilst many rarely exceed six months.

In August 2002 Cancer Research UK published the definitive study on breastfeeding and breast cancer.

It concluded that **the more time a women spends breastfeeding in her life, the less her own risk of breast cancer.**

Scientists have also shown that **the fewer menstrual cycles a woman goes through in her life, the lower her chance of breast cancer.**

Scientists have long been concerned in the West about the lengthening years of fertility in women, a fact that has its roots in our diets. One hundred and fifty or more years ago, a woman was likely to have been fertile from the age of 16 to her late thirties. Without contraception she may have had four children, and these she would have breastfed for nine months or more. The current New York female may have menstrual cycles lasting from her twelfth to her fiftieth birthday, and have two or less children en route. This increases her total number of periods from around 200 to as many as 440. And that's a lot more monthly oestrogen surges and resultant hormone fluctuation. Scientists believe this is also reflected in, for example, increasing incidence of endometriosis and polycystic ovary syndrome.

The Collaborative Group on Hormonal Factors in Breast Cancer, supported by Cancer Research UK, published findings in the *Lancet* in late July 2002 on '*Breast Cancer and Breast feeding*'.

Having reviewed over 50,000 women with breast cancer and 97,000 without, in 47 studies across 30 countries they concluded that the relative risk of breast cancer decreased by 7 per cent for each birth, plus 4.3 per cent for every 12 months of breast-feeding.

These figures seem to apply whether one is studying a developed or a developing country.

In the report the main reason given for these findings confirmed that, 'the more periods a woman has, the greater her overall oestrogen production during her lifetime. Oestrogen is known to have a negative effect on the breast tissue causing it to become dense. And dense breast tissue is risky breast tissue.'

The report finished by stating that there were about 470,000 women in developed countries with breast cancer, and if women had 2.5 children on average and breastfed each for 12 months longer than they currently do, about 11 per cent (50,000) breast cancers would be prevented annually *(Valerie Beal, Cancer Research UK, Epidemiology Unit).*

Worse, **modern women add to their levels of oestrogen by taking the pill or HRT.** Again Cancer Research UK published data that showed women who take the pill increase their chances of breast cancer by 26 per cent. If they take it into their thirties this extra risk rises to 58 per cent. For the 10 per cent of women who take it into their 40s, the figure increases to 144 per cent.

It is worth noting that the original FDA approval for the pill was granted following a single trial on 132 Puerto Rican women, despite five of them dying during the trial *(Science 259, 1993 Marshall).* This resulted in a newer, safer pill in the 70s with a lower dose of oestrogen. However, to this day, there is no single long-term trial showing the pill to be safe.

HRT is a similar though weaker oestrogen-based pill. The late doctor John Lee, who spent more than twenty years looking into oestrogen and its effects on the body, was clear that 'too much oestrogen relative to natural progesterone levels' is the essence of the problems facing women at menopause. He showed that oestrogen at menopause merely fell from 100 per cent to around 65 – 70 per cent, or just enough to switch off egg production. Whereas the real 'faller' was natural progesterone which fell from 100 per cent to less than 3 per cent. Arguably with the increases in blood oestrogen being shown by Cancer Research UK, the last thing a post menopausal woman needs is more oestrogen. Yet women are routinely told they need more oestrogen, and HRT is prescribed to 'alleviate menopausal symptoms'!

In 2002, a seven-year HRT trial, part of the US Women's Health Initiative study, was stopped when the dangers started to emerge. The part of the trial involving a mixed synthetic oestrogen and progesten pill had resulted in a doubling of breast cancer risk.

The part of the trial using an oestrogen-only pill was allowed to continue, but 2.2 million women in the UK may have read that their risk of breast cancer rises by at least 27 per cent solely by taking oestrogen-based HRT.

Other cancers that also might develop were not recorded in this report but The Boston Nurses Study report in 1995 warned of the same risk – 27 per cent increase for breast cancer – but went on to conclude that there was significant risk of other cancers like ovarian too, depending upon length of usage.

The UK Million Women study in 2003 confirmed the increased breast cancer risks, and the German Health minister even went on to say that HRT was 'the new thalidomide'!

Part of the problem is not just the added oestrogen to the body, but the use of synthetic hormone. All synthetic products will have side-effects to some degree, even vitamin pills. And of particular concern is synthetic progesten, often confused by the Medical Profession with natural progesterone. Synthetic progesten has a number of research studies pointing the finger of danger in its direction, whereas natural progesterone actually reduces cancer risks.

If HRT were a herbal supplement, it would have been banned within a week. Interestingly, even the pharmaceutical companies list over 100 potential problems associated with HRT. The one thing they don't tell you is that oestrogen supplementation can be addictive. The *British Medical Bulletin (1992: 48)* talks about problems for women wishing to stop HRT after long-term treatment!

Oestrogen and male cancers

Several studies have linked **Testicular cancer** to xeno-estrogens. For example, in December 2002, Swedish researchers showed that three-quarters of perfumed toiletry products tested contained oestrogen mimics and once in the body, levels of DEHP increased. Perfumes, perfumed body sprays, hairsprays and hair products were the main culprits. Research with pregnant women showed that DEHP affected at least 11 per cent of the male offspring, causing reproductive health problems including undescended testicles, smaller organ size and even to increased levels of testicular cancer.

When discussing **Prostate cancer**, patients are routinely told that the 'cause' is 'high testosterone' alone. This is tosh. If high testosterone caused prostate cancer, the world would be full of

16-year-old male patients.

As men age their testosterone level declines but their oestrogen level increases and it is a combination of the two hormones that lies behind most prostate cancers.

Research has shown that oestradiol can cause enlargement of the prostate gland, while anti-oestrogens, for example, Finistride and ICI, can reduce it. Oestradiol can also convert nice safe testosterone to nasty aggressive DHT, which actually sets off the cancer chain reaction *(Thompson, Texas Cancer Center)*. Research from Singapore National Cancer Centre, the Concord Cancer Institute, Sydney and the Monash Cancer Centre in Australia has confirmed that this 'oestrogen plus testosterone' combination is the usual methodology. So what is the real cause, do you think? Testosterone, or the hormone that activates it by turning it to DHT?

Of course, flooding your body with oestrogen via pills and injections may temporarily stop testosterone production altogether, and thus one of the two precursors of DHT will be removed. But how long is it before the body fights back? The healthy body is in a state of homeostasis – its hormones are balanced. Throw this out, cut one to nothing, and your body will try to correct by doing everything in its power to replace the missing testosterone. Taking oestrogen supplements is no long-term solution. And sadly doctors and patients alike know this now. (See Chapter 10, Professor Ben Pfeifer)

Oestrogen and other cancers

Birmingham University has shown that colorectal cancer is associated with localised oestrogen. Cervical cancers, ovarian cancers and endometrial/womb cancers are too. (In fact, there is a link between Tamoxifen and increased risk of womb cancer). Stomach cancer has been shown to be linked to oestrogenic activity on stem cells by British Columbia University as has brain cancer and gliomas *(MD Anderson)*.

So how could diet help?

The female sex hormone, oestrone, is produced by the ovaries through the C-2 pathway. As we age, men and women produce a different version - the aggressive oestradiol - through the C-16 pathway by aromatase enzymes from their fat stores. Oestrogen-positive breast cancer patients are often given Aromatase Inhibitors to block this pathway.

But you can take your own action to control your oestrogen levels by diet:

* Eating high fat and protein diets increases oestrogen levels.
* Eating excess calories and high sugar content increase oestrogen levels.
* Being overweight increases oestrogen levels
* Localised electrical fields (EMFs) can increase oestrogen levels
* Poor sleeping patterns can increase oestrogen levels

BUT

* Eating certain foods can reduce aggressive oestrogen levels coverting it to less aggressive forms
* Eating certain foods can block the action of some oestrogens even changing the receptor sites
* Having a healthy intestinal 'bacterial' flora can eliminate oestrogens, even synthetic ones, with the help of certain fibrous foods
* Sleeping better and eating certain natural compounds can reduce oestrogen levels

The diet factor

Our diets and the way we live and eat cause excesses of oestrogen. For example:

1. High calories, high oestrogen

A high fat, high sugar and high refined carbohydrate diet provides high calories, and the sugars will flood the blood stream. Worse, we no longer 'graze', we eat one or two big meals a day, concentrating the period of the sugar rush. High sugar rushes cause high insulin levels, as the body has to cope with high blood sugar levels and stop it getting to the brain and causing damage. Insulin surges completely throw out the balance between all the hormones in the body and one in particular also surges – oestrogen. High sugar levels are also linked to cancer promotion. High fat intake also heightens steroid levels, which increase oestrogen levels too.

- A five to ten per cent reduction in daily calorie intake reduces oestrogen levels by 20 per cent.
- Practice portion control.
- Graze – eat six small meals per day.
- Eat slowly.
- Eat whole foods – like whole grains, brown rice, fresh vegetables, greens, nuts and seeds.

2. Being overweight

Right at the start of the book I warned that being more than 7 kilograms overweight can seriously reduce your life expectancy, being linked to increased risk of heart disease and cancer.

One reason for this is that fat is an excellent solvent and will dissolve and store, all manner of toxins and hormones (like oestrogen) your body would rather have excreted. Another reason is that your own fat stores are the raw materials for oestrogen production.

North Carolina University have research that shows reducing your weight does reduce your risk of cancer, and increases your survival time if you have it already. So what are you waiting for?

3. Phytoestrogens

Human oestrogen control

In 1900 we derived 30 per cent of our protein in England from pulses – 100 years on it is just 2 per cent.

Pulses protected us, along with our large consumption of fruit and vegetables. They produced large amounts of phytoestrogens in our blood streams. These substances are much weaker than human oestrogens, competed with it and helped control its levels and effects.

For example, research shows in women with high genistein levels (a phytoestrogen), menstrual cycles are elongated, more regular and reduced in number. This is a good thing. Women in the Far East have blood genistein levels up to one thousand times those of New York women. But we could have these protective levels too. Just remember the foods that have protected us in the UK for centuries: Pulses, broad beans, peas, lentils, chickpeas, plus vegetables like parsnips, turnips, carrots, red peppers, tomatoes and 'greens' like cabbage, Brussels sprouts and broccoli, and herbs. All increase your phytoestrogen levels.

You can think of phytoestrogens as much, much weaker cousins of oestradiol, and decide which one you would rather have sitting on your cellular oestrogen receptor sites. Or like some experts you can think of phytoestrogens as 'anti-oestrogens'. Professor Trevor Powles, former head of the breast cancer unit at the Royal Marsden Hospital and a patron of **CANCERactive,** calls them anti-oestrogens too and is quite clear on their benefits. At the Royal Marsden they are researching the benefits of red clover (high in genistein) with cancer patients. Red clover, the herb of Hippocrates, gives even richer levels of certain phytoestrogens and Professor Powles is confident that they will find a level of usage that is successful with cancers.

Another anti-oestrogenic constituent of vegetables, lignan, is found in high concentrations in the urine of Eastern populations who eat high vegetable diets, especially unrefined grains, seeds, pulses and legumes. The same populations excrete high levels of isoflavenoids (particularly genistein and daidzein). And there is a strong correlation between this and decreased breast cancer rates.

A typical current Western diet of high calories, high saturated fat and high protein, by contrast, has a double negative: Not only does it elevate the sex hormone oestrogen levels, it decreases the 'Sex Hormone Binding Globulin', which would have helped remove them from the body. A diet high in isoflavenoids, flavenoids, lignans and other such phytoestrogens has three research-proven benefits:

- It redresses this imbalance.
- It been clearly shown to block receptor sites on the cell for the mammalian sex hormone oestradiol.
- It can reduce the cancer growth-inducing protein tyrosine

kinase in the cells.

Downgrading dangerous oestradiol

Another important benefit of natural compounds in foods is that they can also 'downgrade' aggressive oestradiol to its safer sisters:

- **Resveratrol** from grapes, **quercitin** from onions, **prunetin** from plums and cherries and **indole-3-carbinol,** from broccoli and cabbages, are all natural substances shown in research to alter the way oestrogen is metabolised in the body, changing it (downgrading it) from the form, oestradiol, that promotes cancer cell formation to its much safer sister-product, oestrone.
- Flaxseeds, when used as a concentrate, have been shown in research to stop the growth of breast cancer, even reducing the size of breast tumours in rats by 50 per cent.

All of these will be covered in more detail in Chapter 24. I will give just one example of the power of natural compounds here.

Indole-3-carbinol (I3C) is emerging as a very important natural compound in the 'treatment' of oestrogen-driven cancers. It has been dubbed 'The safer, natural Tamoxifen'. According to scientists at Leicester University, I3C also seems to alter some of the receptor sites thus preventing the action of oestradiol. It was shown by UCLA to inhibit the growth of oestrogen-positive breast cancer cells by 90 per cent (Tamoxifen scores 60) and also to detoxify the by-products of oestradiol break down (Tamoxifen has no action).

Moreover, the Strang Cancer Research Institute has shown I3C can even breakdown the by-products produced from chemical oestrogens, mimics or xenoestrogens.

I3C affects enzymes involved in the cancer process, and has been shown to stop the growth of cancer cells and also kill them. Not surprisingly, pharmaceutical companies are trying to patent synthetic versions of this natural compound.

Soya is nowadays perhaps one of the most talked about contributors of phytoestrogens in the West, but I would rather you focussed on the 500 other natural vegetables and fruits that have protected us in the Western world for the last 20,000 years – foods we just don't eat in the volumes we used to.

A lot of confusion exists when it comes to soya. Most usually this confusion is caused by a squabble between advocates and adversaries of dairy and soya, frankly, some of whom are paid by the respective industries.

Readers will undoubtedly want to know the truth about soya – my view is that we have plenty of European phytoestrogen-rich foods to eat without becoming hung up on one from the Far East. There are active ingredients in soya that are also found in broad beans and peas, so eat your local, fresh alternatives.

In July 2002, Cancer Research UK published research findings on the clear benefits of soya. A study involving two new pieces of research between Cancer Research UK, The National University of Singapore and the US National Cancer Institute found that a diet rich in soya products could affect the make-up of breast tissue, potentially reducing breast cancer.

Women in the Far East who consume the most soya are 60 per cent less likely to have dense breast tissue. And dense tissue is clearly associated with an increased risk of breast cancer. The study's co-author, Dr Stephen Duffy of Cancer Research UK's Mathematics, Statistics and Epidemiology Department in London says: *"There has always been a question mark over a connection between soya and breast cancer. Some studies have suggested a link but others haven't. This research shows for the first time how the amount of soya a woman eats may have an effect on breast tissue and in turn may potentially reduce her risk of breast cancer."*

In Asian women, menopausal symptoms are almost unheard of, and they have half the levels of oestradiol and oestrone circulating in their bodies. The phytoestrogens in soya have been closely linked to lowering circulating oestradiol levels *(Lee-Jane Lu)* and men get less prostate and women less breast and endometrial cancers. Phytoestrogens from soya and other vegetables have been shown to be especially protective in prostate cancer *(Lancet 1993: 342)*.

But please don't merely swap your large daily intake of dairy for an equivalent of soya. Soya is a new product in the Western world. Soya milk has been with us barely 60 years in the UK. I am not surprised we are seeing more allergies in the young, especially when GM soya is commonplace.

There is one caveat in all this – Asian women take more natural exercise. And as I said earlier, the latest research suggests regular daily exercise lowers oestrogen levels too.

Other 'foods' have strong anti-oestrogen benefits: flaxseed, medicinal mushrooms and resveratrol for starters!

4. *Chemicals, pesticides and oestrogens*

Many pesticides and herbicides have ingredients which, once inside our bodies, can act as oestrogen mimics. Whether we eat them directly due to their residues in our foods, or we eat the animals that ate them, hardly matters. DDT, DDE, dieldrin, lindane, methoxychlor, benzene hexachloride, kepone and more than fifty others are widely used in the world's food production and all have the ability to mimic oestrogen in the body.

The animal fat we consume from meat and dairy brings with it both oestrogens from the animals themselves plus these oestrogen mimics from the toxins in the fields. And fat makes steroids makes oestrogen.

The mimics enter the body and 'lock on' to cellular receptor sites interfering with a host of biochemical processes and making them hard to excrete. Such action has been associated with everything from brain deficiencies to reduced sperm counts, even cellular DNA interference (*Lancet 1993)* and folic acid depletion *(Moscow Cancer Institute).*

Dioxins are toxic chemicals so dangerous their safe levels are measured in trillionths of a gram. They activate cancer genes and suppress tumour-supressor genes. In the USA the worst sources of dioxins are found in river fish, beef and dairy. A longer list extending to all farmed meats for approximately 85 per cent of dioxin 'consumption'.

But again, hope is at hand in the form of natural compounds from foods: For example, UCLA, Berkeley, has shown that indole-3-carbinol can also affect non-oestrogen but cancer-promoting receptor sites on cells, preventing the growth of breast cancer. These sites (Ah receptors) are particular 'attacked' by chemical toxins, like dioxins. Dioxins stimulate cancer by promoting IGF-1, oestrogen and insulin levels. And I3C blocks the receptor site that dioxins attack.

Researchers at Texas University treated breast cancer cells with dioxins and I3C simultaneously and found I3C reduced the negative effects by 90 per cent. Several other studies have shown that I3C can have the effect of reducing chemically promoted breast and prostate cancers by 70 to 96 per cent.

Researchers at Tufts have shown that curcumin (turmeric) can enhance the action of phytoestrogens to inhibit aggressive human and synthetic oestrogens.

So, can you eat-to-beat chemical oestrogen mimics?

There is considerable help at hand from natural compounds. As shown above, indole-3-carbinol and curcumin and plant isoflavones can be extremely helpful, and you may remember from Chapter 15 that beneficial bacteria can break up even synthetic oestrogenic compounds.

5. *Water and oestrogen*

One of the biggest sources of unwanted oestrogen for men and women is tap water in large cities where the water is recycled.

With millions of women on the pill and HRT relieving themselves into a city's waste water, and then little attention paid to filtration of the hormone, recycled tap water has become more than a little risky. Links to male genital problems have been made in several scientific studies (for example, *Athlone Institute, Ireland*).

We have covered water in depth in Chapter 12. To summarise the key points that affect your oestrogen levels: The best solution is to drink glass-bottled mineral water. An alternative is reverse osmosis filtered water with an added re-mineraliser chamber.

6. *Oestrogen in the home*

It is worth noting here that oestrogen mimics surround us. The average American woman has a toxin level in her bloodstream four times that of her male equivalent!

Chemicals in perfumed products, BPA and phthalates in some plastics, parabens, a common preservative, can all be oestrogen mimics.

Cosmetics, from face creams to lipsticks, can all contain oestrogen mimics. Of course, you assume the skin prevents them getting into the blood stream – far from it. Skin is a carrier, not a barrier. The insides of your mouth, underneath your nails, your scalp and your armpits are all good absorption areas. All this makes toxins in hair dyes, nail polishes, toothpastes and deodorants easily absorbed. Worse, chemicals like sodium lauryl sulphate in soaps, bubble bath, shower gels, shampoos etc can increase the permeability of the skin by up to 40 per cent. This just allows more toxins to pass into the bloodstream.

In a German study, endometriosis was linked to chemicals called PCBs and cases of vaginal and cervical cancers have been linked to nonylphenols, which are oestrogen mimics often used in spermicides and contraceptive jellies.

Clearly men are not immune from this – they wash their faces with perfumed soap, use perfumed shaving foam and aftershave or perfumed sprays and deodorants every day.

But it doesn't end there. Your home is a toxic centre – especially if you like cleaning! Bleaches, household cleaners, nice smelling sprays, polishes add to the contamination. Volatile organic carbons may be ingested on dust particles and may come from glues holding carpet or ceiling tiles and even from petrol fumes while filling the car; or from inks in fax machines or computer circuitry if your office is not properly ventilated.

No wonder that women who stay at home have 40 per cent more toxins in their bloodstreams than their sisters who go out to work! It makes Dr Soto's finding that these oestrogen mimics can be cumulative very worrying.

It's very easy to see how we increase our 'oestrogen pool levels'. Unfortunately many governments and leading cancer charities have vested interests and do not condemn these products, so levels of blood oestrogens will just go on rising.

Build your own clean micro-environment – men and women should ensure that they find a reputable provider of toxin-free products for their cosmetic, toiletry, cleaning and bathroom needs. (In our travels we have found one company that seems to do all of this; the only company recommended in the USA by the Cancer Prevention Coalition – Neways, which is now Modere.)

7. *Oestrogen and sleep*

As we observed in Chapter 18, disturbed sleep patterns are associated with increased cancer rates. Night-shift workers, nurses, long-haul airline hostesses, people who sleep in artificially lit rooms – all have higher rates of cancer.

Disturbed sleep reduces melatonin levels in the body, and melatonin has a controlling influence over both IGF-1 and oestrogen levels, as well as having five epigenetic actions against 'mutations' around the genome.

Melatonin levels also decline as we age.

And melatonin levels are depleted by EMFs.

I know of two breast cancer professors in the UK who take melatonin nightly, bringing their own personal supplies in from the USA (which you are allowed to do).

But you can 'eat-to-increase' your melatonin as well! Eating dark chocolate an hour before bed will increase serotonin levels – serotonin is the precursor to melatonin. Green leaves, bananas, peanuts, dates and other protein foods like turkey and fish contain the essential amino acid tryptophan and this increases serotonin levels. Eating magnesium-rich foods and taking a supplement of B vitamins will help production too.

8. *Beneficial Bacteria*

In Chapter 15 I told you about one of the biggest discoveries of this millennium: The crucial and multi-faceted role of beneficial bacteria and the microbiome – not just as directors of our immune systems, but as our own 'foot soldiers' in the removal of toxic products from our bodies. A combination of beneficial bacteria works with certain natural compounds like lignans to break down oestrogenic products in the intestines, binding the resultant molecules to food residues and passing them down the intestine for excretion. The research findings that localised oestrogen is a factor in stomach, colon, and rectal cancers makes the destruction of these good bacteria by antibiotics, chemotherapy drugs, steroids and other chemicals used to 'fight' cancer particularly disturbing.

You should consider taking a daily probiotic containing *L. acidophilus*, *L. rhamnosus* and *bifidobacterium*. You don't need 60 strains and 250 zillion in an expensive pill. If you eat a Rainbow Diet of Prebiotics – whole foods and raw vegetables you will turn 8 billion from your pill into 8 trillion in a few days. It's pectins (apples, carrots) for Lactobacillus and oligopolysaccharides and inulins (chicory, onions) for Bifidobacteria.

While these strains 'hold' any problems, it is important to then add back in a greater diversity for the long-term, especially as you age – sauerkraut, raw milk/cheese, tempeh, sourdough bread, Kombucha and Kefir are helpful. Feed them whole foods and fibre.

9. *Natural Progesterone*

Foods like wild yam are known to limit oestrogen levels. One reason is that wild yam contains natural compounds that are the precursors of natural progesterone. And natural progesterone is a 'balancing hormone' for oestrogen.

It is important to understand that in research **natural** progesterone consistently comes through as a protective, life extending factor.

Synthetic progesterone – more correctly named progestin or progesten, is quite another thing – as the HRT studies have shown. Synthetic progesten has some uses in cancer treatment, but fundamentally the various HRT studies show it to be a dangerous and cancer risk-increasing chemical.

Unfortunately studies into natural progesterone lag way behind the interest levels in oestrogen.

Natural progesterone is not merely a 'balancer' to oestrogen, it is highly protective. For example, Guys Hospital conducted several studies in the mid-1990's concluding that pre-menopausal women who had breast cancer operations during the second part of their cycle, when progesterone is highest, had twice the ten year survival rates of those who had the operation in the first two weeks of their cycle, when oestrogen dominates.

You may want to consider eating more natural wild yam as

you age! Please beware of a number of 'Natural Progesterone' products; since they have been prepared and treated, it is hard to understand how they are 'natural' anymore.

Summary

If doctors are going to give you anti-oestrogen drugs to 'prevent' a breast cancer returning, or a prostate from growing in size, then why not adopt an anti-oestrogen diet too?
The checklist includes:

- Be the right weight for your height.
- Cut your daily calorie consumption.
- Snack and graze – eat 6 small meals per day.
- Cut out sugar consumption.
- Cut saturated fats and trans fats – eat far more plants.
- Eat more phytoestrogens, like pulses, vegetables, greens, yams.
- Eat more 'medicinal' mushrooms.
- Add resveratrol, quercitin, curcumin, flaxseed and indole-3-carbinol into your diet
- Only eat whole foods.
- Eat organic foods.
- Avoid toxic chemicals in the home.
- Drink clean water.
- Take asphalia or melatonin supplements.
- Supplement with multi-strain probiotics daily.
- Exercise daily.

CHAPTER 20
EAT-TO-BEAT INFLAMMATION?

In 2000, the Mayo Clinic published results which showed that small daily amounts of aspirin would reduce the risk of prostate cancer by 40 per cent.

In February 2003 US scientists published a report in the medical journal, *Gastroenterology*, suggesting that aspirin cut risks of cancer of the gullet by 50 per cent.

In April 2003 there was a US desk study confirming daily aspirin prevents breast cancer.

In 2004 the Daily Mail ran the front page headline, *'Aspirin cuts Breast Cancer risk'*. Cancer Research UK were making news with research that showed 'an aspirin a day can slash the risk of developing breast cancer by almost a third'. By 2011 it was researchers at the Radcliffe and Oxford University who were saying that 75 mgs of aspirin a day reduced the chances of developing cancer by about a quarter, cut the chances of it spreading (metastases) by more than half, and increased survival chances by a third.

Aspirin was originally the active natural ingredient found in willow bark and you can still find supplies of willow bark if you search the Internet.

One sad truth about research on natural compounds and/or complementary therapies is that it just doesn't receive anything like the exposure afforded to drug research by the PR machines of pharmaceutical companies, the medical authorities or even governmental and charity links. As a result, expert scientists seem to be repeating the same fundamental pieces of research the world over, and the average oncologist and his hospital medical team knows little or nothing about any of it.

Meanwhile, Herceptin was front page news for months on end – another new study, this time with younger women; or a finding with a different cancer. Woe betide any health authority like NICE that dared to say the drug costs too much and they would rather spend their limited funds elsewhere. Dying patients who were 'denied' Herceptin were dragged onto yet more front pages to protest their need for this 'life-saving drug'.

Not so with natural compounds which cannot be patented and so can never be the source of large pharmaceutical profit and the funding of PR companies, advertising agencies and lobbyists.

Scientists the world over have proved and then confirmed several times over that certain foods reduce inflammation, and with it the risk of cancer. Unfortunately, all too often this research is then promptly forgotten! Let me give you an example:

Back in 2002, as I was writing an article on prostate cancer, I rang a UK charity for a view on the Mayo clinic's findings. The nurses on the 'helpline' had no knowledge of these findings saying that they did not like to recommend aspirin, and anyway the results were new and unconfirmed.

New??!! Unconfirmed??!!

Thirty years ago, in 1982, John Vane won a Nobel Prize and a knighthood for his work on **eicosanoids**. He was particularly interested in one group of eicosanoids called prostaglandins, which in excess can cause inflammation and concluded, even then, that their levels and effects were reduced by aspirin.

Many experts, doctors included, believe hormones are made solely in the endocrine glands. In fact the largest volume of hormones in the body are the eicosanoids, very short-lived hormones lasting less than a couple of seconds at the most, and produced by the nuclear envelope of every cell in your body.

There are over a hundred and thirty known eicosanoids, each producing different responses; some helpful, some negative. Importantly, some eicosanoids, like prostoglandins, are helpful in small quantities but in excess cause significant problems around cells and in surrounding tissues, resulting in inflammation. Inflammation is a known precursor to many cancers and eicosanoids are particularly implicated in this process.

Inflammation is more traditionally associated with conditions such as arthritis, spawning the creation of drugs like Vioxx (now banned, after a death toll estimated at 47,000 people).

These eicosanoids are the final and localised step in the communication process from your brain all the way to your cells. The messaging may be via any chemical – a hormone, a protein and even an electrical chemical. But put simplistically: Stressed brain, stressed breast cell. Happy brain, happy prostate cells.

Of course, the chemical that stimulates the local eicosanoid doesn't have to arrive under direction from your brain. A stressed breast cell could be the result of a number of other more 'random' chemicals too.

Inflammation and stressed cells

How are eicosanoids made? Basically all the fats and oils you eat, whether they are animal fats, fish oils, nut oils or fast food cooking oils are just a part of your body's oil pool, which we will call the 'fatty acid pool'. This pool provides the raw ingredients for the synthesis of all eicosanoids, 'good' or 'bad'. However, the production of bad eicosanoids requires an enzyme to cause the chemical chain reaction. This enzyme, called COX-2, is known, for example, to be stimulated by alcohol and fats in the intestine causing a carcinogenic bile acid, lithocholic acid, to be produced along with inflammation and the formation of polyps, and leading to colon cancer.

The COX-2 chemical pathway has also been shown to be stimulated by chemicals, notably steroids, cortisol and insulin. Science tells us that certain drugs, like **steroids**, commonly given to cancer patients when they are first diagnosed, can actually cause more inflammation at the cellular level. Large meals, high carbohydrate meals, excess sugar or sudden bursts of sweetened soft drinks or fruit juices will all cause **insulin** surges which stimulate the enzyme and turn the environment of your cells negative, significantly increasing the risk of cancer and other illnesses. And **cortisol,** the stress hormone produced under direction from your brain by the adrenal glands, will also stimulate the enzymatic pathway producing more bad eicosanoids and inflammation. Worse, Professor Tian Xu of Yale has shown that two genes are then blocked causing cancer.

Stress increases levels of the hormone norepinephrine which was also shown to increase levels of cancer cells and the inflammatory agents interleukin-6 and endothelial growth factor.

Conversely sulphoraphanes (see Chapter 24) actively reduced the hormone and its effects.

Diet – the good news

As various research studies have found, there are elements of your diet that can be highly protective. For example:

- The active ingredient of **aspirin** has been found in a number of studies to switch off COX-2, stopping it making 'bad' eicosanoids. However, there may be a small problem with aspirin. It doesn't seem to reduce inflammation in every case, just most cases. Andrew Chan of the Harvard Medical School *(J. Nat Cancer Inst 2006. 98; 1494)* believes that aspirin can play an important role in helping fight all cancers, but that the effectiveness may depend upon your genetics.
- This same anti-inflammatory action is also found in aloe vera which contains several anti-inflammatory ingredients. Almonds have a similar and natural analgesic effect.
- Long-chain **Omega-3** (found in fish oils) has also been shown to turn off COX-2 in a number of research studies from around the world.
- **Ginger**, **galangal** and **garlic** also contain ingredients that turn off the enzyme.
- **Vitamin D** has been found to detoxify lithocholic acid *(Howard Hayes Medical Unit, May 2002)* and recent research has shown yet more natural compounds capable of reducing inflammation, notably the **phenols** in **resveratrol**, **olive oil** and **green tea**.
- Finally, the most studied natural compound on the planet, **curcumin**, is known to possess a strong anti-inflammatory benefit. For example, it is now being used in several US medical schools with colorectal cancer.

Eat-to-beat-inflammation

Many cancers go through an inflammatory stage first before becoming full blown cancer. And I have told you that steroids and insulin, cortisol and eating meat and animal fats all increase levels of cellular inflammation.

This chapter started with breast cancer, but many cancers are equally relevant. The most well known inflammatory-driven cancer is colon cancer, where inflammation produces polyps. When colorectal cancer runs in families, regular monitoring to look for the development of pre-cancer polyps is 'officially' the standard practice in the UK. In the clinical trials conducted by Leeds University in 2010 concentrated fish oils reduced polyps and prevented colorectal cancer forming or returning.

As for the 2011 Oxford research on aspirin, the researchers went on to say that there findings were 'so strong' they urged NICE to approve aspirin as part of the UK's cancer treatment programme. If you do take daily aspirin, remember we are talking about only a small tablet, which should always be consumed with food and never if there are sensitivity issues in the stomach or if also taking blood clotting or blood-thinning drugs.

Clearly you may also choose to take turmeric (curcumin) supplements, or resveratol (red grapes) go in the sunshine and increase your intake of green tea and extra virgin olive oil.

You may consider drinking aloe vera which contains six or so anti-inflammatory compounds. Drinking aloe vera has mixed reports. In America some oncologists actively recommend, while others are against. The aloins and anthraquinones may cause some feelings of nausea in a few people (aloe was traditionally used as a laxative). Work by Dr. Bruce Eric Hedendal concluded that drinking aloe promoted a more favourable balance of gastrointestinal bacteria and decreased yeast populations. In his and a great many studies aloe seems to relieve indigestion, irritable bowel syndrome and colitis and promotes improved protein digestion, tryptophan conversion and more. While many have concluded that colon cancer prevention may be increased, I have seen only anecdotal conclusions on its curative effects. There have been two reports that chemicals found in aloe latex may cause cancer. In America Dr. Richard Shulze treats colon cancer patients with a number of herbs including aloe vera.

Some people ask about flaxseed, which has many benefits such as helping to increase blood oxygenation and regulating human oestrogen. However, it is not a substitute for fish oil omega-3; its omega-3 is short chain and only a little (about 13 per cent) converts to long-chain. Fish oils should be the daily focus. 2011 research showed that over the medium to long term they provide higher tissue levels of beneficial omega-3 than eating oily fish.

So eat-to-beat-inflammation? Easy. Fish oils, garlic, ginger, aloe vera, almonds, olive oil, curcumin and green tea head the list of anti-inflammatory foods and herbs. Even a glass of red wine has some inflammation-fighting abilities! It seems to increase plasma levels of omega-3. Then there is good old fashioned chicken soup - boil the bones for four to five hours to release the analgesics - and even 'older' Frankincense.

Finally, a word of warning: Research shows clearly that a diet rich in cows' dairy can produce an excess of inflammatory gut bacteria within just 12 hours.

CHAPTER 21
EAT-TO-BEAT INSULIN?

As we have seen, excess insulin can directly stimulate COX-2 and therefore bad eicosanoid production; and levels of insulin in the body have an indirect effect on levels of cancer – stimulating hormones like oestrogen and Insulin-like Growth Hormone (IGF-1) through the system of hormone balances called homeostatis. Thus insulin is also known to stimulate cell division and the prolonged exposure of cells to increased levels of insulin activates certain genes and changes their genetic behaviour.

Elevated blood insulin levels have been linked with increased risk of colorectal, pancreatic, liver, endometrial and breast cancers so far. Time will probably add to this list.

Then there is the fact that cancer cells have large numbers of insulin receptor sites on their surface, more than normal healthy cells. Cancer cells need lots of glucose and they need all the help they can get and the receptors help drive the glucose into the cells. Research from Harvard comparing two matched samples of mice infected with cancer – one that had normal glucose metabolism, the other had the glucose metabolism blocked – showed that the group metabolising glucose all died, whereas 80 per cent of the blocked-glucose group survived the test period. Cancer cells 'love' glucose.

So, insulin is totally implicated in cancer, as is glucose.

Diabetes

Diabetics have been shown to have an increased risk of cancer. For example in colorectal cancers that increased risk is threefold.

As I explained earlier, poor eating habits produce high levels of glucose in the blood. This in turn stimulates the hormone insulin to be produced. If you become diabetic, the problems do not stop. You may require insulin supplementation but the use of synthetic insulin is uneven during the day, with unused excesses at times.

The medical profession now understands the links between insulin and diabetes. They do not yet understand the relationship to cancer although the research exists.

So, an understanding of diabetes and factors that cause high insulin production is necessary both to help plan a healthy diet and to avoid cancer.

The source of insulin is the pancreas. Indeed, the pancreas makes two hormones: **Insulin**, which takes excess sugar out of the bloodstream before it can reach and damage the brain, and stores it in the liver, muscles or fat cells, and **Glucagon**, which responds to low blood sugar levels by causing stored glucose to be released. A healthy liver is important to this two-way process.

There are two common types of diabetes (although experts now suggest there are as many as eight different 'types' in all). Type 1 diabetes, which can be hereditary but can also occur after viral infection, sees permanent damage to the insulin producing cells in the pancreas and artificial insulin must be given to sufferers or they will go into a sugar-induced coma.

Type 2, or late-onset diabetes, seems to occur typically when people are in their fifties and is usually the result of poor eating habits. However, it is not so 'late-onset' these days with more and more adolescents and children succumbing to it.

For example, Mississippi is the worst region in the USA for late onset diabetes. In 2002 the levels had increased to 8 per cent of all adults. The health authorities blamed the high level of fried food and sweetened orange juice in the diet. Whilst in 1982 about 4 per cent of children (under 12s) in that region had diabetes, by 1994 the figure had risen to 16 per cent!

The UK figures for diabetes are expected to double by 2010 (*British Journal of Community Nursing* 2002: 7). The growth rate of 'late-onset' diabetes in under-fives is currently running at 11 per cent per annum (*BMJ* 1997: 315).

Late-onset diabetes is diet related and had been simplistically linked to calorie intake. However it is increasingly thought to be caused by a complex mixture of a number of factors including high carbohydrate/sugar intake, being overweight, high intake of hydrogenated fats (i.e. trans fatty acids) and, even, milk consumption, as we shall see.

The causes of diabetes – a modern diet

A French scientist, Dr Michel Montignac, developed a theory about the disease in the eighties which, although largely ignored at the time, is now generally believed correct.

Back in the seventies, scientists thought that all overweight people suffered from overproduction of insulin when ingesting carbohydrates, resulting in a storing of the sugars as fat. Montignac felt it was not obesity that was causing the diabetes but simply an overworked, exhausted pancreas.

By 1997 the Harvard School of Public Health had researched a sample of 65,000 women and concluded that those who developed diabetes most commonly ate a diet which was both low in fibre and also high in refined/empty sugars. (*JAMA* 1997: 277). A second study of 40,000 men supported this (*Diabetes Care* 1997: 20).

These findings caused a switch from the theory that a sedentary lifestyle, obesity and stress were causing the problems, pointing the finger of blame firmly at the intake of nutritionally 'empty' sugars and refined carbohydrate; the modern Western diet.

When the Harvard study also found that hydrogenated vegetable oils could bring on diabetes (*American Journal of Clinical Nutrition* 2001: 273) researchers started to understand why the disease was booming in the young. Hydrogenated vegetable oils are commonly used in fast foods and processed foods.

Another surprising contributor was then found to be cow's milk, which anyway contains insulin-like stimulators (IGF1) as we saw in a previous chapter. Finnish research (Diabetes 2000:49) concluded that children had a five-fold increase in diabetes if fed cow's milk during infancy. Mothers, your babies need to eat-to-beat-cancer too; 'breast is best!'

Other causal factors linked to diabetes have been vaccines, beta-blockers and antidepressants such as Prozac.

Interestingly the *Journal of Cardiovascular Risk* carried an article at the start of 2003 linking red wine consumption with protection against diabetes. No further comment from me is necessary!

The pancreas

The pancreas makes insulin and also produces pancreatic enzymes, which are thought by some experts to exert a controlling influence on cancer, by switching cancer stem cells over to normal cells. If the pancreas is stressed by too much glucose in the blood stream causing endless demands for insulin production, it is possible that the pancreatic enzymes production line becomes stressed too.

This theory may well be borne out in reality. Research from the Mayo Clinic *(Gastroenterology 2005)* shows that elderly, late onset diabetes patients have an increased risk of pancreatic cancer.

The ingestion of refined carbohydrates and sugars

Sugar has been 'refined' for over two hundred years in an attempt to prevent it decomposing. It is now 96 per cent sucrose and can create a drug-like dependency in the body. Withdrawal symptoms are common in people who cut sugar from their diets. It also depletes the body of calcium. Corn syrup has similar problems and it depletes the body of B vitamins.

The average individual will consume over 170 lbs of sugar per year (Beasley, *The Betrayal of Health*). Processed and preserved foods are the main culprits as the sugar is hidden.

Our damaging eating habits are worsening. In the UK we start the day with our refined wheat, sugar-laced breakfast cereal (with added salt), and milk; then refined wheat toast and jams. You may even drink processed fruit juice (which is little more than sugared water anyway), and sugar in tea or coffee. In the USA there are refined grain waffles, hash browns and fried, calorie-heavy ham and eggs. The average American breakfast available at drive-ins for less than $7 is a killer. No wonder obesity is running at 26 per cent of US adults and its getting worse!

Snack food is sugar and hydrogenated oil-rich. Consider empty calorie soft drinks, where a fizzy soft drink may contain ten spoonsful of sugar; or chocolate, refined wheat bread, buns, cakes, pasta, ready meals, breakfast cereal, cheesecake and biscuits; or the high street fast food outlets from burger to pizza 'restaurants'.

Natural fibre seems to have been forgotten in all this. Instead we take fibre supplements or enriched bran cereals. BUT. Natural cellular membranes and cellulose plant walls are a barrier which slows down the rate of release of sugar from <u>inside</u> cells. Adding bran fibre to a diet of sugary foods cannot achieve this. It simply cannot stop the release of sugar from sugars!

Whole grains in our diet are also beneficial and protective in other ways. Many natural fibres, apart from aiding our excretion processes and bowel movements, contain compounds that can bind to and regulate fats in the bloodstream. And high-fibre foods are also the feeding blocks for beneficial bacteria in our guts.

Big meals, insulin rushes

It is not just the types of food that we eat that cause surges in insulin – it is the way we eat too.

Modern life means skipping meals and then eating just one or two big meals. Our hunger hormones will not quieten down until about 20 minutes after we start eating. By which time most hungry people will have consumed their whole plate full of calorie-rich, fatty and refined food. This causes great stress on the pancreas.

Glycaemic index

The refining process for grains, rice, processed meals and oils has a lot to answer for. Montignac went on to develop a diet or slimming plan. His basic recommendation was, "eat as much as you like but always foods with a **low glycaemic index (GI)**."

Sugar or glucose is the benchmark with a GI of 100. Refined foods which lack fibre, and over-cooked foods, where the fibre (for example, the natural cellulose walls of vegetables) has broken down, have GIs approaching 100, resulting in a sudden rush of sugar into the bloodstream and an overworked pancreas. Foods like jasmine rice (109) or rice cakes (82) are typical of this.

However, this is why raw vegetables and fruit (with their low GI scores) are so beneficial, as their intact fibre aids a slower and controlled sugar release process. All foods can be assigned a GI but this only measures their 'quality' in terms of sugar release. It needs to be coupled with their 'quantity'. Thus glycaemic load (which is what really troubles the pancreas) is the multiple of the two.

Thus spaghetti (150 gms) when cooked has 48 gms of carbohydrate and a GI of 44. Hence the glycaemic load is 44 x 48 ÷ 100 = 21. So, when looking at the figures below, think also of the amounts you will consume.

Meats and fish have GIs of zero. Fresh, raw vegetables are usually 10 or below unless root crops. Fruits and nuts are usually in the 10–30 spread. Green vegetables around 15, pulses around 30.

Cooking raises the GI load. For example, it takes carrots from

20 to 40 in terms of Glycaemic Load.

GI foods – some examples:

Apple, raw	38	Muesli bar	61
Apple juice	40	Mung beans	39
Apricots, raw	57	Noodles, fresh	40
Apricots, dried	30	Oats	49
Banana, raw	52	Orange	42
Barley, boiled	25	Orange juice	53
Basmati white rice	58	Parsnips	97
Broad beans	79	Peach, fresh	42
Buckwheat, boiled	54	Peach, canned	58
Bulgar, boiled	48	Pear	38
Carrots, boiled	41	Pecans, raw	10
Chickpeas, boiled	28	Oat porridge, whole	55
Cereals, unrefined	40	Potato crisps	54
Cereals, refined	75	Raisins	64
Coco Pops	70	Rice noodles	40
Croissant	67	Ryvita	69
Fish fingers	38	Soya milk	36
Gluten-free muesli	39	Soya beans	14
Ice cream	65	Strawberries	40
Kidney beans	52	Sweetcorn	46
Kiwi fruit, raw	58	Sweet potato	44
Lentils, boiled	30	Wholemeal bread	71
Lychees, canned	79	Yam	37
Milk, fresh	31	Yoghurt, low fat	38
Millet, boiled	71		

It is interesting to note that the Bush people of the Kalahari and of Australia have their staple carbohydrates with GIs of only 10 (e.g. Aboriginals use flour from the wattle seed).

In summary, low GI foods:

- Lead to lower insulin levels and rejuvenate a stressed pancreas.
- Help lower blood fats and cholesterol.
- Reduce risk of diabetes and heart disease.
- Reduce risk of cancer and improve overall health.

Eat-to-beat cancer?

You may wonder why I have suddenly started writing about diabetes. I don't want you to become diabetic, because it will increase your cancer risk. To summarise:

- Diabetes is linked with an increased risk of cancer.
- Poor sugar control leads to high blood sugar levels and causes pancreatic stress, increased insulin production and this leads to diabetes.
- Poor sugar control leads to high blood sugar levels and happy cancer cells.
- Excess insulin takes glucose to cancer cells. If you then become diabetic, the synthetic insulin can do just the same.
- Natural or synthetic insulin in excess can increase levels of oestrogen, bad eicosanoids and cell-promoting IGF-1.
- Type 2 diabetes is indicative of a poor diet – and low nourishment.
- Often type-2 diabetics are overweight, take limited exercise and carry toxins in their fat stores.
- A stressed pancreas may falter in its production of pancreatic enzymes thought by some experts to be crucial in controlling some types of cancer cells.
- Poor dietary foods reduce the excretion of toxins, and the levels of beneficial bacteria.

Can't lose weight – could this be insulin resistance?

There are an increasing number of research studies about the inter-relationship of hormones and illness. Abdominal weight gain can often be a visible indicator of **insulin resistance**, and some estimates put the level of the population affected at 80 per cent. So, you don't have to be in the 8 per cent of the population with diabetes, you may be in a more general 'insulin resistant' category. However, insulin resistance is still a result of poor modern diets and the gut bacteria associated with them.

Calorie Restriction

In Chapter 5, I mentioned calorie restriction – and I will again later.

Limiting calories slows tumour growth and can even stop it. Indeed the various European studies have been confirmed by Harvard *(Nova Science Now Jan 2007)*. They have even produced a video explaining how cutting calorie intake by 30-40 per cent for any organism, can increase longevity by up to 60 per cent.

And the reasons they give are that calorie restriction:

- Reduces insulin levels.
- Reduces metabolic rate and therefore toxin production.
- Increases the body's stress response, increasing survival hormones and strengthening the body's ability to control cell division and repair damaged DNA.

Anything else?

In 2014, researchers at the *University of Toronto* showed a cup of lentils a day lowered the risk of diabetes, heart disease and high blood pressure by modifying blood glucose levels. Apparently, any pulse will do. The French love their lentils!

And researchers at the *Human Nutrition University of Illinois* at *Urbana-Champaign* have found that oregano and rosemary lower blood glucose levels – but they have to be fresh!

Summary

A simple finger prick blood test can show up insulin resistance. And a good nutritionist or naturopath can help you from there. Meanwhile:

- Cut the empty calories, the refined foods, the processed foods and sugar from your diet.
- Graze. Don't eat just one or two big meals.
- Don't rely on 'added fibre'. Eat whole grain, and naturally fibre-rich foods. Eat more fresh and raw vegetables and fruit where the sugar is slowly released as the fibre breaks down.
- Cut bad fats and dairy from your diet.
- Take multi-strained probiotics.
- Eat more slowly. Take 20 minutes from starting to eat before the main course!
- Try and eat fewer calories than you need.
- Don't be overweight.

CHAPTER 22
OXYGENATING YOUR CELLS

Cancer thrives where oxygen is low

As I covered in the first section of this book, take a blood sample from a cancer patient and put it under a microscope. You can usually observe two things: Firstly, the white, immune system cells are 'lifeless' whereas in normal blood they move around. This is a sign that the immune system is impaired. Secondly, the red cells are often clumped together – a sign that both iron and oxygen-carrying levels are low.

Cancer cells use lots of iron and they thrive when oxygen conditions are low.

In 1931, Otto Warburg won a Nobel Prize for this discovery that cancer cells didn't use oxygen.

Since then, German and American scientists have pioneered treatments which aim to get oxygen into cancer cells. Hence the 'alternative' therapies, which use ozone or Hyperbaric Oxygen chambers to try to increase oxygen in the blood system and cells, or high doses of vitamin C, or hydrogen peroxide, or glutathione as cellular pre-oxidants.

Warburg himself concluded that the best way to fight cancer was to deliver oxygen to the cancer cells and to do this you needed highly oxygenated blood in the arteries (as is normally the case) but also highly oxygenated blood in the veins (normally very low in oxygen) to create a 'bottleneck' and a cellular oxygen overload. This is easier said than done. Since veins carry about 70 per cent of the body's blood volume, (arteries carry about 17 per cent, with about 13 per cent inside the organs), you have to somehow get oxygen into vessels that are returning from the organs and tissues immediately they exit the tumour area. The theory of tissue 'oxygen overload' has taxed some of the world's best cancer specialists for the last 70 years.

Certain factors work against cellular oxygen levels. As we have said before, high levels of oestrogen or high sodium levels can both reduce cellular oxygen.

Depression limits blood oxygen; and depressed people develop more cancers.

Certain factors can promote cellular oxygen levels. High potassium, high magnesium and low sodium diets are a start. High vegetable (especially greens) consumption will promote glutathione levels in your body, and this is enhanced by selenium. While pollution is likely to reduce your oxygen levels, fresh air at altitude and exercise will both increase oxygen levels.

Indoors, outdoors

Many people reading this will immediately think of their external environment. Do I live in fresh air near trees and mountains or do I live in pollution, near a main road or factory chimney?

In Chapter 2 I told you that The US Environmental Protection Agency stated in 2006 that indoor air is two to five times more polluted than outdoor air on average, citing 1500 hazardous substances in the average US home. Typically these include airborne pollutants from household cleaning products, and personal care products, second-hand smoke, radon, formaldehyde from pressed wood products, biological agents such as fungi, mites and bacteria and nitrogen oxide from gas appliances. The EPA went on to say that the air in some homes could be 25 to 100 times more polluted than the air outside, and that airborne indoor pollutants from cleaning and personal care products are three times more likely to cause cancer than pollutants outside.

We also use in-house pesticides, from plant sprays to medicated shampoos and mosquito repellants. For example, carbonates have been linked to increased levels of childhood leukaemia *(Insern, France)*; and in-home insecticides containing chlorpyrifos have been affecting testosterone levels *(Epidemiology Jan 2006)*. Not surprisingly, women who stay at home have 40 per cent more toxins in their blood than their identical sisters who go out to work. After all, there are laws governing toxins in the workplace, but at home you are free to pollute your environment as much as you wish. Concerned readers should go to our web site and read an article entitled '*As safe as houses*'.

Never allow anybody to smoke in your home. The biggest

direct hazard to our blood oxygen is smoking, with its carbon monoxide level, which blocks the haemoglobin oxygen-carrying sites. Passive smokers have been shown to be six times more threatened than was originally thought and women are twice as prone to the damaging effects of smoke as negative airway factors have been found to be carried by the X chromosome – women have two X chromosomes, men just one *(Cancer Research UK)*. Children are particularly at risk in homes where a parent smokes.

Polluted air doesn't stop with cigarette smoke. A number of toxins in the air we breathe make us vulnerable to cancer. Motor vehicles emit hazardous toxic chemicals, which collect on dust particles – and we breathe these in. People living near main roads, children living near garage forecourts, both have increased rates of cancer. Sunlight can encourage these polluted dust particles to become even more toxic, making Nice in the South of France on a bad day almost three times worse than London.

These particles collect in the deepest recesses of your lungs and are virtually impossible to clear out. This results in increased levels of toxins in the bloodstream, with further toxins collecting in body fat and organs like the kidneys. Diesel fumes have been noted as the third largest cause of lung cancer in the USA.

Polluted, sunny cities can also have oxygen levels as low as 12 per cent on a bad day compared with the 21 per cent of air normally attributed to oxygen. At seven per cent life ceases. The US Environmental Agency reports that over a hundred million tonnes of various toxic chemicals are released into the atmosphere every year in the USA. *The Nation, September 17 1990* reported that autopsies on one hundred young people in the Los Angeles region showed that all had lungs suffering from toxic air pollution damage.

Increasing your blood oxygen – breathe, eat, exercise

Breathe: Get to the hills! Get outside where there really is clean, fresh bracing air. And walk, briskly if possible; breathe. An important part of Chinese cancer treatment is deep breathing exercise.

The fact is that most of us do not breathe properly. Unless we do something strenuous we tend only to use the top third of our lung capacities, allowing toxic air to sit and stagnate at the bottom of our lungs. This prevents toxins moving out of our bloodstreams and into our lungs to be excreted. Moreover, deep breathing moves the lymph in the thoracic duct and this can increase the lymph flow throughout the whole body, pulling toxins away from the cells.

Eat: Correct iron levels will help too, and many foods, especially green vegetables, are excellent sources of readily assimilated organic iron. They will help you carry more oxygen in your blood stream especially if you live in an outdoor and sunny environment. Russian research on chlorophyll (including chlorella and spirulina algae) has shown the molecule to be very similar to the haemoglobin molecule. One argument put forward is that a good consumption of 'greens' doesn't just provide cancer fighting elements like iron and vitamin K, the action of sunlight combined with the chlorophyll actually increases blood oxygen levels, through photosynthesis. Some people argue that this is why people in the US 'sunbelt' tend to get less cancer; not just because the sunshine helps them generate more vitamin D but because they are farmers with higher vegetable consumption. Some cancer experts are trying to use this theory in a treatment called Photo-Dynamic Therapy.

People with higher blood glutathione levels are 'healthier' according to several research studies. This is especially true for older people. You can increase glutathione levels by a diet rich in green vegetables and fruits – especially organic ones. Glutathione helps the mitochondrial power stations of your cells incorporate oxygen, and in turn this is helped by the mineral selenium.

Exercise: Medical science has proven conclusively that fit people are ill less often. And fit people recover quicker after an illness or an operation.

The magazine *'Integrative Cancer Therapies'* in America reviewed all their research studies where cancer patients had taken exercise and concluded that people with cancer who did daily exercise had 50 per cent less mortality.

Researchers at the University of Bristol have conducted an

extensive review of 52 international studies on exercise and found that physical activity can significantly reduce the risk of cancer, and improve the chances of survival if you do have it. From 37 of the 52 studies on exercise and breast cancer incidence, scientists found evidence that showed typically a 30 per cent reduction in the risk of the disease in women who exercised on a regular basis. Generally, the benefits of exercise were stronger for post-menopausal women than pre-menopausal women.

A 2008 study of girls and young women who exercise regularly shows they cut their risk of breast cancer before the age of 50 by almost a quarter. High levels of exercise between the ages of 12 and 22 offered the most protection. It is thought that exercise reduces oestrogen levels as well. It is quite worrying then, that in a UK report in February 2003, 20 per cent of school children now do not do any exercise in the average week.

There are many more studies, mainly from the USA. The most important conclusions are that:

- Exercise helps prevent cancer.
- Exercise helps increase survival times and prevent cancer reoccurence.
- Exercise has epigenetic benefits. It can modify and correct the expression of your genes.
- The exercise does not have to be strenuous.
- But it does have to be 'daily' – ideally for about 30 minutes.

For example, in 2003 researchers at Fred Hutchinson Cancer Research Center, Seattle, showed that exercise did not have to be strenuous. Women who exercised a little, but every day, reduced their risk of breast cancer 17 per cent. There is even research that shows that physically active people, for example, housework including making the beds, reduce their colon cancer risk by 22 per cent.

Finally, all manner of exercise types can be useful. For example The Center for Integrative Medicine, Thomas Jefferson University Hospital, Philadelphia, studied cortisol levels amongst over 10,000 people. Typically in stressed situations, the brain stimulates the adrenals to produce cortisol, and in Chapter 20, I told you that this can cause cellular inflammation, a precursor to cancer. A doctor might tell you to go home and rest. Researchers found resting would reduce cortisol levels just five per cent, whereas your first ever yoga class reduced levels nearly 25 per cent.

Taking 'exercise'

The Government Health Authority's official recommendation in 2004 was that you should take 20 minutes exercise three times per week. If you want to beat cancer, this advice is undoubtedly poor.

Another problem is that many people find it all too stressful to think about gyms, largely because most people simply do not understand correctly why they should exercise.

Too many people set goals of weight loss for their new-found exercise routines. In the first three months they hardly lose an ounce. This is simply because either they are doing the exercises incorrectly and/or a pound of muscle weighs exactly the same as a pound of fat.

One pound of fat contains approximately 3000 calories. Your first hour on the bicycle in the gym will burn around 400 calories if you can pedal for that long! It is no wonder the pounds don't fall off you at the start! However, over the weeks as you rebuild some lost muscle, an upward spiral starts. For every pound of muscle you add to your body, you burn 30 to 40 calories per day just to maintain it. So by losing three pounds of fat and gaining three pounds of muscle you might feel gloomy when you stand on the scales, but over a week the extra muscle will be burning a 1000 calories or so, even when you have a day off and are sitting watching the TV. Given the daily recommended intake for a woman of 1500–1800 calories and a man at 2200–2800 calories you can see that the benefits will start to grow. Stick at it, weight loss will come over time. And bear in mind that we are not talking about building 'muscles', just converting some of the fat back into the state it was, in your youth.

However, this is not the prime reason to exercise. It is what goes on inside you when you exercise that matters most. You are going to be healthier – reducing certain dangerous hormone levels, moving your lymph, oxygenating your blood, rebuilding your life, your vitality, your vibrancy.

And don't overdo it! Many women may be daunted by images of being surrounded by lycra-clad young lovelies 'going for the burn'. Be reassured. Too much exercise produces even more toxins in the body, burns up certain vitamins and is increasingly thought to be counter-productive. This is part of the reason why so many top athletes are so often ill or end up with diabetes.

So stop worrying. Don't think, *'Exercise to lose weight'*. Think, ***'Exercise for health'***. All those happy hormones produced, less oestrogen, more oxygenated blood, less depressed etc.

Exercise for health should simply be a sensible, controlled and long-term commitment to a healthier you. *"Never confuse motion with action"*, as Ernest Hemingway said. You may see much motion down the gym but the best regimes are planned action programmes for health, not slimming.

You should try to 'exercise' for 20 minutes every day, ideally first thing in the morning. Exercise may be a brisk walk, a swim or T'ai Chi and yoga. It doesn't need to be strenuous. It should involve arm and chest movement, not just leg movement. And you can do something different every day.

The crucial issue is to understand better what you should try to achieve in your fitness programme and weight loss is simply not the number one priority – it will come over time.

i) Oxygenate your cells

Most fitness books talk about the benefits to your heart and circulatory systems and it is true that you should see a gradual improvement in your blood pressure and your peripheral cardio-vascular system. Your heart will become stronger and your blood more oxygenated. This is one of the biggest goals in your plan to beat cancer.

Your lungs will learn to work again. Blood passing past a lung that is using 100 per cent of its capacity will be able to clear out more toxins. In turn it will become more oxygenated.

As the blood system strengthens it will carry this oxygen to the most distant cells much more efficiently than before.

ii) Move your lymph

You have twice as much lymph in your body as you have blood.

It bathes the cells and is supposed to transport wastes and toxins away from the cell, and then to transfer them to the blood stream for excretion. The only problem is that the lymph system has no heart to move it away from the cells and pump it round the body. When you sleep at night, your whole lymph system 'sleeps'. Only you can kick start it again in the morning!

The largest lymph duct is the thoracic duct, which passes across your chest. You must move your lymph daily to clear toxins away from your cells. And you must replace it with clean lymph, which is where exercise and clean water enter the equation.

Yes, of course your lymph will be moved if you take exercise. But other less strenuous pursuits will do the job just as well. Deep breathing and stretching will affect the thoracic duct. Light yoga exercises and graceful T'ai Chi. And swimming and press ups of course. Even yawning and laughing help move the lymph across the chest.

Exercise will also improve your posture, which in turn helps remove restrictions on your lymph and energy flow.

As your peripheral circulation improves, so too will your peripheral lymph system and the net result is that toxins will move more freely away from even the most distant cells. Massage can also help with this lymphatic drainage.

iii) Everyday movement

The basic rule with fitness is to 'think active' – try to be active every day in your life. In one study, a group of Chinese people were found to be burning 3500 calories per week in 'natural' exercise. That's the equivalent of one hour on the bike in the gym every day! But then, US research in *Epidemiology* magazine says that the women with the lowest risk of breast cancer are those taking six or more hours of exercise per week. By all means go to the health club for professional advice but you need to formulate your own plan of what makes you happy and what you think you can realistically do. So ring the changes. Maybe swim, cycle, try yoga or T'ai Chi, join a tennis group, go for a brisk walk and swing your arms repeatedly. Build your own personal programme of activity and be active in your everyday life. It will pay dividends.

iv) Burn visceral fat

A study in 2010 (see **icon** Cancer Watch) has shown that, while it may take six weeks or more to start losing those fat stores around your waist, when you exercise it takes about 20 minutes to start losing visceral fat. This is internal fat; the fat that surrounds your internal organs, holding toxins around your liver, heart, lungs and kidneys. You cannot see it, but the benefits are immediate.

v) Release happy hormones

Exercise also produces endorphins, often called happy hormones. These are addictive – you will increasingly feel more energised, happy, less stressed and lighter in spirit. Endorphins neutralise stress hormones like cortisol and so can change the environment of even your breast and prostate cells, through eicosanoid production, as we discussed. There is some evidence that they decrease levels of oestrogen, as well. Moreover, exercise affects your DNA expression, has epigenetic benefits and helps the biochemical environment of every cell in your body. It's illogical to spend lots of money on chemical antioxidants and toxin-free products if at the same time you allow your cells to float in stressed, toxic surroundings.

vi) Boost your strength hormones

Yes, you may decide you want to lift some weights in the gym. Lifting weights to a point of having tired muscles will cause Human Growth Hormone (Hgh) to be produced. If you are over 50 years of age you are hardly making this hormone any more, but resistance training will produce a shot of growth hormone at almost any age.

Hgh is a powerful neutraliser of free-radicals, and helps to further eliminate fatty deposits and builds lean muscle. In research studies in America with Hgh, people over 50 reported regaining lean muscle mass, losing fat and feeling youthful and re-vitalised. It helps men and women avoid osteoporosis too, without the need for supplements like HRT.

vii) Health and happiness, not slimming

Please understand that you are making a commitment for life. It's not about instant weight loss, it is about overall health and well-being: Moving your lymph, oxygenating your blood, building more muscle tone, increasing the good and happy hormones and, eventually, after 3 to 6 months, sure, you may shed some fat. But please don't go near the scales for three months!

Some days you may go to the gym with your new friends, others you may do yoga in your front room, or walk the dog, or swim, or simply have a massage. Allow yourself a little constructive pampering every now and again!

Drink plenty of water after your exercise to flush out those toxins, and eat protein within two hours of the work out to rebuild the muscle.

Action?

Oxygenating your cells? Take the first step!

If you want to prevent cancer, and certainly if you have it already, it is crucial you give serious consideration to where you live, your in-home environment and how to get a good source of quality oxygen into your lungs on a regular basis.

- Do not smoke, do not have people in your home who smoke.
- Use toxin-free household products, personal products and avoid toxic sprays.
- Do not live near main roads or sources of diesel fumes.
- Live well away from factories or other sources of air pollution.
- Learn to use your lungs and breathe properly.
- Take a holiday at altitude
- Eat plenty of green vegetables, supplement with selenium.
- Be active: Take light, but daily, exercise.

CHAPTER 23
EAT-TO-BEAT YEASTS AND MICROBES

Most people reading this book have a parasite

In my book, *Everything You Need to Know to Help You Beat Cancer*, I covered the view from the World Health Organisation that 20 per cent of cancers are caused by infection. Some experts think this figure is low. Parasites do not have to be three feet long. They can be microscopic like the ones in Carolina that come in the household drinking water as they have become immune to chlorine. Parasites can come with sushi, overseas travel, exotic fruits and even kissing (mucky habit!) The term parasites can also include viruses, bacteria and yeast infections.

Several factors are common. They all deplete you of your nourishment – they do live off your body, after all. And they can produce toxins, some of which may be carcinogenic. And sometimes they can also create unfavourable conditions inside tissues, for example, leading to a lack of oxygen.

- Increasingly, parasites are felt to have a link to cancer. In one study 42 out of 1000 patients in a USA cancer hospital were found to have a liver fluke. This was eradicated and many treated patients recovered. Fluke in British livestock has increased four-fold since 1997.
- Some parasites can produce known carcinogens like aflatoxins.
- 17 cancers are already known to be caused by viruses. As detection methods become more refined who knows how many the final total will be?
- More and more evidence is being produced on the role of a bacterium, *Helicobacter pylori,* in stomach cancers. This bacterium 'hides' from the acid in the stomach by diving into the mucous membrane. This causes the immune system to rush to the other side of the lining, setting up the conditions for an ulcer. In extreme cases of inflammation and in the presence of localised oestrogen a cancer can form.

- Excessive yeast populations are thought to be present in 70 per cent of the UK population, and are often living pretty much undetected. *Candida albicans* is the main culprit. You may have thrush, or cystitis. Or bloating after meals and wind. Typically, males may have yellow toe nails.
- In a case history in America a nurse 'with leukaemia' was cured simply by killing her yeasts. 27 per cent of her child leukaemia ward then achieved the same 'cure'.
- Many 'parasites' simply drain the immune system as it constantly tries to eject them or nullify their toxins. Many parasites are associated with a depletion of B vitamins. Several B vitamins are crucial for their role in the cancer process: For example, biotin boosts the immune system, choline and inositol help de-fat the liver and folic acid is vital for accurate DNA replication.

Many parasites can be detected by a blood test or a stool analysis but the lab technician will only look for those parasites he has been told to look for, so things do get missed. Microbe, virus, bacteria and yeast detection can also be undertaken by 'Alternative' practitioners who use analytical systems like VEGA. Nutritionists, herbalists and homeopaths can then help you work to eradicate these unwelcome polluters. In Germany the use of such 'alternative' systems is far more commonplace than in the UK and is available on the state health service to all patients. In the USA many more people go for parasite checks than do in the UK. In Japan many people take daily anti-parasite supplements (raw fish is a common and increasing source of parasites).

Yeast Infections

US research concluded that women who had had 25 'doses' or more of antibiotics in their lifetimes had double the risk of breast cancer. Researchers decided to go and look at how antibiotics might affect breast tissue.

Another study in the US showed that taking daily cinnamon supplementation could reduce the symptoms of type 2 diabetes in 25 per cent of cases. Researchers decided to go and look at how cinnamon interfaced with insulin and glucose.

Oh dear. Why not talk to a good nutritionist instead. They will tell you what is going on: In one word the problem is, 'Yeasts'.

As we saw in Chapter 15, antibiotics kill bacteria. Not just your infectious ones, but even the beneficial ones in your gut. At night, one of the prime roles of beneficial bacteria is to protect you by devouring the yeasts and microbes you consumed along with your food during the day. One estimate I read said that in a healthy individual the 'friendly' bacteria could devour up to two pounds of these yeasts and microbes a night!

If beneficial bacteria are not present in the right quantities, the yeasts and microbes start to multiply uncontrolled. This can result in all manner of gut problems from Irritable Bowel Syndrome (IBS) to Crohn's, ulcers and even cancers.

Also, yeasts are like mushrooms – they can form colonies and take root, making holes in the gut wall, causing leaky gut. An excess of yeasts can cause toxins in the blood stream making you inexplicably tired, increasing food allergies and far worse. Sometimes yeasts can also cross into the blood stream from where they may pass to almost any area of the body and colonise it. Yeasts are anaerobes – they do not use oxygen to 'live'. So they create a whole non-oxygen world. Your adjacent healthy cells may then be deprived of oxygen. You might expect them to die, but no, they just adapt to metabolise in the absence of oxygen. And this is called a cancer cell.

Now, not every cancer cell or every cancer is 'caused' in this way. As I keep saying – the causes of your cancer can be many and can be as individual as you are. But I am not surprised that antibiotics would be linked to higher rates of cancer – it makes perfect sense. And I'm sure that if the 'experts' checked the figures for other drugs, they might find some similar statistics.

Some yeasts move round the blood stream and stick, using a little carbohydrate, to the surface of cells. Unfortunately this blocks the cells' ability to receive important messages via surface receptor sites. Some of these sites may be insulin receptor sites. So this makes it harder for insulin to remove sugar from the blood stream and it will appear to be failing – and this may be confused with the effects of diabetes. However, it is widely known in hot climates that cinnamon kills yeasts in the blood stream, thus reducing the cell surface blockages and allowing some supposed diabetes sufferers to get sugar out of their blood streams into the cells. One wonders why the 'experts' haven't worked this out too.

Indeed, if you go round the world and look at the warmer countries where yeasts would be more prevalent you see that they have lots of natural foods that protect the populations. The following all kill off yeasts via their daily consumption: **Garlic, chilli, bee propolis, caprylic acid** (coconut), **cinnamon, nutmeg, fennel/anise, oregano, Pau d'Arco** (South American tree bark) etc.

The problem in the UK is that we do not consume anti-yeast foods any more, whether they be herbs or raw honey. And we reduce the numbers of beneficial bacteria in our bodies by caesarian birth, not breast feeding, no longer living on farms, chlorinated water, stress, antibiotics, drugs, pasteurised foods and so on. No wonder 70 per cent of our population has excess yeasts.

You may well have a yeast infection if you have taken antibiotics for a long period; and if you have a yeast infection you must address it.

In the last few years I have visited a number of specialist cancer clinics. In every case, I always go and talk to the people at the 'sharp end', the nurses!

What has astounded me is that they have all been adamant that every cancer patient they treat has a bad yeast infection – women and men. But this should be public knowledge. Back in 1993 *Contemporary Oncology*, a major cancer magazine for doctors in the USA, stated clearly that people suffering from cancer who had radiotherapy and or chemotherapy did not die from their cancers *'but finally succumbed to an infestation of Candida albicans'*. (**common yeasts!**)

Yeast 'poisoning'

Perhaps the best way of thinking of 'yeasts' and similar 'infections' is to regard them as microbes. Yeast infection is microbial infection.

Yeasts may be thought of rather as you would 'fire' – fire is helpful to humans in a controlled form, but devastating if allowed to get out of control. The late Gerald Green was a grandson of Professor Fritz Haber who discovered how microorganisms fix nitrogen leading to an understanding of a number of substances from fertilisers to explosives. Gerald was extremely knowledgeable about such microbes himself and I am indebted to him for increasing my knowledge.

If you have an excess of yeasts in your body, apart from feasting on the nutrients your body and immune system needs, they will create waste products. Some of these are mildly toxic and will reduce your immune defences further. But also *Candida* microbes produce an 'alcohol'. This poisons the bloodstream, making you feel 'hung over' and lethargic, and invoking serious work from your liver to detoxify it. Even worse, it feeds the cancer cells. **This alcohol produces a by-product and cancer cells thrive on it.**

As I covered in Chapter 15, the real breakthrough of the last ten years has been a much better understanding of the role of beneficial bacteria and their interrelationship with food, and microbes in your body's health systems.

For example, we know that *Helicobacter pylori* is a bacterium that causes stomach cancer. It can be treated, although not perfectly, by a combination of three antibiotic drugs – or you can use the herb **goldenseal** with **bismuth** and **acidophilus**, along with a protein diet (no carbohydrate) to increase stomach acid which normally kills it. A little **aloe vera**, sipped slowly first thing in the morning and last thing at night will help calm the inflammation as will **fish oils**.

Recent research has shown that the phenol compounds in both **extra virgin olive oil** and in **green tea** can both prevent and treat *Helicobacter pylori*. Apparently they can still operate in the stomach's acid and were effective even when antibiotics were not. Other studies from the USA show that **curcumin** can kill the bacterium *in situ*.

There are several parasite and yeast 'killers'. Caprylic acid and oregano oil can each kill yeasts with cinnamon being very effective for those already in the blood stream. Fennel and chili peppers do a natural job too. Pau d'arco is also very effective against yeasts and pathogens; in fact it was originally thought to be a cancer killer.

But the best parasite and yeast killer is probably the Chinese herb artemesinin, or sweet wormwood. It has proven more highly effective than drugs against malaria too.

On it's own it is probably not enough, and is most usually found in 'Parasite treatments' along with pau d'arco and black walnut.

An anti-parasite course normally lasts two months (you have to kill the adults, and then their babies a month later after they have hatched) and you and your partner both need to do it (as I said, parasites can be passed by kissing). Other natural remedies include natural foods like pumpkin seed, garlic, anise, butternut, figs, cloves, ginger and pomegranate seeds.

So, when did you last eat raw honey, fennel, pumpkin and its seed, cloves, oregano or pomegranate – all popular in England 500 years ago?

Eat-to-beat yeasts

There is an effective anti-yeast diet which involves:

- Consuming no sugar in any form (lactose, dextrose, glucose, honey etc).
- Consuming no dairy.
- Consuming no alcohol.
- Consuming no yeast products like marmite and mushrooms.
- Consuming no fruit save on an empty stomach first thing in the morning, and never after a meal.
- Consuming no 'soft' vegetables like marrows, cucumbers, squash or courgettes. Both groups can sit on top of the food in the stomach and ferment.
- Taking Pau d'Arco, caprylic acid, garlic, wormwood, oregano and cinnamon, and topping up with multi-strain probiotics.

Junk foods, fast foods, branded fruit juices, processed foods and foods from crisps to breakfast cereals are to be avoided as they often contain both yeasts and sugars. Go fresh and home cooked!

When attempting an anti-candida diet, Green recommended participants avoid certain carbohydrates too, especially refined carbohydrate as this can turn to sugar. For example, he recommended avoiding:

- Bread and all relatives.

- Cereals, hot or cold.
- All snack products from crisps to popcorn.
- All white rice, potatoes, corn and refined wheat products like pasta.
- Most fruit.
- Root vegetables.
- Lentils, chickpeas, dried beans.
- All coffee, caffeine, fizzy soft drinks, fruit juices, alcohol.
- All convenience/junk foods.
- All cows' dairy.
- All processed meat products (bacon, sausages, salami).
- All high salt foods.
- All mushrooms and fungi.
- All condiments.
- All hydrogenated fatty acids and saturated fats.
- Health supplements containing lactose, gluten and citric acid.

His good food choices included:

- Alfalfa and sprouting seeds
- Sweet peppers
- Broccoli, Brussels sprouts, cauliflower, cabbage and greens, kale, chard
- Endive, fennel, garlic, onions, spring onions
- Green beans
- Hot chilli peppers
- Lettuce, spinach
- Parsley
- Radishes
- Olive oil, flaxseed oil, fish oil
- Eight glasses of water per day
- Herb teas
- Whole oats, psyllium seeds
- Free range eggs
- Fresh fish
- Pork, lamb, veal
- Chicken, turkey, game
- Quorn, soya milk, rice milk, sheep's and goat's milk
- Soda bread (wheat free) with no added sugar or salt.

For your information, fresh garlic, when you cut it, oozes like a fresh potato. It does not have a green stem in the middle, nor does it appear as concentric leaves like an onion. It doesn't smell and it is hot on the stomach. Two cloves a day uncooked would be good. (If you buy the 'leafy' variety in your supermarket, you should know that taking the green centre out avoids the stale 'garlic' smell.)

Gerald recommended Pau d'Arco and wormwood, plus half a teaspoonful of freshly ground cinnamon in a glass of water. It helps fight the *candida* in the bloodstream, reduces blood sugar levels and stops the microbes forming the alcohol used by the cancer cells. (Patients with Type 1 diabetes must not use this).

Homeopaths have nosodes (natural potions that stimulate disease responses) to treat yeasts and these too can be very helpful.

And, when you undergo your 'yeast cleanse', you must also aim to strengthen your immune system. The following could be helpful:

- Vitamin C with bioflavenoids: 5 times per day 200 mgs each time
- Vitamin E: total 8 forms, 400 IU
- Zinc: 15 mgs
- Selenium: 200 micrograms yeast-free
- Chlorella

The herbs echinacea and astragalus are also recommended.

If you do need to sweeten things you might consider Stevia. It is a natural leaf sweetener and apart from being considerably sweeter than sugar it has anti-fungal and anti-bacterial properties. (Stevia was originally restricted in both the USA and the UK, but plans to use it in diet soft drinks will change all that!)

In extreme cases of IBS (caused by the bacterium *Clostridium difficile*) patients are finding relief from the use of enemas made from the stools of healthy people. In clinical trials these faecal transplants have been shown to work in over 80 per cent of patients, unlike the drugs, which were shown to work poorly, and even make matters worse.

CHAPTER 24
NATURAL COMPOUNDS IN THE FIGHT AGAINST CANCER

Louis Pasteur, the 19th century French scientist argued that diseases were caused by 'germs'. This has lead to a whole industry whose mentality it is to 'kill the germ', almost at any cost. While people may have heard of Pasteur, few have heard of his then rival, Antoine Béchamp, who argued that the issue was not the germ but the strength or weakness of the organism it attacked. Some 'germs' (for example cholera) would kill many of the pioneers on the wagon train across America two hundred years ago – but not all. Some people's bodies resisted. It is little known that on his death bed Pasteur admitted 'the germ is nothing – the terrain is all'. Better late than never, I suppose, but a quote now totally missed by modern medicine.

What we have seen in this book is that natural compounds have both the ability to kill the germ, and the ability to build the terrain.

Eating a spectrum of foods

This book is not intended as a 'Science Book'; it is an everyday person's guide to natural compounds and the intention is that you should be able to put a spectrum of those compounds into your body each week. I think we all want to know that across the average month we have covered all the bases, and done our absolute best to increase our odds of beating disease.

At the moment the media and some doctors, at best, talk about a few antioxidants like vitamin E, C and beta-carotene, not even understanding the benefits of these in natural form over their synthetic copies.

But these are only a small part of the story. Plants have the ability to synthesise an amazing array of natural compounds, some found in only a few plants, some almost universal. Importantly some of these compounds have antioxidant powers hundreds of times more potent than vitamin E or beta-carotene.

And we are only just discovering this.

Broadly speaking, plant natural metabolites fall into two areas:

- The nitrogen-free compounds: For example, phenolics, polyphenolics, terpenes, polyacetylenes and saponins
- The nitrogen-containing compounds: For example, alkaloids, cyanogenic glycosides, amino-acids and glucosinolates.

The latter group is still poorly understood. For example, many plant compounds contain nitrogen and carbon atoms and can be broken into cyanide molecules by different enzymes. The most 'infamous' of these is B-17, a 'vitamin' that has caused extreme controversy resulting in bans on the transport, usage and prescription of the synthetic form (laetrile) and even attempted restriction of the natural form (amygdalin) contained in sour fruits like gooseberries and pips like apricot kernels. The authorities have actually banned the planting of bitter almond trees! The stupidity of this can be seen in the sheer volume of other 'cyanide containing' plant compounds; there are probably more than 4000 natural compounds that 'technically' could be split to provide a cyanide molecule – are we to ban them all? Impossible; the most common high street version of vitamin B-12 and the one most doctors use for injections is cyano-cobalmin, the more naturally occurring one is methyl-cobalmin. B-12 is part of over 300 essential chemical reactions in a healthy body. No one in their right mind talks about B-12 'containing cyanide' or banning it, but they do about B-17. The fact is we need and use these cyanide combinations – they keep us alive and they protect us.

In 2009 a group of scientists from UCLA Santa Barbara published a report on the action of isothiocyanates. *(Carcinogenesis 29, 12, 2360-80)*. In this they studied how cruciferous vegetables (cauliflower, broccoli and cabbage) could prevent cancers like breast and prostate. The report also talks of 'the healing power' of these vegetables, and that 'broccoli and broccoli sprouts have the highest levels of particularly active isothiocyanates called **sulphoraphanes**'; (sulforaphanes, if you are American). The paper went on to look at how these natural compounds could heal, or correct, at a cellular level in both breast and prostate cancers.

Then there are the **polyphenols** where research is accelerating rapidly. Those in green tea actually target metabolic pathways that shut down the proliferation and spread of tumour cells, as well as inhibiting the growth of blood vessels in tumours. They also restrict the action of IGF-1; and a group of polyphenols in apples, called procyanadins, reduce pre-cancer lesions – the early stages in the development of cancer. Other research shows polyphenols can hijack the cancer cell signalling process, switching it off and leading to cancer cell death. Two natural phenol compounds (called chlorogenic and neochlorogenic compounds) found in colourful fruits with stones like plums and peaches have been shown to stop breast cancer cell growth according to research by Doctors Byrne and Cisneros-Zevallos in the *Journal of Agriculture and Food Chemistry*. Phenols are both preventative and corrective chemotherapy agents according to *The American Association For Cancer Research on Frontiers in Cancer*. Natural compounds that 'contain cyanide'? We need them.

We have covered several studies in Cancer Watch on pomegranates, the juice of which seems to be able to both prevent and reverse prostate cancer. Researchers at the University of California, Riverside, have also shown that it contains compounds that can block metastases. In a presentation to the American Society for Cell Biology's 50th annual conference the researchers showed that phenylpropanoids, hydrobenzoic acids, flavones and conjugated fatty acids in the fruit had the potential to stop cancer cells developing, to prevent metastases to nearby bone cells and even to kill prostate cancer cells. The compounds increased cancer cell adhesion and thus stopped migration to other tissues.

Then there are many studies on the anti-mutagenic abilities of extracts of pulses, cereals, vegetables, seeds and herbs. These have shown that, even with mutations caused by aging or genotoxins like X-rays, pesticides and chemicals, certain natural compounds have the ability to repair damage already occurring around the core DNA – this could have incredible importance, not least to patients having radiotherapy and chemotherapy.

Hopefully, one day your doctor will have the knowledge to tell you exactly how you can keep your healthy cells from damage when he is trying to kill the cancer cells.

But the sad truth is that, whether it comes to killing the germ or to nourishing the terrain, we have lost our way in the UK. We just do not eat these epigenetic, bioactive natural compounds in the volumes we did, or should do. And it is no surprise, in my opinion, to see our cancer rates and five-year survival figures worse than average in Europe.

This chapter contains a selection of natural compounds you might like to include in your weekly menu. Some are 'Natural Foods' and others are 'Natural Compounds'. I have chosen just an indicative twenty something. It could have been 100. There are over 4000 plant, vegetables and fruits containing flavenoids already identified!

What is most relevant is that often the 'active ingredient' is the pigment – the metabolite that confers part of the plant's natural colour. Bees seem to know this. Their hives and honey are full of natural compounds from the colourful pigments that attracted them. So if you want to be healthy, you need become bee-like and accumulate these colourful natural pigments in your diets too!

An explosion in research

Every month in Cancer Watch I seem to report on research from America about a natural compound, which has benefits against cancer. To me it is not in the least bit surprising that The American Cancer Society has talked about an 'explosion' in research into complementary therapies. It is exactly what I have been telling people. And it is particularly pleasing that they report that there is 'overwhelming' evidence that **diet, exercise and weight control can increase survival times, helping people 'live longer' and 'stay cancer free'.** The report *(the Nutrition and Physical Activity Guidelines for Cancer Survivors)* was published in May 2012 and a spokesperson, Coleen Doyle, ffrom ACS said 'the research was overwhelming and gives us the confidence that these things really matter'.

Around the same time, I covered several studies in Cancer Watch. Firstly, one from Windsor University in Canada on the ubiquitous dandelion. Oncologist Dr. Caroline Hamm had noted that her patients drinking dandelion tea seemed, in some cases, to be recovering from their cancers. So she asked a biochemist, Siyaram Pandey, to see if there was more to this weed than meets the eye. Sure enough, in his first experiments with leukaemia cells he food that dandelion root extract caused apoptosis. The cancer cells died. Importantly, the healthy cells in the blood samples were left untouched. The work was then extended to other cancers and the same results were noted. More work is now being undertaken and the research team has asked for approval to go to Phase I clinical trials. Of course, we are not naïve: No herb has ever been approved for use as a cancer agent on the other side of the Atlantic, so I pass this on for interest only.

But my real hobby horse is 'vibrancy'. The rainbow of colourful foods that surround us; the vibrancy being the result of natural pigments.

So it was no surprise to receive a study by researchers at Ohio State University Cancer Center on blackberries. They fed blackberries to one group of rats but not to a similar group. Both were then given oesophageal cancer-inducing factors. The group consuming the blackberries developed 60 per cent less cancers, a result lead researcher Gary Stoner described as 'astonishing'. A follow-up study measured the gene activity in the rats and showed considerably less in the blackberry-eating group. Yet more studies were conducted using several colourful foods and to quote Stoner, *'What is emerging in cancer chemoprevention is that using single compounds alone is not enough'*. **Although the blackberries seem to provide several benefits, he advocates eating yet more beneficial foods at the same time – such as grapes, medicinal mushrooms, broccoli, cruciferous vegetables and flaxseed.**

Finally, researchers at the City of Hope in Los Angeles (October 2011; *The Journal of Nutrition*) showing that eating blueberries could reduce the growth and metastasis of a very aggressive form of breast cancer (triple-negative cancer), for which there are few effective drugs. Tumour size reduced by 60-75 per cent. Molecular analysis revealed that blueberry consumption altered the expression of genes that are important to metastasis. The 'dose' required of blueberries to achieve these results was equivalent to two cups of fresh blueberries per day. This finding is potentially MASSIVE. It's epigenetics at work.

Now you may receive a quizzical look from your oncologist if you tell him about this research. He may even sigh and shake his head. Just ask him a simple question, *'Do you think it was the anthocyanins, the resveratrol or the pterostilbene in the blue colour that was responsible for this result?'*

Chemoprevention, epigenetic correction, eating a variety of pigmented foods, an explosion in research, 'overwhelming' evidence, the science of Salvestrols and much, much more. In America natural compounds in foods and their ability to protect and correct is ever more studied and has a name: Phytomedicine. By now, even the most conservative UK sceptic must acknowledge that a vibrant 'Rainbow Diet' can help you prevent and correct. It's all in the pigments!

Anthocyanins

Background: Dr Ferenczi may have cured himself and a number of patients with his beetroot diet because beetroot contains anthocyanins and these are known cancer cell killers. Typically these compounds are blue in alkaline and deep red in acidic conditions and are formed from anthocyanidins and their precursors pro-anthocyanins, usually in combination with various sugar molecules. There are a great many anthocyanins and they have many different functions for the plant. They are antioxidants, protect the plant against UV-light, are a defense mechanism and are very important in pollination and reproduction, attracting insects.

Sources: the main sources of anthocyanins are beetroot, blackcurrants, dark olives, elderberries, figs, deep red plums, red grapes, blueberries, blackberries and some vegetables, such as aubergine, red onion, red cabbage, avocado and hawthorn. The volume in certain fruits, especially if organic, can be 1-2 grams per kilo.

Eat-to-beat cancer benefits: Used as a staple in Russian soup, beetroot and these other foods have antioxidant properties. Anthocyanins have been the subject of many experiments – there are more than 200 articles in *PubMed* on the benefits of anthocyanins. Benefits include:

- They seem to provide protection to DNA.
- They reduce the growth rate of cancer cells, and tumours.
- They have anti-oestrogen activity.
- They have anti-inflammatory benefits.
- They increase white cell levels and stimulate the immune system.
- They inhibit cancer enzymes and can directly kill cancer cells (apoptosis). For example, researchers at Ohio State University have shown that eating these purple foods slowed the rate of growth of colon cancer and actually killed up to 20 per cent of the cancer cells.

The biggest problem is that research is difficult because anthocyanins seem to interact so freely with other plant compounds. Also, like quercitin, these plant compounds are broken down extremely rapidly in the body making it hard to follow all the various metabolites and what they are up to!

Aubergines contain anthocyanins and also a number of dark blue/mauve pigments. They are a staple part of the French and Mediterranean Diets. Researchers from the Royal London Hospital conducted a double-blind, placebo-controlled study using an extract (BEC5) from aubergines. Doctors treated both invasive, and non-invasive non-melanoma skin cancers and showed that it killed off the skin cancer and left healthy cells untouched. *'In our experience, BEC5 is... safe and effective... a cost effective treatment for both primary and secondary skin cancer'*. Microscopic analysis showed the death of cancer cells and that the cancer did not reoccur.

Oligomeric Proanthocyanidins (OPCs)

Information: OPCs are more powerful antioxidants, reportedly 20-50 times more powerful than vitamin E. They scavenge and neutralise free-radicals. Much work is being undertaken with these products in cancer studies, although they already have other known benefits and effects:

- Prostate cancer: 35,239 males were followed over a 10 year period in the VITAL cohort study (May 2011). Those with "high average use" of an individual grape seed extract supplement experienced a 62 per cent lowered risk of prostate cancer compared to non-users. Even average users of grape seed extract supplements experienced a 41 per cent lowered reduction.
- Haematologic cancers: 66,227 men and women in the same VITAL study who had ever used grape seed supplements saw a 43 per cent lowered risk of haematologic cancers.
- Skin cancer: A study carried out by Maryam Asargi et al, *(Department of Dermatology, University of California at San Francisco, San Francisco, California; June 2011)* involving 830 people compared various combinations of vitamins. The group taking grape seed extract had an incredible 74 per cent reduction in squamous cell carcinoma.
- Grape seed extract activates an important cellular protein which regulates apoptosis (cellular death). The extract helps the cell recognise that it is flawed; 78 per cent of leukaemia cells were killed in the first 24 hours of research. *(University of Kentucky)*
- OPCs strengthen heart and blood vessels and help in artherosclerosis, high blood pressure, high cholesterol and poor circulation and varicose veins.
- They limit complications occurring due to diabetes – e.g. macular degeneration, eye and nervous conditions.
- They promote wound healing.
- They may inhibit destruction of collagen.
- But, they may thin the blood and so may double up with drugs trying to achieve the same ends – be careful.

Sources: Commonly found in grape seed extract and in pine bark in slightly different forms. Proanthocyanins are also found in tea, red wine, cranberries, apples and pears. Pycnogenol (from French Maritime Pine Bark) is highly promoted in the USA.

Eat-to-beat cancer benefits: The US National Cancer Institute

records a number of anti-cancer studies including:
* Breast and prostate cancer prevention.
* Reduction of damage to breast tissue after radiotherapy.

Ellagic Acid

Information: Ellagic acid is an extremely stable polyphenol. Dr Daniel Nixon at the Hollings Cancer Institute, at the Medical University of South Carolina began studying ellagic acid in 1993. It is a proven antioxidant, anti-carcinogen, anti-mutagen and anti-cancer initiator.

Sources: It is found in some 46 different fruits and nuts, for example pomegranate, red raspberries, blackberries, strawberries, blueberries, cranberries, pecans and walnuts.

Eat-to-beat cancer benefits: Ellagic acid is a proven anti-cancer agent. Initial studies and clinical tests have shown that ellagic acid can protect the *p53* gene. Recent published data from MUSC includes the findings that:
* Ellagic acid has anti-bacterial and anti-viral properties.
* It can prevent Human Papilloma Virus infected cells developing, and cervical cells infected with HPV experience apoptosis (normal cell death).
* It slows the growth of abnormal colon cells. It increases the rate of metabolism of carcinogens and prevents the development of cancer cells.
* It affects and inhibits the action of acrylamides, known as potent carcinogens. And, as a powerful antioxidant, it neutralises the affects of aflatoxins produced by parasites within the body.

And all these benefits seem to come from eating just **half of one cup of red raspberries per day!**

Resveratrol

Background: Resveratrol is the exciting new kid on the block. It is a polyphenol and comes in two forms, cis- and trans-. Both forms are found in the skins of a number of fruits and plants, where its prime function is to protect against potential invaders like moulds and fungi. Its claimed benefits from research include lowering inflammation, improving bone health, reducing macular degeneration, dementia and Alzheimer's progress and stimulating levels of hormones called sirutins that normally protect the body when on a calorie restricted diet. Sirutins are linked with longevity. The World Health Organisation have said resveratrol can reduce 'bad' cholesterol and reduce cardiovascular risk by 40 per cent.

Sources: Typically, red grapes and red wine – especially organic varieties, as pesticides kill the moulds and fungi that cause its promotion. Much smaller amounts (about 10 per cent of these levels) also occur in blueberries and bilberries and even smaller amounts in raspberries and blackberries.

Eat-to-beat cancer benefits: Research is coming thick and fast from Harvard Medical School, Memorial Sloan-Kettering, MD Anderson, Cornell and more.
A great deal of new research suggests it:
* Fights yeast and fungal growth.
* Is anti-inflammatory and acts against COX-2 *(Sloan-Kettering)*.
* Stops tumour cell growth *(Harvard)*.
* Reinstates action of the *p53* gene *(Cornell)*.
* Causes apotosis: Kills cancer cells.
* Suppresses metastasis *(MD Anderson)*.
* Enhances both chemotherapy and radiotherapy performance *(MD Anderson, Missouri School of Medicine)*.
* Attacks cancer cells in the body through increasing levels of two proteins, perforin and granzyme B *(Missouri School of Medicine)*.

Researchers from the Faculty of Pharmacy at the University of Calabria in Italy *(The FASEB Journal report)* have shown that resveratrol blocks the effect of oestrogen on cells by reducing the receptor sites and can help to prevent the malignant growth of breast cancer.
The Caribe School of Medicine in Bayamon, Puerto Rico have

248

shown resveratrol enhances drug action against breast cancer and that reveratrol, quercitin and catchetin treatment restricts blood supplies to tumours and prevents cancer cell signaling.

Resveratrol is one of Professor Potter's Salvestrols. He believes resveratrol is another pro-drug and research shows that when it comes into contact with the CYP1B1 gene unique to cancer cells, it is converted to piceatannol which causes the cancer cell's death.

At the MD Anderson Cancer Center in Texas, professors have described it as a 'wonder compound – both a preventative and chemotherapy agent'.

Pterostilbene

Information: There is little research on this natural compound as yet – but what there is seems extremely promising. It is an aromatic hydrocarbon and the 'cousin' of resveratrol (being the methoxylated version). It was originally praised for its anti-fungal and glucose-lowering benefits. US Department of Agriculture researchers have found that it acts in a similar way to the drug cipofibrate, using cellular receptors to lower LDL cholesterol and triglycerides. However, unlike the drug, it has no side-effects of muscle pain and nausea.

Sources: It is part of the blue pigment in blueberries, cranberries, loganberries, and grapes. It was originally isolated from red sandalwood.

Eat-to-beat cancer benefits: Researchers from Taiwan (*Journal of Agriculture and Food Chemistry*) found that pterostilbene is potent in generating powerful antioxidant enzymes which can reduce colorectal cancers. It seems more potent than resveratrol in the colon.

Rutgers University and the US Dept. of Agriculture have said that the compound is a powerful antioxidant and seems to mop up free-radicals especially those that lead to polyps and colon cancer. Further work by Agnes Rimando at Oxford and at The University of Medical Sciences Poznan, Poland, has shown a cancer cell killing ability with breast cancer, plus an ability to turn off an enzyme called cytochrome p450. Cytochrome P450 enzymes activate a variety of compounds known as "procarcinogens", which can turn substances such as cigarette smoke and pesticides into carcinogens. Hence pterostilbene seems to be a great protector.

Curcumin

Background: The active 'ingredient' of the orange/brown spice turmeric. Research suggests it inhibits microbial action in the intestine and stomach, it is an anti-inflammatory, boosts cellular glutathione levels, is a powerful antioxidant, and can prevent and treat cancer. American cancer centres have done a lot of work on curcumin in the last three years.

Sources: A member of the ginger family, it has been used in Ayurvedic medicine for years. Levels to obtain benefit are way in excess of those you would achieve by having a few curries though!

Eat-to-beat cancer benefits: In America, *Memorial Sloan-Kettering, Tufts, Emory School of Medicine, UCLA and MD Anderson* all seem to be fans and have shown that curcumin seems to inhibit a multitude of cancer pathways:

- This spice can stop the action of the enzyme COX-2 known to produce cellular inflammation. Such inflammation can be a precursor to cancer, especially in the intestine.
- It has also been shown to inhibit vascular epithelial growth factors, essential in forming a blood supply to tumours.
- It has been shown to stop metastases in prostate cancer *(Ludwig-Maximilians University, Munich)*.
- It has been shown to kill B-lymphoma cells.
- Tufts have obtained results with breast cancer, using curcumin and isoflavenoids to limit environmental damage.
- Kentucky University have shown it inhibits leukaemia cells.
- Sloan-Kettering used green tea spiked with curcumin in their research and concluded it was a 'cancer beater' – it seems to prevent tumour formation and stops the development of essential blood supplies. In fact curcumin seems to work synergistically with both green tea's active ingredient EGCG and resveratrol.

250

There are twenty or more studies where it causes cancer cell death and even more where it prevents tumours forming a blood supply.

Piperine

Information: An alkaloid found in black pepper *(Piper nigrum)* and long pepper and responsible for its pungency. It has effects on the brain and nervous system and has been studied in relation to Alzheimer's. It seems to enhance cognitive function and is protective of brain function. Long used in Ayurvedic medicine. 2009 research showed that it can increase the bioavailabilty of many natural compounds if used in conjunction with food.

Eat-to-beat cancer benefits: Researchers at the University of Michigan Comprehensive Cancer Center in 2009 found that piperine and curcumin could each stop the development of breast cancer stem cells. 2012 research showed it inhibited angiogenesis (the formation of tumour blood supplies). Piperine enhances the effects of curcumin. The National Cancer Institute in America talks of its thermogenic properties and states that 'co-ingestion of piperidine enhances the bioavailability of various nutrients, including beta-carotene, curcumin, selenium, pyridoxine and coenzyme Q10. In addition, this agent may exert anti-inflammatory and anti-tumor activities and may enhance the production of serotonin'. Piperine and resveratrol were shown to increase tumour sensitivity to radiotherapy *(BMB Rep. 2012 Apr; 45(4):242-6)*.

Green Tea

Information: Of course, green tea is not native to the Mediterranean, where infusions of leaves and herbs are more the norm. But it contains important polyphenols which the lack of processing leaves unaltered, while the drying process concentrates. Polyphenols are powerful antioxidants, protect against heart disease, lower 'bad' fat LDL levels and stop artery plaque building. Apparently, you may need to drink more than 10 cups per day for the full benefits. Some of the polyphenols, called catechins, are five times more potent than vitamin E. They

251

help in limiting the effects of diabetes, and green tea even helps in weight loss *(University of Geneva)*.

Sources: India and Asia – *Camellia sinensis*.

Eat-to-beat cancer benefits:
- One catchetin in green tea (EGCG) has been shown to be effective against UV-induced skin cancer.
- It can also inhibit the spread of cancer *(Nature 1997, Jankun)*.
- EGCG has been shown to limit oesophagael cancer even amongst smokers and drinkers, by 60 per cent *(Shanghai)*.
- EGCG has been shown to block an enzyme that multiplies cancer cells, causing their death.
- It also promotes beneficial bacteria in the intestine.
- People consuming 5 cups per day have 40 per cent less cancers of the blood and lymph nodes *(Tohoku Medical School)*.
- The Mayo Clinic claimed their research showed 4-7 cups per day could 'stop leukaemia in its tracks'!
- Research from Perth, Australia, shows drinking one cup per day reduces ovarian risk by 60 per cent and prostate risk by 33 per cent.
- Researchers from Newcastle University have shown that the action of beneficial bacteria in the gut makes chemical by-products from the chemicals in green tea, and the by-products are even more effective with 'significant anti-cancer and anti-Alzheimer's benefits'.

There are studies on colon, breast, prostate and other cancer, and even studies that show it enhances radiotherapy and chemotherapy, whilst reducing side-effects.

Olive Oil

Information: Olive oil also contains polyphenols. And extra virgin olive oil seems to be particularly healthy, as it is made from pressing olives without the use of heat or chemical treatments. Cancer benefits start with the issue of good cholesterol, good fats and less free-radicals.

Eat-to-beat cancer benefits:

- *The Journal of Agriculture and Food Chemistry 2007*, covered research on how extra virgin olive oil can both prevent and treat *Helicobacter pylori* infections linked to stomach cancer.
- Olive oil polyphenols have also been shown to reduce inflammation by inhibiting the COX-2 enzyme.
- The University of Ulster have shown another ingredient, oleocanthal, is particularly important in reducing inflammation.
- Danish scientists have shown that olive oil reduces oxidative damage to cells and DNA. *(Copenhagen University Hospital)*.
- Natural compounds in extra-virgin olive oil suppressed the cancer promoting gene HER-2 *(Catalan Institute of Oncology, Dec 2008)*.
- Rats fed on olive oil diet have less pre-cancerous cells and less tumours than the control group *(Barcelona 2008)*.
- Researchers at Universitat Autonoma de Barcelona have shown that long-term usage of olive oil protects DNA from free-radical damage, deactivates certain dangerous proteins and lowers overall risk of cancer.

Carotenoids

Information: Carotenoids are a group of more than 600 naturally occurring pigments and are powerful antioxidants found in fruits and vegetables. They also improve communication between cells and empower the immune system. Most can be converted into vitamin A, but not all (e.g. Lutein). Carotenoids are destroyed by cooking. Best absorbed when eaten with fats.

Sources: Various – and typically carotenoids provide the *Rainbow Diet* with some of its most vibrant colours.

For example:

Alpha-Carotene - found in carrots, coriander and green beans

Beta-Carotene - found in apricots, cantaloupe melon and broccoli

Beta-Cryptoxanthin - found in persimmon (Sharon fruit), papaya and tangerines

Capsaicin - found in chilli, sweet red bell and jalapeno peppers

Lycopene - found in tomatoes, guava and watermelon

Lutein - found in turnip, kale and spinach

Zeaxanthin - a strong yellow pigment found in fruits and vegetables

Eat-to-beat cancer benefits:
- Many have been found to inhibit cancer development but this inhibition is reversible, meaning that stopping a diet rich in carotenoids may allow the cancer to grow again.
- Shown to prevent breast cancer; and importantly to prevent the return of breast cancer by blocking the action of oestrogen in cells.
- Lycopene can bind fats in the blood stream, reduce prostate risk and symptoms by up to 40 per cent *(Harvard)*.
- Lutein and Zeaxanthan are found in the retina and lens of the eye. Slow macular degeneration.
- Carotenoids facilitate communication between cells and help maintain cells in the differentiated (rather than stem cell) state *(Linus Pauling Institute)*. (See also vitamin A and beta-carotene.)

There's a great deal of research into the effects of carotenoids. One way that carotenoids inhibit cancer growth is related to their ability to improve intercellular 'communication' by increasing the production of a protein (connexion 43, C43) which sits between cells. Cancer cells lack the C43 protein, which means they also lack a vital growth control system. A diet rich in carotenoids can help return the situation to normal, especially when combined with selenium – a constituent mineral of C43 found in brown rice, fish and Brazil nuts.

Two studies, one from **Albert Einstein College of Medicine,** New York and the other from **Harvard** in 2009 showed that eating colourful red, yellow and orange vegetables not only reduced the risk of developing breast cancer, but helped prevent it returning. In both cases the groups eating the carotenoids almost halved their risk. *(International Journal of Cancer, 2009 Jun 15; 124(12):2929-37. Cancer Epidemiology; Biomarkers and Prevention. 2009 Feb; 18(2):486-94).*

Shhwartz and Shklar at Harvard University studied the ability of carotenoids to inhibit tumour growth in breast, lung, oral and skin tissue. They found a positive response to treatment within 1 to 5 hours.

Stahelin and colleagues from the University of Basel researched the role of a number of antioxidants, including carotene in 3000 men over a period of 15 years. They found that there was an increase in cancers of the stomach and bronchus in subjects with low plasma levels of carotene.

Another example from research concerns vitamin A, mainly created in the body from carotenoids consumed. Known to drive many cancers from breast, to colon, to prostate and even some brain tumours, oestrogen causes its damage by binding to cellular receptor sites. Scientists at the **University of Chicago** have shown that a metabolite of vitamin A (retenoic acid) can compete with and block this damaging action. Whereas oestrogen causes random and rapid cell growth to occur, the vitamin A was found to normalise proceedings.

Capsaicin

Information: One of the active ingredients in spicy peppers. One of a number of compounds called vanilloids. Already used in the treatment of muscle strain and of psoriasis. Promotes endorphins (happy hormones) in the body, reducing stress hormones.

Sources: Chillis

Eat-to-beat cancer benefits:
- Research indicates that the natural compound can kill microbes in the stomach.
- It is also effective against certain types of skin lesions and skin cancer.
- 2007 research by Nottingham University showed that this natural compound could actually knock out an enzyme which is unique to the power production system of a cancer cell, and is not found in healthy cells. Scientists are hoping to prepare a drug based on this compound.

Indole-3-Carbinol (I3C)

Information: In 2004/5 the pharmaceutical company Hoechst started to patent indole-3-carbinol and a number of its close relatives. It claimed that eventually these new compounds will be used to treat all manner of illnesses from arthritis, to MS to cancer, and even replace Tamoxifen with a better alternative. I3C is a member of the glucosinolates family. This family contains other indoles and also isothiocyanates such as sulphoraphane.

Sources: Greens such as broccoli, kale, cabbage, bok choi, Brussels sprouts and cauliflower contain Indole 3 glucosinolate; upon chopping or mastication it releases I3C. Cato the Elder, a Roman Statesman around 200 BC, wrote, *'If a cancerous ulcer appears on the breast, apply a crushed cabbage leaf and it will make it well'.*

Eat-to-beat cancer benefits: There is a problem. I3C is unstable, and its attributes may well be more due the performance of its metabolites. One in particular called DIM (Diindolylmethane) has many well-researched benefits and supplementation with this rather than I3C seems to provide more controlled blood levels of active ingredient. Research suggests I3C and/or DIM have the following actions:

(i) General:
- I3C acts as an antioxidant, neutralises free-radicals.
- Inhibits Human Papilloma Virus (HPV).
- Inhibits certain aflatoxins, and prevents aflatoxin-induced liver cancer, leukaemia and colon cancer.
- DIM is anti-inflammatory.

(ii) Specific to oestrogen-positive cancers:
- I3C/DIM reduces and even reverses oestrogen-driven cancers:
  - by converting highly active oestrogen variants into safer 'sisters'; and neutralising carcinogenic by-products.
  - by regulating a binding protein, and modifying oestrogen receptor sites on cell membranes thus preventing oestradiol action.

I3C has been dubbed (by UCLA and others) the 'safer, natural Tamoxifen'- it inhibits breast cancer cell proliferation by 90 per cent, whilst Tamoxifen scores 60. I3C also neutralises the by-products of oestradiol breakdown, whereas Tamoxifen has no effect.

UCLA and Strang have shown that it can have a big effect on neutralising the attack from chemicals such as oestrogen mimics and dioxins, and their dangerous breakdown products.

(iii) Action not involving oestrogen; all cancers:

* DIM restores the *p21* gene, preventing synthesis of DNA for new cancer cells and stopping cancer cells forming or growing.
* DIM has also been shown to decrease HIF-1 alpha and stops tumours forming a blood supply *(May, 2008 Biochemical Pharmacology Journal)*.

2010 research from Ohio State shows that orally taken supplements of I3C can cause destruction of the Cdc25A molecule. Cdc25A is responsible for the rapid cell division in cancers like breast, prostate, colorectal, oesphageal, liver and non-Hodgkins. Cdc25A is present in abnormally high levels in about half of all breast cancers. With supplementation, tumour size declined by 65 per cent. Although the research was done with mice the researchers concluded that I3C supplementation could potentially block the growth of many cancers, not just breast.

Please note: Some people are sensitive to I3C/DIM. Some people have a genetic mutation preventing some of the actions.

Sulphoraphanes (Sulforaphanes)

Information: Sulphoraphanes are sulphur containing isothiocyanates and have been dubbed the most exciting natural anti-cancer agents; the ultimate in epigenetics. The Dept. of Molecular Biology at UCLA Santa Barbara has shown how they work at a cellular level both in prevention and in cancer cell death. Once inside the cell they act as signaling agents to wake up over 200 genes, that were suffering from toxins, age or poor health factors. They turn on glutathione production and block oestrogen receptors. Sulphoraphane also exhibits anti-diabetic and anti-microbial action. Research shows that the action of sulphoraphanes seems to be enhanced by selenium.

Sources: Brassica (cabbage, kale, Brussels sprouts), broccoli, watercress and radish. And especially sprouting seeds. Chewing the vegetables causes the release of this natural compound; concentrated supplements are best.

Eat-to-beat cancer benefits: Researchers from Penn State College of Medicine have shown that isothiocyanates, used in conjunction with selenium, can 'shut down' the protein AK13 which causes cancer cell division in melanoma. Research has shown that sulphoraphane (SUL) can inhibit the development of breast cancer cells. Research presented in the *Proceedings of the National Academy Oct 2007*, showed that sulphoraphane activates cancer-fighting enzymes beneath the skin to fight melanoma and skin cancers. The researchers used broccoli seed extract. Several other cancers have been studied and in all sulphoraphanes seem to have the ability to consistently 'shut down' the cancer process. Another mechanism appears to be the ability of sulphoraphanes to turn off the inflammation and pre-cancer stimulating effects of the stress hormone norepinephrine.

Researchers from the Institute of Food Technology in Norwich studied people with a faulty PTEN gene. In healthy people PTEN produces a protein, which blocks tumour growth. But even where it was faulty, sulphoraphanes were shown to block the growth and spread of prostate tumours, even causing cell death.

Finally, broccoli sprout consumption inhibited *Helicobacter Pylori* infection and growth.

Garlic

Information: Garlic crops up time and time again in the fight against cancer, whether we are looking at Asian diets, or Mediterranean diets, glycoproteins or yeast control. The bad news is that **fresh, chopped or crushed garlic is essential.** Cooking ruins the effect and, in tests, some garlic pills are pretty useless too. There are several active ingredients. Most garlics have active sulphur ingredients. Although many reports talk about the active ingredient being allicin, other anti-cancer agents, like alliin and the enzyme allinase, appear to be produced on cutting or crushing.

Eat-to-beat cancer benefits: Garlic has strong anti-cancer benefits.

- It seems to restrict the blood supply to cancer tumours and thus stops them growing.
- Garlic is particularly protective in stomach, gastric and colon cancers and, across several epidemiological studies, it has been linked to reduced rates of growth in a wider range of cancers, from lung to oesophageal. For example, in the Iowa Women's Health Study *(Steinmetz 1994)* of 127 foods, tested with 41,387 women, garlic was the only fruit or vegetable that produced an effect; one or more servings of fresh garlic a week was linked with 35 per cent less colon cancer and 50 per cent less distal colon cancer.
- In a 1998 study in China *(You et al)* people taking large quantities of garlic every day (up to 60 gms per day!) had fewer than half the cancers of those taking only a little.
- It is possible that allicin works as an antioxidant, and it is certainly effective in reducing blood cholesterol levels. Allicin is also a very strong natural weapon against microbial infection, particularly bacteria, viruses, yeasts and intestinal amoeba. Allicin interferes with enzymes necessary for the growth of these microbes and also enhances a liver enzyme, which detoxifies aflatoxins before they cause damage. Allicin thus wards off infection and allows the body's natural defences to be stronger.
- Allinase seems to promote this action and in tests, allicin has been shown to inhibit cancers of the breast, liver and colon.
- Allicin appears to bind to breast cell receptor sites preventing the action of cancer agents. Prostate cells exposed to the garlic chemical SAMC grow at only 25 per cent of the normal rate.
- Garlic also seems to protect the body against the side-effects of radiotherapy, particularly DNA and chromosome damage.
- Professor Wargovich of the University of Texas has been working on two other active ingredients: dialylsulphide and S-allyl-cysteine. These have been shown to reduce animal cancers by 50 to 75 per cent and, in another test on animal cells, to totally protect against a deliberate attempt to induce a particularly virulent oesophageal cancer.
- Some garlics contain good levels of selenium and these varieties

have been particularly successful in treating breast cancers. Garlic is a good source of glycoprotein polysaccharides.

- Garlic also contains good levels of tryptophan, which is the precursor of serotonin, which in turn is the precursor of melatonin. Melatonin, as we saw earlier, is an excellent and very powerful neutraliser of free-radicals.

Fish oils

Information: Dr Benjamin Frank (*Nucleic Acid Therapy in Ageing and Degenerative Disease*) showed, nearly thirty years ago, that we need to produce about one to one and a half grams daily of nucleic acid. Dr Frank believed that nucleic-acid-rich foods could retard or even reverse the ageing process.

Top of his list was fish, which he believed should be eaten at least seven times per week. He also suggested freshly made fruit or vegetable juice and good water intake. Apparently **all** his patients benefited from his diet.

Fish oils have been shown to prevent heart disease and dementia, increase IQ in children, prevent cachexia, lengthen telomeres and thus aid longevity, cancer prevention and control.

The origins of these long-chain polyunsaturated fats are the microscopic algae and plankton that the fish feed on. Sadly, of course, fish farming methods may mean less consumption of these vital nutrients. This is why the best fish is 'deep-sea caught'.

Eat-to-beat cancer benefits: Fish oils contain omega-3, vitamin A and vitamin D, and most contain good levels of selenium and some vitamin E. Importantly, the omega-3 is long-chain omega-3, which is known to reduce inflammation in tissues. Thousands of years ago we consumed one unit of omega-3 for every unit of omega-6, 9 and others in total. Now a New York twenty-something consumes just one unit for 50 of the other oils. But your body really needs it. Research shows that omega-6 can actually accelerate the growth of human prostate tumours. (*Cancer Research UK*). Omega-3 can balance this.

Inflammation, especially in colon cancer, depends on the enzyme COX-2. Levels of the enzyme are high in 85 per cent of colon cancers (*Dubois, Vanderbilt*), and also in breast cancer.

Work is underway on drugs which block COX-2. **But why take drugs when the fundamental answer lies in increasing your intake of fish oils?** The *International Journal of Cancer (March 2002)* reports on 250 women with breast cancer and the findings that **women who are cancer free have much higher omega-3 fatty acid levels in their breast tissue!**

Three 2010 studies summarise this:

* Researchers at UCLA, San Francisco *(JAMA)* have shown that patients with high levels of omega-3 in their blood stream experienced a slowing in the shortening of their telomeres. Telomeres are protective proteins at the ends of DNA strands that shorten over time and this shortening is linked to the ageing process. This especially occurs during cancer.

* In a large 35,000 study on women between the ages of 50 and 76 *(Vitamins and Lifestyle study, VITAL)* researchers from the Fred Hutchinson Cancer Center in Seattle have found that regularly taking a fish oil supplement may lower the risk of breast cancer by approximately a third. "*This study is one of the largest studies that have come out showing that there may be a role for fish oil in the prevention of cancer, specifically breast cancer,*" said Lorenzo Cohen, of the M.D. Anderson Cancer Center at the University of Texas-Houston. This followed a similar study, analysis and conclusion by Harvard for prostate cancer.

* Researchers from several UK Cancer Hospitals worked with patients diagnosed with an inherited disease producing intestinal polyps, the pre-cursors of colorectal cancer. A concentrated form of omega-3 significantly reduced the size of the polyps and prevented the onset of colorectal cancer.

There are, literally, hundreds of studies like these from Harvard to Perth. Take your fish oil supplement, daily.

Polysaccharides, or glycoproteins

Information: Four Nobel Prizes for Medicine in recent years (1994, 1999, 2000 and 2001) have been won with research on how cells communicate, and the importance to our health and well-being.

Three had implications for cancer prevention and treatment.

In 1994 Gilman and Rodbell won for their discovery of 'G-proteins' and how cells handle signal substances from glands, nerves and other tissues to make changes.

In 1999 Gunter Blöbel and his team looked at how proteins have specific protein signals built into them so that they reach the correct destinations.

And by 2001 Hartwell, Hunt and Nurse had won for showing an understanding of the cellular messages involved in the cell cycle – its growth and division into two identical daughter cells – and how mistakes might result in a cancer development.

Blöbel also found out why your immune cells could not recognise some cancer cells – and it was all to do with imperfect membrane structures being coated by carbohydrate molecules.

These protein messages often involve complex sugars, and so it is common in the USA to call them 'supercarbs' or monosaccharides (which is actually wrong as most are polysaccharides). In fact most are a combination of 'sugars' and 'peptides' (small proteins of less than 30 amino-acids in length). Importantly, you can't make these sugar chains – and nor can you break them. So you must consume them whole, and they will not suddenly flood your body with unwanted glucose.

Sources: Aloe vera; arabinogalactins (found in carrots, leeks, radishes, corn, pears, red wine, coconut meat, tomatoes, curcumin and echinacea); brans (slow cooked oatmeal, whole barley, brown rice); breast milk; garlic; pectins (apples, pears and citrus fruit eaten whole). Shiitake mushrooms contain 1:3 beta-glucan polysaccharide and medicinal mushrooms in general are strong suppliers of polysaccharides (reishi, cordyceps, maiitake, shiitake); psyllium seeds. MGN-3 (or Biobran) is made from rice bran and enzymes from shiitake mushrooms. It is one of the most powerful immunomodulators currently available. Breast milk is another big source of glycoproteins – nourishing brain cells and boosting the immune system in babies.

Eat-to-beat cancer benefits: Even very small amounts can make a big difference. Eat the right polysaccharides and they will help clean up your membranes, stop the carbohydrates sticking and the immune system can spot the good, the bad and the ugly and will itself be greatly boosted. Pharmaceutical companies are working on drugs to enhance this process – you can eat the foods.

Professor Gilbon-Garber has shown that the invasive process of bacteria, viruses and indeed cancer cells which involves the above 'bonding' process to membranes, can be inhibited by glycoproteins in mother's milk. Because these molecules used in her experiments are all-natural, no side-effects occurred. Many experts believe that the discovery of polysaccharides could turn out to be more important than vitamin C or antibiotics.

Medicinal Mushrooms

Information: Mushrooms have long been used in medicine. The earliest records go back over 4000 years in China and they have been used to treat a wide variety of illnesses including cancer. In particular they are used to 'normalise', or balance, the blood. Their use is not confined to South East Asia, and they have long been used especially in Southern Europe for illnesses from arthritis to diabetes. (We have an old man who sits in the market at Le Muy in Provence every Sunday, selling various mushrooms and claiming they cure all manner of illnesses – claims that were handed down through the family for generations!)

Research shows that medicinal mushrooms contain high levels of glycoproteins and polysaccharides (Beta Glucan Polysaccharide being a particularly active 'health' contributor). Not surprisingly then, they have a significant effect in boosting the immune system.

Sources: The benefits largely depend on the particular mushroom consumed. In South East Asia Shiitake, Maitake, Cordyceps, Reishi, Coriolus Versicolor and Phellinus linteus have all seen extensive research into their benefits. But Girolles, Chanterelle, Morel, Porcini, Pleurotte (oyster) mushrooms and many more are in plentiful supply in Europe even if the research can be more traditional and anecdotal than scientific.

Eat-to beat cancer benefits: It all depends which mushroom extract you choose, how concentrated it is, and whether you use complementary doses of vitamin C and other such natural compounds. Research on medicinal mushrooms shows they can:

- Increase survival times in research trials with breast, lung and prostate cancer patients.
- Shrink cancer tumours by up to 70 per cent (some extracts even caused cancers to disappear).
- Stimulate the immune system, for example increasing macrophage activity or stimulating B- and T-lymphocyte production.
- Reduce blood supply to prostate cancer tumours.
- Reduce side-effects of radiotherapy and chemotherapy significantly (like nausea and hair loss).

Memorial Sloan-Kettering sent out a press release in 2011, in which they said that maitake mushroom extracts can stop cancer in animals, not directly, but through boosting the immune system. I received a copy. I wonder how many British Doctors received one? In people with myelodysplastic syndrome the bone marrow does not work normally and they produce low levels of red and white blood cells. Memorial Sloan-Kettering is also running a Phase II clinical trial to see if maitake mushrooms can sort this out. If so it could be a huge boost to people with all manner of blood and lymph cancers.

Even button mushrooms have their benefits: Research from Perth University in Western Australia showed that women who ate 10 gms of button mushrooms a day, developed one third of the **breast cancers** of non-eaters! The reason given was their content of linoleic acid, which acts like an aromatase inhibitor and restricts the production, and action, of oestrogen. (The same study noted that if these women also drank green tea, their breast cancer rates fell to just 1 in 10 of the norm!)

A study by UCLA in 2009 showed that breast cancer patients who ate medicinal mushrooms two times per day, prevented their cancers returning. Again this was concluded to be due to the mushrooms' anti-oestrogen activity.

I will now just look at some research, including clinical trials, on four medicinal mushrooms. Far more can be found on our website.

Maitake mushrooms: contain grifolan, a beta glucan polysaccharide which has been shown to activate macrophages. Another ingredient, termed d-fraction, stimulates the immune system at the cellular rather than blood stream level. It has been shown in clinical trials to enhance the effect of cancer drugs whilst reducing side-effects such as nausea and hair loss. Maitake has been found in the Kobe College of Pharmacy to destroy tumours and to be helpful against **leukaemia, stomach and bone cancers.**
The New York Medical Center has shown that an extract of Maitake mushrooms can shrink tumours of **bladder and prostate cancers** by as much as 75 per cent. In certain cases the tumours disappeared. Researchers believed this was because the active extract stopped a cancer-driving enzyme. They also used the extract in conjunction with interferons, which can boost the immune system. *(British Journal of Urology – Dec 2009)*

Shiitake has been used in medicine for years as a blood 'balancer' and particularly for lowering cholesterol levels. The National Cancer Center in Tokyo isolated lentinan, one of the active ingredients, and showed that the extract could reduce tumours in mice by 80 to 100 per cent.

Phellinus linteus. In 1993 Korean scientists successfully extracted an anti-tumour medicine from *Phellinus linteus*, following the 1968 research study by Dr Ikegawa *'Anti-tumour activity of some basidiomycetes, especially Phellinus linteus'*. *Phellinus* has been used in Chinese Medicine for thousands of years for everything from rheumatism to arthritis and gout. Biochemistry Professor Tae Woong Kim of the Korean National University says that the mushroom extracts kill cancer cells with no known side-effects or toxicity.

Several other studies *(e.g. Leo JLD Van Griensven and Huub Savelkoul)* have shown that beta glucans from these mushrooms can alter cytokine and T- and B-cell activity. Research shows an effect in solid tumours but also in fighting blood cancers where the white cells themselves were in trouble (like **leukaemia**).

The Boston University School of Medicine have found that where the mushroom extract was added to doxorubicin (a prostate cancer drug), the drug performed much better, with many more cancer cells killed *(British Journal of Cancer August 2006)*.

Previous studies from the same University in 2005 (Drug Discovery Today) showed that **Reishi**, *Ganoderma lucidium*, restricted blood vessels to **prostate cancer** tumours and stopped cancer cell proliferation.

Nitrilosides

Information: There are at least 1200 species of plants in the world that are nitrilosidic and the natural compounds are often described as nitrilosides or beta-cyano-genetic glucosides. Sadly, in the UK we are eating less and less of those that were indigenous to us like gooseberries, blackberries, blackcurrants, quince, millet, maize, barley, watercress and pulses.

Sources: Flaxseed, linseed; bamboo shoots, grains: barley, buckwheat, maize, millet, blackberries, black and redcurrants, cassava, cranberries, gooseberries, loganberries, quince, raspberries, strawberries, yams, papaya; brown rice, pulses: lentils and many pulses like kidney beans and fava beans. Nuts: For example, pecan nuts, macadamia nuts, cashews, walnuts, almonds. Beans: For example, lima beans and field beans; sprouts like alfalfa or Mung bean; watercress, sweet potato. The seeds of lemons, limes, cherries, apples, apricots, prunes, plums and pears.

Eat-to-beat cancer benefits: There is a group of approximately 14 natural compounds, which are water-soluble and are dubbed 'vitamin' B-17, or amygdalin. B-17 has been used as a cancer treatment for a number of years. Amygdalin was first isolated in 1830 and used as an anti-cancer agent in Russia as early as 1845. But it was reborn by the father/son team Ernst Krebs senior and junior, who prepared a purified form (calling it laetrile) and, with others in the late fifties to seventies, sought to explain its action.

Cancer cells differ in a number of ways from normal cells. In a cancer cell there is a unique enzyme called glucosidase, which breaks down B-17 into hydrogen cyanide (which kills it) and benzaldehyde (an analgesic). In normal cells, where glucosidase is virtually non-existent, another enzyme, rhodinase, renders the B-17 harmless. Poorly-informed people talk about B-17 containing cyanide but, as we have seen so far in this book, hundreds, if not thousands, of plant compounds can 'contain cyanide'. Proponents clearly believe B-17 is a seek and destroy missile targeting only the cancer cell mitochondria.

Well, maybe. Every day you produce several hundred cancer cells. Get them early with a rich B-17 diet and this could be true. However, as cancers develop they often form protective protein coats around the cells to ward off the immune system. These protein coats will protect the tumours from B-17 too.

Various cancer clinics have thus developed 'metabolic therapy packages'; these include bromelain (from pineapple), papain (from papaya) and two pancreatic enzymes trypsin and chymotrypsin to break down this protein coat, plus vitamins A, E and B complex, plus high dose vitamin C and high dose minerals.

The difficulty then becomes, "which bit worked?" Having personally talked to leading B-17 therapy users in the USA and Europe, none doubts its efficacy, but all felt it was not as potent as high dose vitamin C or pancreatic enzymes and that clearly a significant contribution was being made by the other participants in the therapy package.

2014 research is PLOSONE, by Makarevic et al showed that amygdalin stopped bladder cancer cell progression *in vitro.*

Laetrile is the synthetic form of B-17 and therefore it is a drug. There are no Phase III clinical trials on laetrile, so obviously it is not approved as a drug. Dr Contreras of the Oasis of Hope Hospital in Mexico is one of the foremost advocates of B-17 therapy. He has dubbed it 'nature's chemotherapy', and uses it on all cancer treatments but notes that it does not work for brain tumours, sarcomas or liver cancer. He knows of no one who has died from taking B-17.

Krebs recommended eating ten apricot seeds per day for life as a preventative measure (the seeds, or kernels, have the highest levels of B-17); cancer treatments use four to six 500 mg tablets per day or intravenous injections. It is not a vitamin.

One issue is overdosing as cancer patients most usually have toxic livers, and an enzyme, glucorinide, in the liver will have to detoxify any excess B-17. **A maximum of five kernels at any one time in a two-hour period is recommended for prevention or cancer patients,** and cancer treatments have to be properly supervised. I met a gentleman in Australia who had prostate cancer and had been to a talk on B-17. He was taking 50 kernels for breakfast and wondered why he felt sluggish and livery!! Excess B-17 and cyanide by-products have been known to build up in the liver. Each of us has different liver detoxifying capacities and the cancer patient has an already impaired liver. Cyanide poisoning of the liver can result if excess is consumed by someone with an impaired liver. **1 gm of vitamin B-17 is the maximum recommended dose to be taken at any one time and the US Nutrition Almanac recommends a maximum of 35 seeds per day.**

I apologise for dwelling on B-17 longer than other natural compounds but I am frequently asked about it. Bitter vegetables like watercress, pulses and gooseberries plus seeds and nuts are important elements in the 'Rainbow Diet'.

Isoflavones and phytoestrogens

Information: Isoflavones are widely found all over the world in herbs, plants and vegetables being an alternative term for flavenoids. Flavenoids have been shown in research to exhibit a number of anti-cancer benefits with colorectal, laryngeal, prostate, ovarian and breast cancers, for example.

Some of them have oestrogenic power – phytoestrogens, are similar but not identical in chemical composition to oestrogen; however their action in the human body is much, much weaker than the human hormone and as such they have been dubbed protective and even called 'anti-oestrogens'.

Isoflavones and phytoestrogens have been very protective to people in the UK for thousands of years. **Red clover**, the herb of Hippocrates, has a long history of use as a medicinal herb. It's an excellent blood purifier that gradually cleanses the bloodstream and corrects deficiencies in the circulatory system. It is found as a central ingredient in a number of herbal anti-cancer formulas, including the Hoxsey formula, Jason Winter's tea, and Essiac tea.

Sources: Flavenoids are abundant in plants, vegetables, fruits, herbs and pulses. Typically many people talk about phyto-estrogens in pulses like broad beans, peas, flageolets and lentils, chickpeas and hummus; or in red clover.

Eat-to-beat cancer benefits: There is a lot of mythology and argument. Several US 'experts' and even the FDA had dismissed red clover as useless in dealing with cancer. Some even think it dangerous. Red clover contains four main oestrogenic isoflavones, daidzein and genistein and compounds called coumestans, for example, biochanin and formononetin.

- Red clover is being studied with breast cancer patients at the Royal Marsden.
- Researchers at the National Cancer Institute have confirmed that there are indeed anti-tumour properties in red clover.
- Georgetown University in Washington, DC have found that genistein increases repair protein levels in the cell, and this helps prevent damaged messages being passed on. These repair proteins are regulated by genes such as the BRCA genes and only low levels are found in cancer cells.
- According to the NCI, genistein has the ability to prevent tumours from developing the blood supplies they need to survive, thus starving and killing them.
- **Genistein,** like other phytoestrogens, has also been shown to have the ability to block receptor sites on cells, preventing the much more active human oestrogens, like oestradiol, binding there. Genistein is used by Plaskett in his therapy and by a number of clinics to treat hormonally driven cancers.

Genistein levels in red clover are about ten times the level found in soya. Little of the other active ingredients are found in soya.

Pulses formed an important part of the UK diet 200 years ago but no longer. Pulses do contain protein and oils and these are frowned on by the more extreme cancer therapies, like Gerson, where even modest levels of fat and protein are forbidden. Pulses can also contain phytic acid, which prevents the absorption of certain minerals. Fortunately this rises to the surface on boiling and can be skimmed off.

Soya is an incomplete protein source and lacks vitamin B-12. Fermented soya products have a less effective anti-oestrogenic action. Some mass-market soya milks are GM originated. You should also beware of mass-market soy sauces as they have high sugar and salt content. Shoyu and Tamari, brewed in oak casks are more natural but still high in salt, albeit sea salt.

Cancer Research UK contributed to a study which looked at soya consumption and cancer in Eastern women. Women who consumed the highest amounts had 60 per cent fewer cancers than those who ate the least.

Asian women, who have far, far fewer cancers than Western women, have up to a thousand times the isoflavone levels in their bloodstreams when compared to their Western equivalents, and many studies have concluded that this is a vital and protective factor.

Citrus isoflavones were studied in a limited way with brain tumours and showed some positive results; isoflavones have been shown in small scale studies to aid the effectiveness of radiotherapy.

Chlorella and spirulina

Information: The earliest life forms; over 30,000 species inhabit the earth where there is a natural water supply. At one extreme are microscopic blue-green algae, at the other 150 foot long strands of kelp.

Probably the best known are spirulina and chlorella, having many properties in common although, unlike other algae, chlorella has a nucleus.

They are excellent sources of vitamins and minerals, enzymes (including digestive enzymes) and amino-acids (with all eight essential acids). However, they have notable other benefits.

Eat-to-beat cancer benefits: Spirulina and chlorella are both excellent sources of polysaccharides. Chlorella contains mannose, arabinose and galactose amongst others. These help communication between cells and your immune system to identify rogue cells.

A large number of Japanese studies have shown how both boost white immune cell levels – interferon and particularly T-cells.

Chlorella seems to enhance levels of *lactobacillus* in the gut aiding the immune system and general nourishment.

Both have excellent levels of beta-carotene (about ten times the level of carrots), organic iron and vitamins D and K. In chlorella, B vitamin levels are excellent, especially B-12, although folate levels are low.

Chlorella, supported by the action of intestinal bacteria, helps in detox diets since it can help bind heavy metals and some pesticides making elimination easier.

A particularly interesting development is in the use of such chlorophyll-rich algae as agents in Photodynamic Therapy. Russian work shows that the chlorophyll, which produces oxygen when light is shone on it, can destroy cancer cells; and US research *(Waladkami, Clemens, 1990)* has shown how important green vegetables and phytochemicals are in the restriction of cancer development.

There is an increasing body of opinion that chlorophyll (which has a similar molecular structure to haemoglobin) can circulate in the bloodstream and even help to oxygenate (and kill off) cancer cells by photosynthetic action. The sun belt that runs through the USA is also the area where people have the highest vegetable intake, and the lowest cancer rates.

Quercitin

Information: Another flavenoid, it is also a phytoestrogen and features in both the Gerson and Plaskett therapies and is increasingly being shown in research to have many benefits. Quercitin is metabolised very quickly in the intestines and liver after ingestion and very little is found in the blood. This has greatly hindered research to date. Now more studies are looking

271

at the effect of its metabolites. One hypothesis is that even small doses are very important to humans, and the speed of its metabolism and destruction was no problem 100 years ago because quercitin is so widespread in fruit and vegetables and we ate fruit and vegetables all the time continually 'topping up' the levels of quercitin in our bodies.

Sources: Commonly apples, onions and tea. But also (in descending order of concentration) capers, the herb lovage, red grapes, citrus fruits, rhubarb, green vegetables including broccoli, cherries, raspberries, chokeberries, and in small amounts in tomatoes and honey.

Eat-to-beat cancer benefits:
- Specifically it is an antioxidant, an anti-histamine and an anti-inflammatory agent.
- It has also been found to be an effective 'hyperthermia sensitiser'. Hyperthermia can kill cancer cells.
- UCLA research found that quercitin used in conjunction with ultrasound can effectively kill both human prostate cells, and skin cancer cells (*British Journal of Cancer* (2005) 92, 499-502).
- This makes it a potential adjunct in the treatment of various cancers that are sensitive to heat stress or hyperthermia (e.g. leukaemia, colon, prostate, melanoma etc). Its formula is related to the group of compounds called anthocyanins.
- The Mayo Clinic report that their research shows that quercitin blocks the androgen pathways in prostate cancer, slowing or stopping prostate cancer cell growth. They believe quercitin could provide a non-hormonal alternative to prostate cancer therapy.
- Research by the Italian Cancer League has shown that it prevents the growth of prostate cancer cells. And the skin of apples has been shown to inhibit colon cancer.
- It stops the proliferation of cancer cells in vitro, especially if vitamin C is present *(Kandaswami)*.
- Quercetin and genistein are the most potent anti-proliferating flavenoids in colon cancer *(Kuo)*.

- Quercetin has potential in the treatment of leukaemia *(Teofil)*.
- Quercitin is a phytoestrogen and there are two studies suggesting positive effects with breast cancer and lung cancer, but these need confirmation.
- The University of Maryland and the Cedars-Sinai Centre report that quercitin flavenoids seem to enhance several chemotherapy drugs, but may be themselves damaged by chemotherapy drugs. They may also have the same effect as certain antibiotics. Whether this means there is a clash with antibiotics, and quercitin should not be taken at the same time, or it actually enhances the antibiotic effect is not fully understood yet.

Fucoidan

Information: Although not strictly a common ingredient of the Rainbow Diet, it is present in the diet of the Okinawans, and consumption is highest in the prefecture of Okinawa with the lowest cancer rates! Fucoidan is a sulphated polysaccharide and an important anti-cancer agent; a strong body of research evidence shows it causes cancer cell death.

Sources: Brown Seaweed, rockweed, kelp, Fucus brown algae which reached up to 60 cms in length. The slimy constituent of sea vegetables is a high source.

Eat-to-beat cancer benefits: Best taken as a natural supplement, although some are used as human food.
- *PubMed* has a number of research studies showing, for example, a decrease in stomach cancer caused by *Helicobacter Pylori*; the suppression of lymphoma cells.
- Helps curb malignant tumour growth by causing self-destruction or apoptosis *(Bromedical Research; Takara Shuzo)*
- Fucoidan enhances immunity; for example increasing T-cell formation and action against cancer cells *(Hong Kong Uni, 2008)*
- Fucoidan restrains blood supply development in tumours *(Fuknoka University 2003)*
- Stops leukocytes entering the brain in cases of meningitis

(Satens Serum Inst. 2000)

- Aids phagocytosis of cancer cells *(Dept. Pathology Cincinnati, 2003)*
- Causes cell death in human lymphoma *(Aisa et al 2005)*
- Inhibits metastasis *(Liu et al; Anticancer Res. 2005)*
- Induces apoptosis in leukaemia cells *(Hangi et al Nutrition Cancer 2005)*

Bee propolis

Information: Bee propolis has always had a healthy image. After all, honey was one of the staple foods in the Middle Ages and is known to have significant anti-viral and anti-fungal benefits. Propolis is a natural compound produced by bees from the buds of plants and mixed with wax and resin. It is used to repair the hive, and to protect it from predators like viruses, bacteria, fungi and various microbes and diseases. It maintains the temperature and health of the hive *(Park et al 2002)*.

Not surprisingly, it can be extremely useful in fighting various infectious diseases. A range of safe and positive effects has been identified – for example, it is highly effective with:

- Wound healing.
- Skin infections.
- Tissue repair.
- Gastro-intestinal problems.

The actual content of bee propolis depends on the geographic location of the bees and the time of year *(Banskota et al 2000)*. Propolis often comprises more than **180 natural compounds, many of which are concentrates of powerful antioxidant plant flavenoids and phenols.** The bees seem to understand the importance of The Rainbow Diet! Bee propolis is now also known to have:

- Anaesthetic benefits
- Immuno-modulating benefits
- Anti-inflammatory benefits
- Antioxidant benefits
- Cardiovascular benefits

- Cancer prevention and treatment benefits

Sources: Brazilian bee propolis (Green Propolis from *Baccharis dracunculifolia*) has been the subject of many serious clinical studies, and according to *PubMed*, accounts for over 26 per cent of all new research. Because the 'ingredients' of bee propolis can vary greatly, I will confine the rest of this piece to Brazilian green propolis. (Much of the research detail comes from an article published in the *International Journal of Cancer Research 3 (1); 43-53 2007)*.

Eat-to-beat cancer benefits: Brazilian bee propolis has significant and varied anti-cancer benefits, some of which will surprise many orthodox experts. Furthermore, it has been shown to enhance the benefits of chemotherapy and radiotherapy, having a protective effect on healthy cells and an enhancing effect on chemotherapy action.

(i) **Anti-inflammatory action**

Propolis has been shown to inhibit prostaglandin, leukotriene and histamine release *(Khayyal et al 1993; Mirzoeva and Calder 1996; Hepsen et al 1999)*. In each case the response was as good as the recommended prescription drug *(Menezes et al 1999)*. Propolis was even found to overcome formaldehyde induced arthritis. Typical active ingredients were the flavenoid hesperidins *(Hata and Beyer 2004)*.

(ii) **Anti-yeast; anti-bacterial; anti-viral**

Various research studies have confirmed bee propolis effectiveness against all the principle strains of *Staphylococcus, Escherichia coli, salmonella, E coli, Candida albicans* and even *HIV*. A number of flavenoids seem particularly important, especially kaempferol, pinocembrin and galangine. Controls were taken using prescription drugs such as AZT, the anti-AIDS drug. Moronic acid in propolis had significant anti-HIV effect, out-scoring the AZT drug.

(iii) Wound healing

Propolis has been found to have antiseptic, anaesthetic and healing powers. It has been shown to have a healing effect in the tissue repair of oral mucosa *(Bretz et al 1998)* – hence the use of Manuka by Christie Hospital, Manchester, after orthodox therapies for patients with mouth or throat problems. It is also effective as a 5 per cent mouthwash after dental surgery *(Carvahlo 1994)*. Post operative wounds – for example after cancer surgery – in subcutaneous tissues were more quickly healed with a compress of propolis, honey and comfrey ointment *(Magro-Filho 1987)*.

(iv) Immune stimulant

The ester of caffeic acid (CAPE) is one of the main active compound of propolis, along with the flavenoids quercitin and hesperidine. They seem to have two actions. Firstly, they inhibit cellular growth and secondly, they increase the presence of certain white immune cells like T-lymphocytes, also increasing hydrogen peroxide production without any simultaneous and damaging nitrite production, which usually occurs with macrophage activity. *(Than et al 2003; Ansorge et al 2003)*

(v) Free radical scavenging

The many flavenoids give propolis its powerful antioxidant benefits. *Matsushige et al; 1996* isolated a compound from propolis to show that it had a stronger antioxidant benefit than vitamins C and E.

(vi) DNA protection

CAPE, even when used in low doses, can prevent cellular mistakes in healthy cells and induce apoptosis (cell death) in cancer cells. Thus it seems to have a double benefit of protecting healthy cells whilst killing cancer cells. *(Chen et al 2003)*. This selective effect was previously shown by *Su et al; 1995*.

(vii) Anti-tumour effect

The ability to protect healthy DNA was confirmed by *Banskota et al; 2001*, and by *Suzuki et al; in 2002*. They both also noted that propolis had anti-tumour activity. The ability to kill cancer cells has been shown both *in vitro* and in animal *in vivo* studies. The particular ingredient responsible is Artepillin C, which leads to cancer cells' DNA fragmentation *(Kimoto et al; 1998)*. Kimoto has also shown that intra-tumoural injections of 500 mgs of Artepillin C produced apoptosis and an increase in immune defences.

CAPE and another 20 ingredients of propolis were tested by *Nagaoka et al; 2002*. Four were found to cause cancer cell death. Where CAPE was taken orally by mice with lung tumours, a reduction of tumour size of 50 per cent was noted. Researchers similarly tested another group of mice using the drug cisplatine. No difference in effectiveness was noted, but the mice taking the drug had significant weight loss, a side-effect not noted with propolis *(Nagaoka et al; 2003)*. It was concluded that CAPE had a cytoxic effect, and could also block the invasive metastasis noted with these tumours.

(viii) Enhancement of orthodox chemotherapy approaches

Propolis has biological effects that act in synergy with chemotherapy drugs such as 5-fluoracil *(Suzuki et al; 2002)*.

Importantly, *Santos and Cruz, 2001* showed that the antioxidant properties of propolis could reduce the side-effects caused by chemotherapy drugs without any detriment to the therapeutic effects.

Suzuki researched two drugs in experiments with mice and cancer (mitomicine C and 5- fluoresce) and showed that the combination of drug plus propolis had by far the greatest regression effects, especially in advanced stages, over the drugs used on their own. The propolis usage resulted in higher levels of white and red cells and less side effects. The conclusion of the research was that propolis increased the bio-availability of the drugs. The desired effect could therefore logically be achieved on smaller doses and with even fewer side-effects.

Orsolic and Basic (2005) used mice with breast tumours to show antioxidants can enhance the performance of both radiotherapy and chemotherapy, by using water soluble bee propolis. This supports the work of Chan, noted above, that CAPE has a cytoxic effect and can cause cell death, whilst protecting the DNA of healthy cells. 'Chemotherapy agents used in anti-metastatic activity have their benefits enhanced' was again the conclusion. The authors recommended clinical trials should take place as all the indications were for greater effect in radio- and chemotherapy, whilst minimising blood cell declines and other side-effects.

Padmavathi et al (2005) studied the drug paclitaxel with propolis, in DMBA-induced mice breast cancer and concluded that the two in combination suppressed breast cancer, decreased lipid peroxidation, and increased the activities of antioxidant enhanced super oxide dismutase and vitamin C. They concluded that the combination of paclitaxel and propolis offers maximum effect in DMBA-induced breast cancer.

Overall

I have provided an extended look at bee propolis.

Firstly, because it is a 'super-concentrate' of a **rainbow diet** of natural compounds. The bees have done it for you. It is what this book is all about. They have partaken of 180 natural compounds from all manner of plants whose pigments and colour attracted them.

Secondly, because, yet again, these natural compounds have research that shows they can provide wonderful health benefits.

Thirdly, because it can help you beat cancer.

Fourthly, because it can increase the effectiveness of radiotherapy and chemotherapy, whilst reducing the side-effects and protecting healthy cells. Something too many oncologists in the UK deny is possible.

Eat-to-beat cancer?

Now, do you believe me? Of course, there will always be someone who quibbles with this or that study. But the sheer volume of studies now coming to the fore is hard to argue with. And in this book I have a fifth of what is on the CANCERactive website. Adding these bioactive natural compounds into your diet, in a way that they can combine synergistically and enhance the effects of each other, is going to increasingly be shown as the way our diets worked 200 years ago. Then we ate honey, and herbs like parsley, sage, rosemary and thyme, and lovage and feverfew. And basic vegetables like turnips, beetroot, watercress, cabbage, broccoli, sprouts, peas, broad beans, tomatoes, potatoes, parsnips and carrots. And fruits like apples, pears, quince and black and red currants, gooseberries and berries from the hedgerows.

This 'rainbow' diet of vibrant colours protected us and nourished us – it almost certainly 'corrected' and healed us too. And what we can learn from the French Paradox and all the research I have put to you in this chapter is that it is very, very powerful.

While the French Paradox diet shows they eat more fat (both good and bad), the vibrancy of the rest of the diet corrects the excesses. So too, if they err and consume a little added sugar. The protective and corrective epigenetic benefits are found in at least 60 common food compounds and I have listed some of these in Appendix II.

This highlights the current problem in the UK. We go for a 'junk meal', but then we do nothing to nourish, protect and correct in return. The message of the Rainbow Diet is clear. It doesn't matter if you stray from the path of food righteousness a little, as long as you eat a lot of different corrective foods to compensate. Diets shouldn't be restrictive, and the Rainbow Diet isn't. It is a diet of what to add into your weekly meals, not a diet of what to leave out. Nowhere is this shown better than in *'Rainbow Recipes'* our new book.

CHAPTER 25
EAT-TO-BOOST YOUR IMMUNE SYSTEM

How do I boost my immune system?

It is one of the questions most asked of our charity staff. People who want to prevent disease know that a strong immune system will give them better protection. People who have something wrong with them understand that their immune system has failed them.

I'd make a terrible doctor. You see, if I had just diagnosed someone sitting in front of me as having a cancer I'd be saying, *'Right, before I send you off for surgery, radiotherapy or chemotherapy, let's sort out two things:*

Firstly, what might have caused your cancer – and so could still be there maintaining it? We'll then do our best to remove the threat.

Secondly, let's do everything in our power to re-boot your immune system so it is as strong as possible, before you have any debilitating orthodox therapies'.

While the full answer to the first question is outside of the scope of this book and better answered with *'Everything you need to know to help you beat cancer'*, I hope that by now you feel that bioactive natural compounds and 'good diet' can correct causes like 'poor diet', some infections and even some toxins. And where it cannot correct, it could well hold the symptoms at bay. Good diet is a clear part of the way you can boost your immune system. But other factors are important.

Boosting your immune system: a summary

1. **The liver** is the organ of detoxification in the body and in cancer patients it becomes toxic. To recap:

   * Fats and cholesterol 'clog it up' anyway.
   * There may be dead bacteria, microbes or even parasites.
   * The cholesterol can collect around dead cells and form

gallstones – there may be thousands of these particles, most only the size of grains of sand. One US estimate was that 99.99 per cent of cancer patients had gallstones blocking the bile ducts so the liver could not excrete the toxins into the waste system properly.
- Then there is the lactic acid from cancer cells. Plus the drugs from steroids to chemotherapy that must be detoxified. And then there may be lots of dead cancer cells.

You need to:
- Strengthen your liver – milk thistle, magnesium, curcumin, vitamin K, dandelion, artichoke may all help
- Clean it out – a detox of olive oil and Epsom Salts should do the trick
- Dilate the bile ducts to enhance excretion of toxins – boldo tea or a series of coffee enemas might help.

You also need to clean up your lymph.
- Lower bad fat consumption anyway – it blocks the flow.
- Consume eight pints of good quality water a day
- Move your lymph everyday. Half an hour of light exercise like yoga, T'ai Chi or swimming to move the lymph in your thoracic duct.

2. **Exercise** improves the immune system. Apart from moving the lymph to take toxins away from cells; it oxygenates the blood, strengthens your body, increases levels of happy endorphins and Human growth hormone, both of which can reduce levels of 'bad hormones' and neutralise free-radicals. Plus it starts to dissolve visceral fat, the fat you cannot see but the fat that is holding toxins around your internal organs. Half an hour every day is the level you need and it does not have to be strenuous.

3. **Eat a Rainbow Diet** across the week. A rainbow of colour and foods from red peppers, raspberries, pomegranates and cherries; to oranges, papaya and apricots; to yellow pineapples, grapefruit, ginger and nuts; to greens, onions, apples; to blues and red-purples like beetroot, plums, figs, aubergines. And, yes,

there are some supplements you can add to this like resveratrol, grape seed extract and curcumin.

4. **Sunshine** can boost the immune system because it causes the production of vitamin D from cholesterol under your skin. Sunshine boosts your whole immune system. If you cannot get at least 30 to 40 minutes in the sunshine every day, think about supplementing with 1000 to 5000 IUs of vitamin D3. And don't forget the vitamin K which helps the action of vitamin D. You can derive enough from a good helping of greens (assuming you have good gut flora present). If unsure you can supplement with vitamin K.

5. **HUG yourself.** Rebuild your gut and your health with the HUG protocol. **Your gut microbiome controls the strength and memory of your immune system.** You cannot get better until your gut gets better. Hold; Eliminate; Replenish; Heal (Page 142).

6. **Antioxidants**

A) Research shows that vegetables and fruit provide more antioxidants from their natural compounds than are derived from synthetic vitamin supplements – providing you EAT WHOLE FOODS and that they are ORGANIC.

Top natural food sources for the everyday antioxidants are:

Vitamin E: 2 tablespoons of sunflower seeds (11 mgs); 20 almonds (8 mgs); 1 tablespoon wheat germ (3mgs).
Vitamin C: 1 large red pepper (224 mgs); 100 gms raw broccoli (90 mgs) 150 gms papaya (90 mgs); 1 large orange (65 mgs).
Beta-carotene: 1 cup carrot juice (24 mgs); 1 medium sweet potato (10.0 mgs) 5 dried apricots (6.2 mgs); 1 cup cherries (6.2 mgs); half cup cooked spinach (5.7 mgs).
Zinc: 6 oysters (55 mgs), 1 medium steak (8 mgs); 4 tablespoons sunflower seeds (96mgs); serving of All Bran (4 mgs).

Selenium: 4 cracked Brazil nuts (150 mcgs); 4 slices of wholemeal bread (60 mcgs); 2 tablespoons sunflower seeds (15 mcgs); 1 free range egg (15 mcgs); 1 chicken breast (10 mcgs).

Lycopene: Tomatoes – 1 tin tomato soup (65 mgs); 5 tablespoons tomato paste (22 mgs).

B) You may still wish to supplement.

The best immune booster in US research was grape seed extract. But as an OPC it is not as powerful as pine bark extract, which was not included in the research. Another good immune booster is curcumin, which has significant other cancer-fighting properties too.

The best herbs are echinacea, cat's claw and particularly astragalus. Tinctures seem especially effective for herbs, rather than pills.

Other supplements to consider are:

(i) **<u>Minerals</u>:**

Zinc: 15 mgs per day

Selenium: 200 mcgs per day

(ii) **<u>Vitamins</u>:**

Vitamin E – Natural, 8 forms, **Total Vitamin E** – 400 IUs per day, **Coenzyme Q10** 30 – 50 mgs per day

You may take a B complex if you are worried about whether or not you have healthy gut flora to release the biotin, niacin, choline and B-12 you need from your whole food. Instead of common beta-carotene supplement consider **chlorella**.

C) You may also consider boosting your polysaccharide levels with the foods I mentioned before, like whole brown rice to medicinal mushrooms. Above all, boost your natural fibre intake. A supplement called **MGN-3 Biobran** has some impressive research behind it as do beta-glucans in supplements like **Immiflex.**

7. **Take fish oils.** The importance of reducing inflammation is not just confined to certain cells but aids the whole immune system. In 2011 research it was found that daily fish oil supplementation was far superior in omega-3 delivery than merely eating oily fish everyday. Olive oil has a supercharging effect on the benefits of long-chain omega-3 from fish oils and *vice versa*. Curcumin, resveratrol, aspirin, garlic and ginger are also important.

8. **Laugh** – laughter boosts the immune system and moves your lymph. So see friends, watch old movies you like, old comedy shows, and go and see a show. Cut all the people and things out of your life that make you feel guilty, stressed or depressed. Let no one put you down.

CHAPTER 26
FOOD FOR THOUGHT

Cooking tips

While many extol the benefits of raw food, others believe juicing helps to break up cellular structures and release minerals and enzymes. Many believe lightly cooking, blanching or steaming helps digestion and absorption.

Research from The University of Grenada in 2016 shows that flash frying vegetables in Olive Oil locks in more of the nourishment. For example, while boiling vegetables loses polyphenol content, levels go up if you sauté in extra virgin olive oil, according to the study.

Spit roasting is common in the Mediterranean – it leaves little fat content. Roasting is good as long as it is done slowly with the temperature below 120°C, especially for potatoes, to avoid acrylamide formation.

Wood or coal barbecues are poor ideas: Smoke and flames burn the meat and increase levels of highly carcinogenic nitrosamines. Use an electric grill, or 'fake' charcoal (but it's really gas) grill. Best to grill by wrapping the fish in foil before putting it on the barbecue.

Fried food is linked to higher rates of hormonally driven cancers, and men who eat fried food regularly have a three-fold increase in cancer risk.

Microwaves polarise general opinion but not mine! In one study, Kirlian photography (which shows the energetic forces naturally occurring around a body or a plant) showed a strong field around broccoli both in its raw state and after steaming – but absolutely no energetic aura after just one second in a microwave. Every atom in every molecule in your food has electrons spinning in specific defined ways. In a microwave the atoms are energised to heat the food and it is absolutely impossible to expect all the electrons to be in the places they should have been when you turn off the microwave. You are eating irradiated, genetically modified food. William Kopp studied German and

Russian papers on the subject and concluded that microwaved food is nutritionally deficient, and increases the number of cancerous cells circulating in the bloodstream. Beware, some restaurant chains only serve microwaved foods. Many restaurants use microwaves to defrost food.

Slow cooked stews are actually full of nourishment with the temperature lower than would allow nitrosamines or acrylamides to form.

'Wok cooking' in South East keeps the oil to a minimum. (In Asia water, and oyster or fish sauce are more often used, not oil.) Vegetables are served crisper and retain higher nourishment values because they are cooked for shorter times.

Eating tips

- Eat 5-6 meals a day – not one or two big ones. 'Graze' don't stuff.
- Prepare some healthy snacks in the morning to eat during the day – slice vegetables to dip in olive oil/balsamic dressing; or a bowl of sunflower, pumpkin, sesame and linseeds with a few chopped nuts.
- Eat some raw vegetables as a snack about 20 minutes before you eat your lunch or dinner. Your hormones will then tell you to feel less hungry when you come to the main meal and you absorb up to 40 per cent more vitamins and minerals by eating them this way.
- Don't drink water shortly before, during or after the meal – you don't need to. And it will dilute your digestive enzymes and reduce the nourishment taken from your food.
- Eat slowly and think about the food – don't watch TV or read the paper – you will eat too fast, and may produce stress hormones that can affect the digestive process.
- Food is for enjoyment – it is not fuel.
- If you ever say, 'I'm starving', you are ill. Few people in the Western world know what 'starving' is.
- Chew well or the carbohydrates will not be digested – they need the ptyalin from your saliva glands. If you don't digest your carbohydrates properly you will not get full nourishment, and you may become constipated.

- Only put food that is whole in your mouth. Your body deserves nothing less.
- Eat less than you need to fill you up. Your stomach will tighten after a couple of days and you will eat less.
- If you feel hungry, drink a glass of water. It will curb your hunger.
- If you believe you may have yeasts, fruit should always be consumed first, at the start of the meal and on an empty stomach. Otherwise digested soft fruit and sugars can sit on top of a meal in your stomach and colon and ferment. People on anti-yeast diets need to avoid this complication as the fermentation aids the growth of yeasts. Very sweet fruits are also to be avoided in this scenario. For healthy people without a yeast problem fruits may be eaten at any time.
- Vegetables, pulses and oats, for example, contain soluble fibre. This is essential to the alimentary canal, where it dissolves, transports and helps excrete toxins and excess hormones. Organic, whole, brown rice should be your staple carbohydrate as it is particularly good at cleansing your system.
- Green tea (especially decaffeinated) is a strong antioxidant and helps to balance any acidity in the food you have eaten. Red wine has similar benefits. It's OK to drink a glass of red wine!
- Do not eat carbohydrate and protein at the same time. In the wild, our natural environment saw us find tubers and eat them, or gorge at a fruit tree, or capture an animal. We didn't take them all back to the cave and eat them on the same plate. Your digestive system is not designed for this total simultaneous consumption.

Let me explain: The carbohydrate and protein mixture passes to the stomach where it needs an alkaline environment for maximum efficiency. Carbohydrate on its own clears the stomach in about one hour. Protein on the other hand passes to the stomach where it meets its digestive enzyme pepsin and this requires an acid environment. Protein on its own can be digested in about one and a half hours.

But mix the two and the stomach doesn't know whether to be alkaline or acid, with the result that the food is improperly digested and takes up to eight hours to pass through. This results in inefficiency throughout the intestinal system. Digestion of protein is also further hampered in the over-50s who anyway produce less acid.

It is particularly important to people over 50 that they avoid mixing protein and carbohydrate on the same fork! Levels of acid in the stomach can anyway decline by 30 per cent after 50 making digestion and absorption of key vitamins a problem.

Meal making tips

- Get planting – why not plant some fruit trees in a sunny area? Wisley Royal Gardens have fruit trees for all sizes of gardens.
- Grow some vegetables and fruits yourself. Runner beans, perpetual spinach, gooseberries, raspberries are all very easy.
- Have a little herb garden – you can even do this in pots on a patio or balcony.
- Sprout some seeds – buy Mung beans, or even broccoli seeds and put them in a covering of water on a little tray for three days in the window.
- Find a supplier of organic meat – chicken, game and so on.
- Eat more spices – flavour vegetables with turmeric, or saffron.
- Eat more salads – can you grow your own? Add olive oil or walnut oil – throw out the mayonnaise.
- Make your own breakfast – organic muesli from whole grains, dried fruits, sunflower seeds, pumpkin seeds, crushed pecan nuts and a few psyllium seeds or linseeds.
- Find a supplier of organic fruit and vegetables.
- Make your own bread without refined wheat, sugar or salt.
- Buy a good juicer and make your own juices using nourishing vegetables and fruit like carrots, ginger, and apples.
- Buy a reverse osmosis, remineraliser water filter to provide water for cooking and washing utensils.
- Talk to the local restaurant for the phone number of a supplier of glass-bottled mineral water for drinking.
- Make your own nourishing soups.

CHAPTER 27

THE RAINBOW DIET: EATING A SPECTRUM OF BENEFITS

The Ten Truths

From the outset I have told you ten truths about cancer:

1. Your cancer is as individual as you are – there are many causes.
2. It is not an item – it is a process.
3. It has many stages, many facets.
4. There will never be a magic bullet that can tackle all the causes and stages, simultaneously.
5. For thousands of years we have developed 'illnesses', almost without 'knowing'. Our inbuilt body systems are usually strong enough to correct and heal them. One Danish study reported that we each may develop cancer 6 times in our lifetimes.
6. This illness and healing struggle doesn't stop the moment a doctor tells you that you have cancer.
7. The factors that caused a cancer in your body could still be maintaining it.
8. Your defences are almost certainly weakened, and unable to cope.
9. The principles of prevention and correction are much the same – but the major difference is that there are fewer steps to tackle in prevention, more to tackle when correcting.
10. A multi-step development process demands a multi-step programme to tackle it.

'Protection' and 'Correction' using natural compounds

The only potential multi-stage protective and corrective programme available to you is consuming a spectrum of natural compounds in food – unless someone in power somewhere is contemplating cancer patients taking 50 different drugs to combat 50 different possible causes and steps in the cancer process!

Only food and natural compounds have the width to tackle all the steps necessary to both protect and correct.

Each of us has two options. Either work for a biochemistry degree, then a nutrition degree; accurately plan the multistep process that is cancer and then take specific corrective steps against the stages you may have. Or, adopt the width of the Rainbow Diet!

Only food and natural compounds have the spectrum of benefits capable of delivering.

Only food and natural compounds have the ability to be used in combination and volume without side-effects or debilitating consequences.

And finally many natural compounds seem to have a synergistic effect enhancing the effect of each other and often following different pathways to healing.

And before self-styled 'quack-buster' professors rush to put pen to paper in Medical Journals, or overweight nurses think to throw more books at us, they should know that many micro-biologists and biochemists in universities and pharmaceutical companies are actively working at this very moment on natural compounds and trying to make synthetic versions they can patent and therefore profit from. I can list any number of natural compounds that are being concentrated and reformulated right now – from vitamin D to quercitin – how many do you want?

The pharmaceutical companies know that natural compounds are capable of repairing damaged DNA, of reducing levels of bad oestrogen, of preventing tumour formation and of killing cancer cells. They know natural compounds can help their drugs identify cancer cells, help the immune system identify cancer cells and even help reduce side effects.

Eminent professors will agree that a 'Good Diet' will prevent cancer. Why won't the same people own up to the fact that a spectrum of natural compounds that covers all the bases can be corrective, too, not simply protective, if you can eat enough of them?

But what is enough? Already we have seen that just one glass of organic red wine a day has a significant effect, and half a cup of raspberries. Preventing, and correcting.

Let us change the paradigm. When research on natural compounds takes place it nearly always studies just **one** ingredient – at best, a couple of vitamins. And that's why when studies on high doses of vitamin C in Arizona show that a number of cancer cells have their oxygen levels increased and it kills them, 'orthodox medical experts' rush to belittle the findings and the compounds by saying, '*It's not a cure for cancer*'.

No, it isn't – but then nor is Herceptin, or Tamoxifen.

Let's get it clear – to effectively beat cancer – whether preventing or healing – the best approach involves width, a spectrum, a rainbow of pigments, active ingredients, natural compounds to work together and cover all the bases. Vitamin C used as part of a much bigger package will do a job but not the whole job.

In my view natural compounds

* are easier to obtain,
* are much cheaper,
* have few or no side-effects,
* have been through 'clinical trials' for 200,000 years,
* have the necessary WIDTH to do the job, when taken in combination.

A multi-step programme?

In Chapter 1, I told you that I would show you by the end of this book how a spectrum of natural compounds could tackle the various stages of cancer – protecting and correcting. Healing the daily illnesses. Let's see if I have done this. (You can cross-reference any of the following, by using the glossary/index at the back of the book).

* **Providing important factors to perfect DNA copying**
  For example: Folic acid (Sources: leafy green vegetables, avocado, pulses, carrots, apricots) is able to help here.
  For example: Anthocyanins protect the DNA and reduce copying errors (Sources: Purple colour foods like beetroot, blackcurrants, dark olives, elderberry, figs, deep red plums, red grapes,

blueberries, blackberries, aubergine, red onion, red cabbage).

* **Providing important factors to correct DNA mis-copying**

For example: Genistein promotes levels of repair proteins in cells.

For example: Resveratrol repairs and boosts repair genes (red grapes, blackberries).

For example: I have told you how bee propolis protects healthy DNA whilst helping attack cancer cells.

* **Avoiding excesses of factors that increase free-radicals**

For example: I have told you how smoking, trans fats, saturated fats, acrylamides, microwave cooking and other poor diet factors can cause increases in free-radicals.

For example: I have told you about calorie control. And the effect of sirtuins and resveratrol.

* **Providing more antioxidants to neutralise free-radicals**

For example: I have told you that OPC's (pine bark, grape seed) are 20-50 times stronger antioxidants than most high street antioxidant supplements. They are also found in apples, pears and cranberries. Lemongrass is another powerful anti-oxidant.

For example: I have told you about many natural compound antioxidants like curcumin, and the benefits of sleep and melatonin.

* **Removing the toxic chemicals and heavy metals from your body and cells**

For example: I have told you of the benefits of beneficial bacteria in conjunction with chlorella and lignans.

For example: I have told you about selenium.

For example: I have told you about indoles and dioxin elimination.

* **Boosting your immune system and helping it 'see' rogue cells**

For example: I have told you about how polysaccharide-rich foods like medicinal mushrooms can boost your white cells and help inter-cellular communication.

For example: I have told you of the benefits of grape seed extract and how astragalus helps your immune system 'see' the rogue cell. But I have told you how it doesn't work without vitamin D molecules, and maybe vitamin K.

For example: I have told you of the benefits of having healthy gut flora and the possible need to supplement with multi-strain probiotics, chlorella and flaxseed.

* **Keeping your cells and immune system alkaline**

For example: I have told you how eating potassium and magnesium rich foods (lentils, whole potato, broad beans, peas, whole grains, nuts, bananas) and avoiding sodium foods can achieve this.

* **Avoiding parasite and microbial infection**

For example: I have told you the natural compounds that can kill most parasites (cloves, wormwood herb, fennel, garlic).

For example: I have told you the natural compounds that can kill *Helicobacter pylori* like goldenseal herb, curcumin and olive oil.

For example: I have told you which natural compounds kill yeasts (coconut, garlic, oregano) and given you a diet.

* **Minimising pathogens in the blood stream**

For example: I have told you about several natural compounds like quercitin, which is an natural antibiotic (onions, apples, honey)

For example: Ellagic acid is anti-bacterial and anti-viral (sources: pomegranate, raspberries, walnuts)

For example: Pau d'Arco is anti-viral, anti-bacterial, anti-fungal.

* **Reducing inflammation – a precursor of many cancers**

For example: I have told you how the COX-2 enzyme can be turned off by fish oils, aspirin, aloe vera, ginger and phenols, for example in olive oil and green tea

For example: I have told you about the many active

ingredients in bee propolis

* **Preventing a blood supply to the developing tumour**

   For example: I have told you the benefits of sulphur compounds like sulphoraphanes and garlic; and also about isoflavones.

* **Lowering aggressive oestradiol levels**

   For example: I have told you about indoles (sources: Greens, cabbage, broccoli).
   For example: I have told you about melatonin and asphalia.
   For example: I have told you about phytoestrogens and genistein (sources: red clover and pulses).

* **Keeping blood and cellular oxygen levels up**

   For example: I have told you the benefits of regular daily exercise, supported by vitamin C and especially foods that contain glutathione (Sources: most fruits and vegetables especially green ones).

* **Strengthening your liver, and therefore your immune system**

   For example: I have told you about the benefits of a liver flush using Epsom Salts and olive oil.
   For example: I have told you the benefits of magnesium, soya lecithin, and of coffee enemas and of the herbs boldo and dandelion in the elimination of toxins.

* **Increasing your pancreatic enzyme production**

   For example: I have told you about chromium picolinate and about a low glycaemic/whole food diet.

* **Killing cancer cells**

   For example: I have told you about vitamin D and its ability to change the cancer cell and its process back to those of a healthy cell.
   For example: I have told you about niacin, and sodium butyrate produced by beneficial bacteria and how these chemicals can kill cancer cells. And how sulphoraphanes can stop cancer cells forming, and kill ones already in place,

especially if helped by selenium

For example: I have told you about nitrilosides (sources: bitter natural foods like quince, almonds, macadamia nuts, gooseberries, papaya, bamboo shoots, yams and sprouting seeds).

For example: I have told you about research on chapperal; on capsaicin (source: chilli peppers) and on sulphoraphanes (Source: sprouting seeds)

For example: I have told you about quercitin and its ability to heat up cancer cells and kill them.

* **Increases survival rates**

For example: I have told you about the big research studies – the China Study and Su.Vi Max studies on antioxidants vitamin E, C, beta carotene and zinc and selenium and how they reduce mortality from cancer.

Phew! In fact I've told you about much more than this – about the wonderful width of benefits that natural compounds have – but do not forget the great reduction fertilisers, pesticides and herbicides have on their levels.

A fundamental truth

We've seen that the diet therapies of Gonzalez and Pfeifer are quite rigorous and disciplined, as are some exponents of Gerson and Plasket. They cover all the bases. John Boik did exactly that too – perfect if you are a scientist or doctor.

But the rest of us are just ordinary folk trying in our own ways to get a little reassurance and discipline into our diets, and give ourselves the very best odds of beating a cancer. And I believe the answer is exactly the same as these professionals employ – and that is width. A discipline that is simple to use, and goes right across the many stages of cancer.

And for this reason I am far more in favour of the French Diet with hints of the Macrobiotic discipline than the Vegetarian, South East Asian, or whatever. For me the French Diet, and particularly the Mediterranean Diet, has a corrective enormity. It also acknowledges a fundamental truth that comes out of the studies on these natural compounds. And that is that there are foods around us, in our local environments, that we have eaten fresh and in season for thousands of years, **and they work with our bodies to protect and correct us all day long.** They heal our illnesses.

We no longer consume:

- Radishes, red peppers and raspberries.
- Turmeric, oranges and honey.
- Fresh nuts, ginger and seeds.
- Spinach, broccoli, watercress, Brussels sprouts and quince.
- Oily fish, clean water.
- Beetroot, cherries, pomegranate.
- Blackberries, seeds and figs.
- Herbs like oregano, marjoram, sage and thyme.
- Mushrooms, of several varieties.
- Onions, spring onions, garlic.

And this is why I find the Government's standard of '*Eat 5 portions of fruit and vegetables a day*', completely meaningless. According to research people rarely eat more than two a day in Britain and think chips count as one of these helpings and even pizzas with tomato sauce! My personal shorthand is not five a day or 25 a day. I believe you just need to put some colour back into your life. Vibrancy on your plate to put vibrancy in your life.

Research in 2013 from Harvard Medical School and Brigham and Women's Hospital in Boston, *(Annals of Internal Medicine)* certainly endorses this point about vibrancy in your life. Apparently middle-aged women who follow a Mediterranean diet increase their life spans, avoiding physical or cognitive impairments and chronic illnesses in older age. Researchers concluded that those who closely followed a Rainbow Diet were 'Healthy agers' and more likely to live past age 70 without heart disease, diabetes or other chronic diseases.

CHAPTER 28
THE RAINBOW DIET: THE SHOPPING TROLLEY

The Ten Commandments?

First read out loud:

1. I will try to avoid salt and sugar, and processed and packaged foods.
2. I will try to avoid dairy.
3. I will try to avoid fizzy soft drinks, fruit juices and smoothies, sweeteners and refined products.
4. I will put only whole foods in my mouth.
5. I will supplement – but I will only use natural supplements.
6. I will grow more of my own foods.
7. I will eat more fresh foods; living foods – especially those that are locally grown and in season.
8. I will try to find a supplier I can trust to supply organic food without pesticides.
9. I will only drink clean water.
10. I will fill my kitchen and my plate each week with the colours of the Rainbow.

Be inspired. There is so much to choose from and to enjoy.

Eat a Rainbow

No longer will you struggle to eat five portions of fruit and vegetables a day. No longer will you feel guilty if you've eaten something naughty. Instead you are going to have two large flat plates or bowls sitting in your kitchen – one of vegetables and the other of fruit. And each is going to have a rainbow of wonderful colours in them.

Reds for ellagic acid in raspberries, and lycopene in tomatoes. Orange for carotenoids and carrots, peppers and apricots. Yellow for honey and propolis. Greens for polyphenols, indoles, and sulphoraphanes, or apples and onions for quercitin, herbs for their cancer killing powers and anti-microbe strength. Blues for pterostilbene and blueberries. Indigo and Violet: try aubergines, beetroot and dark plums for anthocyanins; cherries, blackberries and grapes for resveratrol. All washed down by a glass of red wine or a cup of green tea.

Research from Illinois University has shown that these natural compounds frequently affect different anti-cancer enzyme pathways; while research from Ohio State University has shown that these bioactive compounds have more effect, the more you eat. So, eat lots of different colours and lots of each colour. And take a daily dose of sunshine (30 minutes should be enough).

The shopping trolley

The best way to plan your healthy diet is to prevent yourself being weak-willed. Pre-plan and only bring healthy foods into your home. *"It is not the mountains we conquer, but ourselves"*, according to Sir Edmund Hillary. Sometimes we just need a little help towards that self-discipline.

Now I realise not all of these products are from the UK and locally grown but I wanted you to see a real width of possible products so you could choose for yourself. Here is a look at what your shopping trolley might contain:

RED:

Red peppers, tomatoes, tomato puree, pomegranates, raspberries, strawberries, red currants, cranberries, radish, red grapes, chilli peppers, watermelon.

ORANGE:

Oranges, apricots, peaches, turmeric, carrots, mangoes, papaya, yams, bananas, satsumas, clementines.

YELLOW:

Mushrooms, ginger, saffron, yellow peppers, fresh sweetcorn, squash, bamboo shoots, lemons, limes, melon, pineapple, nectarines, grapefruit, honey. Nuts – fresh Brazil, pecan, macadamia, walnuts, cashews.

GREEN:

Watercress, spinach, broccoli, greens, cabbage, kale, Brussels sprouts, chard, courgettes, avocados, green tea, fennel, green beans, runner beans, cauliflower, celery, apples, pears, asparagus tips, chives, spring onions, cucumber, lettuce, endive, leeks, green peppers, broad beans, peas, sprouting seeds, alfalfa, plums, green grapes, kiwi fruit.

PURPLE/BLUE:

Aubergines, red plums, figs, beetroot, blackberries, blueberries, blackcurrants, lentils, red kidney beans, wild and brown rice, Japanese mushroom, pumpkin seeds, cherries, dates.

WHITE/BROWN:

Oats, barley, buckwheat, millet, rye, clean water, potatoes, onions, garlic, parsnips, turnips, whole grain pasta, sunflower seeds, sesame seeds, psyllium seeds, lychees, swede, butter beans, chick peas, hummus, coconut milk, deep-sea caught fish, oysters, rice milk, soya milk, goat's milk, eggs, wheatgerm*.

HERBS and SPICES: Mint, sorrel, sage, thyme, coriander, nutmeg, cinnamon, lemon grass, saffron.

OILS: Extra virgin olive oil, walnut oil.

OTHER: Dried fruits, Quorn, red wine (Cabernet Sauvignon is best – especially organic), apricot kernels, eat the grape seeds.

POSSIBLE SUPPLEMENTS IF YOU THINK YOU NEED THEM
Multi-strain probiotics
Chlorella
Fish oils
Total (all 8 forms) vitamin E
Coenzyme Q10
Selenium
Zinc
Aloe vera
Resveratrol
Grape seed extract

Vitamin D3
Turmeric/curcumin
Quality mineral supplement
Occasional herbs – like astragalus, echinacea, cat's claw

NOTABLE OTHERS

You may like to include:

- Flaxseed/linseed, for omega-3
- Sodium bicarbonate, for alkalinity
- Organic apple cider vinegar for alkalinity
- Bee propolis
- Essiac (all 8 ingredients)

You could sprout your own seeds and grow your own wheatgrass (from kits); your salt can be Himalayan or Dead Sea; and your pepper black.

Just remember the school definition of the colours of the Rainbow: Red, Orange, Yellow, Green, Blue, Indigo, Violet.

(*You may prefer to avoid wheat)

CHAPTER 29
THE RAINBOW DIET: THE PROGRAMME

The Programme

The aim is to keep it simple. The aim is to bring only the good foods home. The aim is not to chastise yourself if you had baked beans and a sausage with the kids at tea. This is for fun. It's an indication of what you might attempt across a week.

The target is 100 points per day (especially for those with cancer). Eat what you want but beat the target, everyday. Have fun.

Daily Starting Score

This is your start point each day. You can get a head start if you watch out for the following:

1) If you do 30 minutes 'exercise' every day award yourself: + 15 points
2) If you filter your tap water with a reverse osmosis filter, and drink glass bottled water: + 15 points
3) If you sleep in a completely darkened room: + 5 points
4) If you are correct weight for your height: + 5 points
5) If you are 4 kgs overweight: – 3 points
6) If you are 10 kgs overweight: – 20 points
7) If you smoke at all: – 20 points
8) If you take a daily Probiotic multi-strain supplement: + 5 points
9) If the majority of your food is organic: + 10 points
10) If you have 30 minutes of sunshine – or supplement with vitamin D3 (1000 IUs):   + 5 points

Points for foods

All points have been assigned on a balance basis. For example, baked beans have the benefits of tomato (puree) and pulses, but the negatives of lots of sugar and salt and being canned.

Whole grain pasta is beneficial and achieves a positive score.

Normal pasta is worthless.

Fresh is best

Give yourself 3 points extra if you eat something organic, although strictly speaking, everything you eat should be organic.

This is meant to be a fun programme, so we have not assigned detailed weights or volumes.

The principle is that you can have your piece of lamb, if you really enjoy it, but put a tomato stuffed with garlic and parsley with it; perhaps some unrefined wild rice and lentils. This is how you pick up points and how you add in protective agents and eat to beat cancer.

It's not one single ingredient but the totality of the meal that matters.

10 Points (1 serving e.g. large serving spoon)

FRESH (IDEALLY LOCALLY GROWN) VEGETABLES AND FRUIT (LOW GI)

Alfalfa and sprouting seeds	Leeks
Apples	Lettuce (various)
Apricots	Olives
Berries	Onions
Beetroot	Parsnips
Broccoli	Peaches
Cabbage	Pears
Cauliflower	Pomegranates
Celery	Raspberries
Chard	Radishes
Cherries	Redcurrants
Chives	Spring onions
Cucumber	Sorrel
Endive	Spinach
Garlic (1 clove raw)	Squash
Ginger	Swede
Green beans	Tomatoes
Kale	Turnip
Kelp	Watercress

10 Points (continued)

FRESH NUTS
e.g. Almonds
     Brazils
     Cashews
     Pecans
     Macadamia nuts
     Walnuts

SEEDS
Pumpkin
Sesame
Sunflower
(N.B. Alcohol outside meal score -5)

OILS
Flaxseed oil
Linseed oil (linseeds)

CARBOHYDRATE AND GRAINS
Fresh boiled potato
Brown unrefined rice, wild rice
Oats, millet, barley, buckwheat
Unrefined grains

PULSES
e.g. Broad beans
     Butter beans
     Chickpeas
     Kidney beans
     Lentils
     Peas

DRINKS
1–2 modest glasses red
wine especially Cabernet
Sauvignon with meal

FLESH
Deep-sea caught oily fish

OTHER
Home-made muesli
Home-pressed fruit juices
Mushrooms – have
several types on your
plate

5 Points

IMPORTED FRUITS AND VEGETABLES AND DRIED FRUITS
e.g. Avocados
     Bamboo shoots
     Bananas
     Cranberries
     Currants and raisins
     Dates
     Dried fruits
     Figs
     Grapes

5 Points cont'd

Spicy chillies
Lemons
Lychees
Mangoes
Melons
Papayas
Peppers
Satsumas
Yams

OTHERS
Aloe vera
Eggs – poached, boiled (free range and organic)
Garlic (cooked)
Canned tomatoes

HERBS
Basil, fennel, coriander
Home-made bread (no salt, sugar – add seeds)
Honey
Hummus
Psyllium seeds
Spices – turmeric, chilli, cinnamon, nutmeg, saffron
Supermarket high grade muesli, or non-baked cereals

FLESH
Deep sea oily fish

2 Points

OTHER
Baked potato
Canned fish
Canned fruit
Coconut milk
Green tea – 1 cup
Natural oat bran
Organic lean chicken, turkey, game (max 1 serving per day. Any further serving – 5 points.)

2 Points cont'd

Potatoes (fresh) or mashed (no milk)
Quorn Soups (chilled)
Soya and soy milk
Spices – chilli, cinnamon and nutmeg Sweetcorn Tomato puree
(not ketchup)

OTHER FRUITS

1 orange (max. per day)

0 Points

Bagels
Baked beans
Herb teas
Jams
Marmalade
Muesli bars, cereal bars
Organic bread
Organic meat, poultry, game
Processed fruit juices
Shoyu and tamari soy sauce
Smoked fish
Soups

0 Points cont'd

Stir-frying
Sunflower, safflower oils
Tomato ketchup
White wine
Wholemeal bread

–5 Points

Alcopops
Any processed food, ready meals (e.g. instant noodles, packaged
soups), frozen meals
Beer, spirits, liqueurs
Biscuits
Bread, waffles – white or malted
Cakes

−5 Points cont'd

Chips
Chocolate snack products
Coffee
Crispbreads
Crisps, peanuts (salted)
Fizzy soft drinks
Mayonnaise
Pasta
Pizza
Processed breakfast cereals
Refined wheat, grains, sugar, rice
Salt
Smoked meats
Sweeteners
Tea

−10 Points

Any dairy/milk product/yoghurts
Bacon, pepperoni, frankfurters, sausages, dried meats, pâté, rilletes
Barbecued food
Fast food (e.g. burgers, chicken portions, chips)
Fried foods
Hydrogenated vegetable oils
Margarines
Microwaved food
Pickled foods
Chinese foods

Why not invest in a copy of our new book *'Rainbow Recipes'*, which I have co-authored with nutritional expert and Chef Barbara Cox?

CHAPTER 30
THE RAINBOW DIET: A POSTSCRIPT

'Food colours could hold the key to new cancer drugs'

Thus ran the heading in a UK Newspaper in 2010. Let me quote Dr Monica Giusti, from Ohio State University in Columbus. 'All fruits and vegetables that are rich in anthocyanins have compounds that can slow down the growth of cancer cells'. She went on to suggest that synthetic food dyes should be replaced by the use of anthocyanin-based pigments instead. What a good idea!

In a number of research studies at Ohio, experiments using a variety of foods have shown that cancer cell growth could be 'significantly' reduced and foods with the highest levels of active ingredients were most effective – what a surprise!

Scientists are now investigating concentrating the chemicals to provide a 'new generation of drugs'.

A search of the research shows that this is already happening and companies are currently looking at:

Anthocyanins – their use in killing cancer cells.

Indoles – to reduce levels of aggressive oestrogen, block receptor sites on cells and neutralise by-products of oestrogen.

Polyphenols – how they can repair DNA; and how they can kill rogue cells.

Polysaccharides – how they can improve communications between cells, especially enhancing the immune system to recognise and attack cancer cells.

Astragalus – how it can expose cancer cells to be recognised by the immune system.

Feverfew and some 18 other herbs – to isolate the active ingredient and concentrate it to kill cancer cells.

Wormwood and Pau d'Arco – both being studied for their active anti-viral ingredients.

Capsaicin – being studied for its ability to kill cancer cells directly.

Resveratrol – being studied for its ability to replicate calorie restriction benefits in the body, repair DNA and treat diseases from Alzheimer's to brain tumours.

And probably a hundred more.

While the pharmaceutical companies are concentrating these natural compounds you can be eating the benefits, today. And anyway, if they are herbs, concentrates already exist – they are called tinctures.

The truth is that the pharmaceutical companies, through their actions are clearly endorsing the benefits of these natural compounds – they deliver.

Why wait for the synthetic versions? You can start eating the powerful, organic natural versions of these compounds now. And the more you eat the greater the effect.

'Eating different natural compounds multiplies the effect'

The University of Illinois has been studying lycopene (from tomatoes) and indole-3-carbinol (from broccoli). Each is known to have a positive benefit with prostate cancer. John Erdman, Professor of Food Science, says that they are quite different substances and don't have to be eaten together to have an effect. But when combined, there effect seems to multiply up. They work on completely different anti-cancer pathways, but eating both in the same meal seems to have a much greater effect. We have seen this synergistic effect throughout this book.

Natural compounds can outperform drugs

In the same studies, Erdman concluded that the combined effect of broccoli and tomatoes had better results than the oestrogen-inhibitor Finasteride.

But then indole-3-carbinol is producing better results than

Tamoxifen, Pterostilbene produced better results than cipofibrate, ellagic acid was better than HPV-preventing drugs, and the herb Feverfew produced better results than the leukaemia drug cytarabine.

Christie Manchester has a novel way of treating infections of the mouth and throat after chemo- and radiotherapy. No more are they thinking of providing drugs. Instead they are turning to the natural anti-bacterial powers of Manuka honey.

In 2010 Spring **icon** we covered two news stories. One was for a 'breakthrough' biologic drug that cost $60,000 per year. It doesn't cure cancer, but it reduces tumour size by up to 30 per cent.

The other story concerned yet another study on medicinal mushrooms. American research confirmed previous Japanese studies that one medicinal mushroom, could completely overcome cancer tumours and the average effect was a 70 per cent reduction in size. Which would you rather have? The 70 per cent reducing food or the 30 per cent from the expensive drug?

I could list many more examples. Western cancer bodies are preoccupied with drugs. The pharmaceutical companies have an increasing, near total, control over cancer treatment. No longer are they trying to find a cancer cure. The new goal is cancer survival; the business is cancer management.

If an active ingredient is found in a food we are repeatedly told that drugs need to be formulated to concentrate the active ingredient and give it more power – I believe the answer to this is another natural food, rhubarb!

Can you imagine anything more stupid than this: A friend of mine, a British oncology professor, wants to test food effects on prostate patients to see if they will delay the need for surgery. Foods like broccoli. So he wants to dry them and put them into pill format. But the powers-that-be say 'No, that's now a drug. The pill must be made by a drug company.' And, of course, no drug company will do it for him.

This explains why the scientists at Leeds University did their polyp research not with omega-3 fish oil but using a 'drug', which was a concentrated form of omega-3.

The Rainbow Diet and cancer

On the very day the first edition of the Rainbow Diet went to print, the *British Journal of Cancer* reported a new Harvard Medical School study with the heading *'Mediterranean Diet Cuts Cancer Risk'*.

Lead author, Dr Dimitrios Trichopoulos, professor of cancer prevention and epidemiology at Harvard University, said "Our results show just how important diet is to cancer. Of the 26,000 people we studied, those who closely followed a traditional Mediterranean diet were less likely to develop cancer."

Importantly he added the following; a statement that lies behind my belief on the Rainbow Diet and nourishing your body with a WIDTH of ingredients: "Although eating more of one food group alone didn't significantly change a person's risk of cancer, adjusting one's overall habits towards the traditional Mediterranean diet had an important effect. Consuming more good fats (like those found in olive oil) rather than bad fats (like those founding chips, biscuits and cakes) had a the greatest effect, reducing cancer risk by 9 per cent.

The research also showed that making two changes to your diet, such as eating more peas, beans and lentils and less meat, could cut cancer risk by 12 per cent.

And the more changes made, the bigger the effect!"

Only recently another Harvard professor was talking about how we develop illnesses all the time – almost without knowing it – but provided we had the right nutrients in our bodies we corrected the problems.

You will see many more studies supporting the Mediterranean diet, and lifestyle. But you can smile in the knowledge that the real benefits come in the countries on the Northern shores, and the epicentre of low cancer and low heart disease isn't even on the Mediterranean!

One such study, released in June 2010, and published in the *American Journal of Clinical Nutrition (Trichopoulos et al)*, shows that post-menopausal women on the full diet were 22 per cent less likely to develop breast cancer than those who erred from the diet.

The Rainbow Diet and stress

I have explained that emotional stress can definitely cause cancer, contrary to what other UK charities tell you – whether simply through the eicosanoid system or through the damages to two genes discovered by the Yale team. Anyway, scientists working in epigenetics are quite clear about the message-blocking and gene-silencing capabilities of hormones like cortisol and epinephrine.

But even if stress didn't cause your particular cancer, it is important to understand that when you develop cancer your stress hormone levels increase. This is linked to heightened levels of inflammation throughout the body. It is one way the cancer helps drive its metastases.

UCLA have looked at this in great detail. They showed that *'people who went on Stress Management courses survived significantly longer'*. Stress Management can mean counseling. But other complementary therapies were listed in the UCLA report from numerous studies they have completed over the years. Transcendental Meditation is recorded as a powerful way to reduce damaging stress hormones, as is yoga (as we previously mentioned). Fish oils get a recommendation, but underpinning all, according to UCLA, should be *'a colourful, Mediterranean Diet'*.

Of course, you don't have to have cancer – the findings above would be good for anyone who feels stressed.

The Rainbow Diet and diabetes

At the start of the book I explained that my personal knowledge was confined to the studies crossing my desk about cancer, but that I felt the Rainbow Diet could be useful with all sorts of illnesses. I was therefore not surprised to come across this study on diabetes in May 2010.

Type-2 diabetes rates are growing dramatically in the modern world. Medical recommendations are usually 3-fold; To lose weight, to take drugs and to follow a low-fat, low cholesterol diet.

Researchers from the Naples Department of Geriatric and Metabolic Diseases, in Italy decided to study the medical recommendations regarding the Rainbow Diet in light of the

313

latter's good fat and protective foods content (fish oils, olive oil, nuts, seeds, lignans, carotenoids and lycopene).

They took 215 newly diagnosed Type-2 diabetes patients and put half on the medically recommended low-fat diet, and the other half on the Rainbow, Mediterranean Diet. Both groups were overweight.

After four years only 44 per cent of those on the Rainbow Diet needed prescription drugs, compared to 70 per cent of the group on the low-fat diet.

What was equally interesting was that, although both groups consumed the same number of calories on a daily basis and took the same levels of exercise, the group eating the Rainbow Diet lost significantly more weight.

As if to prove my point about how these studies are often ignored and repeated, in 2012 in Cancer Watch we covered a very similar study prepared jointly by the Second University of Naples and the Warwick Medical School in Coventry, England (Annals of Medicine). The newly diagnosed type-2 diabetes patients were divided into two matched groups, one given standard NHS recommended diet and the other the Mediterranean version. The latter group 'went significantly longer' before needing any drugs and those needing drugs required only half the level of those on the NHS recommended diet. Their conclusion was that the diet is better than the doctors' recommendations for type-2 diabetes.

The Rainbow Diet and depression

A review of 10,000 men by the University of Las Palmas, Spain, showed that the Mediterranean Diet could cut depression in adults by 30 per cent.

The Rainbow Diet and heart disease

A 'New Diet' involving a high intake of fruits and vegetables, whole grains, poultry fish and nuts combined with relatively low fat dairy products, and less sugar and red meat would help decrease the levels of cholesterol in the body according to Dr Marilyn Granville, a nutritionist. 'People should try as many different colours as possible; they need to eat a rainbow'.

Apparently, sugar enters the blood stream quickly causing high blood glucose and cholesterol, and this causes a problem when it oxidizes. High intakes of fruit and vegetables prevent this oxidation.

The 'New Diet' has been called the Dash Diet (Dietary Approaches to Stop Hypertension) and follows research entitled *'Circulation: Cardiovascular Quality and Outcomes'* in the *American Heart Journal*. This showed that eating a rainbow of fruit and vegetables reduced the risk of suffering heart disease by 18 per cent, and a reduction in LDL, or bad cholesterol, by 8 per cent *(The Independent, Sept 2010)*.

Epigenetics Rules. OK?

In Cancer Watch at CANCERactive over the last 5 years we have received no research on any drug tackling Triple Negative Breast Cancer. But we have received research on six bioactive natural compounds showing epigenetic benefits with TNBC – vitamin D, curcumin, indole 3 carbinol, bioactive compounds in blueberries, carotenoids and sulphoraphanes. No one is talking about any of these as a cure – but it's an important start and clearly something to consider in your Complementary and Integrative Treatment Programme.

As we have seen through the course of the book, even Pharmaceutical companies recognise that damage around the DNA can be reversed and are looking for drugs that can have a positive effect. To quote from one study, *'We have long thought that we inherited diseases from our ancestors as a result of the genetic imprints. But an emerging new science called **epigenetics** helps us to see that we do have control over the destiny of our health. An improved diet that is very high in antioxidants and phyto chemicals like sulforaphane can actually signal the genes and the DNA to be expressed in a healthy way instead of being expressed in a disease.*

According to the National Cancer Institute, women born now, have an average risk of 12.2 per cent of being diagnosed with breast cancer at some time in their lives. By becoming informed about the latest research and making small changes in their diets, women may have a better opportunity to impact those statistics

315

in a positive way'.

You can potentially undo the damage in chronic illness – you are not doomed.

Obviously, while research is growing in a turbo charged way, the full picture is not there yet. But there's hope. One 2004 study from the *University of Buffalo*, having shown concentrates of supforaphanes inhibited the growth of human breast cancer said this " .. research indicated a potential use of this compound as a chemotherapeutic agent in cancer treatment". Jokingly, scientists talked of wishful thinking – hooking up women to sulforaphane drips instead of chemical IV drips!

Live Younger. Longer?

Harvard Medical School in its *Harvard Health* newsletter described 2013 as being a 'watershed year' for research into the colourful Mediterranean Diet.

One study followed 10,000 middle-aged women for 15 years and showed those who adhered most closely to the colourful Mediterranean Diet were 40 per cent more likely to reach the age of 70, and at the end of the study were free of 11 chronic illnesses, wherever they lived in the world *(Annals of Internal Medicine, 2013)* Another research study *(BMJ, December 2014)* showed that following a colourful Mediterranean Diet was linked to telomere length (the binding ends of your DNA) and this is linked to longevity. Telomeres shorten as you age, but the Rainbow Diet keeps them longer. So, you really can '**Live Younger, Longer with the Rainbow Diet**' – see more on our website, www.the-rainbow-diet.com.

Eat a rainbow

If you wanted any more evidence that there's science and sense behind the Rainbow Diet, now Oprah Winfrey and Men's Health in America have developed *'Eat the Rainbow'*. Never mind Harvard Medical School, Oprah says it's right!

So what are you waiting for? Go on, 'Eat a Rainbow' – take some sunshine into your life, look for organic fruits and vegetables from a good local supplier – and even grow a few yourself. Enjoy a long life of protection and correction, without even knowing about it!

I am absolutely convinced from the research that is coming thick and fast out of cancer centres from Tokyo to California, that we have already entered the new era of bioactive compounds and 'Phytomedicine'. Traditionalists in Britain my protest but the truth is that the research is already there and this is simply too big now to be ignored. It is also something which empowers the patient. It allows you to take back your life – to do something positive towards your own survival, increasing the length of survival and preventing the return of the cancer.

You can do it for yourself.

And, frankly, I have seen little or nothing in my research that even suggests possible conflict and contra-indication with modern drugs. That is just the usual mythology, often started by people with vested interests and those that put profits before people.

The truth is that Hippocrates got it right. Doctors swear the oath and then immediately ignore his message. *'Do no harm but let your food be your medicine and your medicine be your food'.*

Eat a Rainbow Diet: Put some real life back into your food and put some real food back into your life.

APPENDIX I

Liver Cleanse / Gallstone Flush

Ingredients:

$^1/_2$ cup extra virgin olive oil
1 very big grapefruit (providing $^3/_4$ cup of juice)
4 tablespoons of Epsom Salts
3 cups of water
Ornithine tablets.

Preparation:

Set aside 3 days.

Day 1:

Eat a no-fat breakfast and lunch.
Eat and drink nothing after 2.00 pm.
Mix the Epsom Salts in the water (easier if water is warm), then cool.

6.00 pm	Drink a quarter of this liquid.
8.00 pm	Drink a further quarter of the liquid
10.00 pm	Mix the olive oil and pulp-free grapefruit juice and shake vigorously.
	Drink the liquid through a straw before 10.15 pm. The original recipe suggests you take four Ornithine tablets to help you sleep but doesn't specify size.
	Retire immediately and massage your stomach.
	Focus your mind on your liver and imagine the toxins leaving it, along with the stones.
	Sleep.

Day 2:

Upon waking and not before 7.00 am take the third quarter of the Epsom salts mix. Two hours later take the last quarter.

Expect diarrhoea for two days; don't eat before lunch time on day two and keep food to salads and fruit, plus baked potatoes for days two and three.

You may need to repeat this treatment after a few weeks. 2000–3000 small stones may be passed.

Please note – This recipe is derived from William Kelley's cancer treatment. It has thousands of testimonials, none report pain, only success; but nobody at **icon** has any first hand experience of it. And although a number of our readers have now tried the 'treatment' and been happy with the results, we are merely **told** it works!

APPENDIX II

Factors with Epigenetic effects

1. Known factors linked to methylation, DNA expression blockage and gene silencing

Homocysteine
Stress
Poor Diet
Hormones (such as oestrogen, cortisol)
Environmental Toxins (smoking, hormone mimics such as BPA and phthalates, heavy metals such as lead, cadmium, mercury, arsenic; certain drugs, solvents and chemicals like formaldehyde and dioxins and pesticides like carbendazim.)

2. Factors known to protect and correct

i) Core Epigenetic compounds

Vitamin D
Curcumin
Resveratrol
Fish/krill oils (Omega-3)
Catechins (EGCG)
Conjugated Linoleic Acid (CLA)
Coenzyme Q10
Indole 3 Carbinol/DIM
Sulphoraphanes
Anthocyanins (deep purple of beetroot, plums, aubergine)
Quercitin
Grape Seed Extract
Pine Bark Extract
Modified Citrus Pectin (MCP)
Folate, B-12, biotin
Melatonin
Pomegranate
Soy/Genistein
Lycopene
MSM
Pterostilbene
Coffee Diterpines
Apigenin

Silibinin
N-acetylcysteine
Vitamin E
Choline
Piperine
Sodium Butyrate
Niacin

ii) Others

Minerals (an extremely diverse range, for example selenium, zinc, iron and particularly trace minerals such as boron.)
Exercise
Beneficial bacteria

INDEX

A

abdominal weight gain 219
abiraterone 79
N-acetyl cysteine, orthodox therapies and 152
acid bodies 14, 98–102
acidophilus 235
acrylamides 125, 247
aflatoxins 122, 231
aggression 60
AIDS 174–5, 176
AK13 258
alcohol in diets 56, 70
alkaline bodies 98–102, 295
allergies, GM foods and 129
allicin 258–9
S-allyl-cysteine 259
almonds, against inflammation 210
aloe vera 176
    against cancer 176–7
    against inflammation 210, 235
    orthodox therapies and 152
aloins 211
alpha tocopherol 149
alternative therapies *see* complementary/alternative therapies
aluminium 108
Alzheimer's disease
    from aluminium 108
    glutathione and 161
    piperine for 251
amygdalin 240, 266
animal fats see saturated fats
anthocyanins 127, 244–5, 309
anthraquinones 211
Antibiotic Resistant Marker gene 130

antibiotics
    breast cancer risks from 232
    IBS developing from 140
    killing beneficial bacteria 139–40
    in meat products 135, 140
    quercitin and 273
    resistance 130
    in tap water 110
antidepressants, diabetes and 215
antioxidants
    for boosting immune system 283–4
    foods for 127, 128, 294
    with orthodox therapies 150–1
    pterostilbenes 249
    reduced risk of cancer by 77, 148–9
    in SE Asian diet 57
    supplements 144
apples 1, 128, 241
apricot seeds 267
arabinogalactan 175
arabinose 270
argenine 184
aromatase inhibitors 196
arsenic in water 108
artepillin C 277
Asian women, isoflavone levels in 269–70
aspartame 124
Asphalia 183
aspirin
    cancer prevention 78–9, 207, 210
    against inflammation 211
astragalus 174–5, 309
    for glioma x

immune system and 173, 174–5, 238

orthodox therapies and 152, 175

atoms in body, balancing 27–35

attitudes to life 187

aubergines 245

B

bacteria

bee propolis against 275

beneficial 25, 57, 101, 204–5

bad fats intake and 42

destruction by chlorine 106

green tea and 252

immune system and 137–8

importance of 137

killing off 139–40

oestrogen levels and 196

role 235

types 138–9

resistant to antibiotics 130

balance and harmony of body 27–35

bamboo shoots 57

barbecues 287

barley grass, for liver strengthening 41

Batmanghelidj, Dr 104

Beard, Dr John 85

Beare, Sally 53

BEC5 245

Béchamp, Antoine 239

bee propolis 273–8

bees

attracted by colourful pigments 242

death of 133–4

beetroot

diet 244

for liver strengthening 41

berberis root 167, 168

beta carotene 153–4

chlorella and spirulina 270

foods for 127, 283

polyunsaturated oil inhibiting 119

supplements 143, 148

beta-blockers, diabetes and 215

Bifidobacterium 139, 142

bile, production by liver 38

bile duct blockage, liver flush for 121

bioactive food components 81–3

Biobran 89–90

Biocare 283

bioflavanoids, for boosting immune system 238

biotics *see* bioactive food components

biotin 156, 189

birth defects from chlorine in tap water 106

Bishop, Beata 91

bismuth 235

black pepper 90, 250–1

blackberries 243

bladder cancer

chemotherapy and supplements for 151

chlorinated water and 106

nitrates causing 109

blessed thistle 171

Blöbel, Gunter 262

blood

arterial plaque blocking 251
in cancer patients 13–14
detoxification by liver 37
oxygen levels 221–30
    depression and 60, 222
    increasing 223–30, 296
supply to tumours prevention 258–9, 273, 296
types, diet and 53
see also specific cells, e.g. red cells
blood cancers
    grape seed extract for 246
    green tea for 252
    mushrooms for 264, 265
blood pathogens, eating to avoid 295
blood root 178–9
blood system cancers, Hoxsey Therapy 169
blood tests, for parasites 232
blueberries 78, 243–4
B-lymphocytes, stimulation 89–90
B-lymphoma cells 250
Boik, John 15–16, 96, 150
boldo tea, for liver strengthening 41
bone cancer, mushrooms for 265
boron supplements 144
bouillabaise 68
bowel cancer, chemotherapy and supplements for 151
brain deficiency, oestrogen mimics and 201
brain tumours
    mobile phones and 23
    nitrates and 123
    nitrites and 109

oestrogen and 195
sweeteners and 124
toxins and 133
vitamin B-17 therapy 267
see also glioma
Brazilian bee propolis 274–8
bread 290
breakfast cereals 125
breast cancer
    antibiotics and 232
    aspirin and 207
    bee propolis for 277
    blueberries for 243–4
    calcium and 162
    carotenoids for 253–4
    chemotherapy and supplements for 151
    COX-2 and 260–1
    diet for 78, 241
    exercise and 225
    garlic for 259
    growth hormone production and 76
    indole-3-carbinol for 256
    lignans and 198
    melatonin and 181
    mushrooms for 263, 264
    obesity and 45
    oestrogen and 191–4
    pancreatic enzymes for 86
    piperine for 251
    pterostilbene for 249
    quercitin for 272
    resveratrol for 248
    sulphoraphanes for 257
    thyroxin and 185
    types 13
    vitamin A and 153

vitamin D and 159
vitamin E and 160
breast feeding 56
  beneficial bacteria and 142
  against diabetes 215
  glycoproteins and 262
  immune system and 139
  protection against breast cancer
  191–2
breathing properly 223–4
broccoli 78, 257, 311
  microwaving 287
bromelain 267
bronchial cancer, carotenoids and
255
Brusch, Charles 170
buckthorn bark 167, 168
Bupleurum scorzoneraefolium **see**
thorowax
burdock root 167, 168, 171
Burke, Dan 79
Burke, James 168
Burzynski, Dr 97
Bush People's diet 49, 53, 191,
218–19
butcher's broom 179

C
C43 protein 254
cachexia 75
caffeic acid 275–7
caffeine depressing uptake of
minerals 124
Caisse, Rene 170–2
calcium
  cancer and 162

depressing uptake of minerals
114
loss in vegetables 131
-magnesium balance 33–5, 100
sugar depleting 216
calcium fluoride 107
calorie restriction 49–50, 184, 220
calories in fat 226
cancer *(general only)*
  acid-loving tumours 99
  antioxidants and 138–9
  blood supply to tumours
  prevention 258–9, 273, 296
  breakdown of tumours 92
  causes 11, 12
  dairy foods and 113–15
  diabetes and 213–19
  diet for 78
  diet preventing xii
  gallstones and 39
  herbs and 165–80
  how do we develop it? 9–10
  individual to patients 13
  insulin role 213
  liver function and 39–40
  low oxygen and 221
  as modern disease 9
  natural compounds for 239–79,
  291–3
  nourishment curing regular
  occurrences 3
  parasites and 231
  as a process 15–16
  pro-drugs for 80
  protein marker 79
  rainbow diet for 312–13
  statistics 45
  stem cells and 81–2

ten truths about 291
in Thailand 56–7
vitamin D deficiency and 34
vitamins and minerals and
143–64
what is it? 9–17
as whole body disease 13–14
see also rogue cells
cancer cells
acid-loving 99
apoptosis 273
energy production by 14, 75, 99
natural compounds killing off
79, 296–7
yeasts and 233
Cancer Therapy: results of 50 cases
92
Cancer Watch xi
CANCERactive xi, xiii, 74
Candida spp. 232, 235
canola, GM, cancer risks from 129
caprylic acid 57
capsaicin 255, 310
carbohydrates
protein and 289
refined 65, 196, 216–17
carbonates 222
carctol 179
Carman, Judy 129
carotenoids 78, 253–4
carrots 78
cascar 167
casein 114
castor oil 92
catechins 251
cat's claw see Uno de Gato
Cdc25A 257
cells *see specific cells, e.g.* stem cells

cereals 125, 241
cervical cancer 195, 203
cheese 69
chemical messages, disrupting 24
chemicals 201–4
blood oxygen levels and 222
in home 21, 191, 202–4
legislation 21–2
statistics 21
chemotherapy
bee propolis with 277–8
for glioma x
with herbs 173–6
killing beneficial bacteria
139–40
mushrooms with 264
supplements and 150–2
chi *see* astragalus
chicken 55, 135
chicory, beneficial bacteria and 142
children
diet, deficiencies in 47
farming family, better immune
systems in 139
organophosphate levels in urine
134–5
chillis 55, 57, 255
Chinese cabbage, organic 128
Chinese food 126
chips, causing cancer 125
chlorella 270–1
for boosting immune system
238, 284
for displacing heavy metals 25,
145
for increasing blood oxygen
levels 224
for liver strengthening 41

for vitamin B12 53
chlorine, in water 106
chlorogenic compounds 241
chlorophyll, blood oxygen levels
and 224
chlorpyrifos 222
chocolate for better sleep 204
choke berry, for glioma x
cholesterol levels
'bad' see LDL
garlic for 258
'good' see HDL
high 120–2
mushrooms for 265
choline 156–7
neutralising free-radicals 42
chromium picolinate, in Gerson
Therapy 95
chymotrypsin 267
cinnamon supplements 232, 233–4,
238
citrus isoflavones 270
clinical trials
limitations 19
patient selection 88
Clostridium difficile 140–1
clover 127–8
see also red clover
coconut 57
Coenzyme Q10 158
in Gerson Therapy 95
for glioma x
supplements 146–7
coffee 69
enemas 41, 92, 96
see also Gerson Therapy
immune system and 124
colitis 211

colon cancer see colorectal cancer
colorectal cancer
beta-carotene and 154
calcium and 162
chlorinated water and 106
COX-2 and 209, 260
curcumin and 210
dairy foods and 113
diet and 77, 78
fish oils for 260
folic acid and 154
garlic for 258, 259
inflammation in 210–11
lack of beneficial bacteria and
141
magnesium for 163
oestrogen and 191,195, 204
prostaglandins and 118
pterostilbene for 249
quercitin for 272
supplements and 148
vitamin A and 153
vitamin D and 159
colostrum in Gerson Therapy,
defatted 95
colourings in meat products 135
complementary therapies 74
contraceptive jellies 203
contraceptive pills, oestrogen levels
and 193
Contreras, Dr 96–7, 267
cooking tips 287–8
copper in water 108
corn, GM, cancer risks from 129
corn oil 116
corn syrup 216
cortisol levels
endorphins and 228

exercise and 225–6
inflammation from 209
stress and 59–60, 100
cosmetics 191, 202–4
coumestans 269
COX-2 209, 210, 213, 250, 253, 260
crisps, causing cancer 125
crocin 68
crop rotation 128, 131, 146–7
cross-breeding 128
curcumin 250–51
    cancer prevention 78
    for glioma x
    against *Helicobacter pylori* 235
    immune system boosting 284
    against inflammation 210, 211
    neutralising free-radicals 42
    studies on 2
    supplements 144
Curcumin Complex 90
    immune system and 173
    against oestrogen 202
cyanide, poisoning liver 268
cyanide-containing plants 240
cyanocobalamin 97, 155, 240
CYP1B1 gene 249
CYP1B1 protein 79
CYP17 protein 79
L-cysteine, orthodox therapies and 152
cytochrome p450 249

D
d'Adamo, Peter 53
daidzein 269
dairy foods *(general only)*
    avoidance 102
    cancer risk and 113–15
    damaging cells 100
    diabetes and 215
    lacking in SE Asian Diet 55
    myths about 33–5
    substituting 115
    toxins in 201
    see also milk
dandelion
    against cancer 242–3
    for liver strengthening 41
Dash diet 314
DDT 133
DEHP levels in toiletries 194
dehydration 104
dehydroepiandrosterone 184
depression
    blood oxygen levels and 60, 222
    diet and 77
    exercise and 228
    rainbow diet for 314
detoxification (Gonzalez') 89
detoxification (Kelly's) 86
detoxification (Gerson Therapy) 92
d-fraction 265
DHT from testosterone 195
diabetes
    cancer risk and 213–19
    cinnamon supplements for 232
    diet and 76
    insulin receptor sites and 233–4
    OPCs for 246
    rainbow diet for 313–14

dialylsulphide 259
diesel fumes 223
diet *(general only)*
 for boosting immune system
 282
 calorie restriction 50
 cancer prevention and 51–8,
 312–13
 changing 312
 to deplete toxins 25
 against depression 314
 diabetes and 214–15, 312–13
 getting nourishment from
 137–42
 against heart disease 314
 high calorie/high oestrogen
 196–7
 for increasing blood oxygen
 levels 224
 killing infections 12
 nourishment in modern-day 2–3
 against oestrogen 195–201
 paucity of advice 73–6
 preventing cancer development
 xii, 4–5
 against yeasts 236–8
 see also foods; *specific diets,*
e.g. South East Asian Diet
dietary typing 86
dieticians 75
dieting, tips for 50
digestion, liver function and 38
digestive system, beneficial bacteria
and 138
diketopiperazine, produced from
aspartame 124
dioxins 22, 201–2
 indole-3-carbinol for 256

 neutralisation 25
DNA
 perfect copying 293–4
 rogue
 see genetic mutations
doctors, lack of knowledge on
nutrition for cancer 1, 73, 74–5
drugs *(general only)*
 in combinations 19–20
 quality control 21
 toxicity 19–21
 see also clinical trials
Duke, Dr James 168

E
Eat Right for Your Type 53
eating tips 288–90
echinacea 175
 for glioma x
 immune system and 173, 238
Efferth, Dr Thomas 165
eicosanoids 118, 208–10, 228
electromagnetic fields see EMFs
electronic fields around body,
damage to 28
ellagic acid 247, 311
 supplements 144
EMFs
 increasing oestrogen levels 196
 melatonin levels and 23, 101,
 182, 204
 as toxins 23
endometrial cancer
 oestrogen and 195
 phytoestrogens and 200
endometriosis, oestrogen levels and
192

endorphins
   from capsaicin 255
   from exercise 228
endothelial growth factor 210
energy production, liver function
and 38
environmental balance with body
59
environmental toxins 100, 110,
145, 191, 222
Enzyme Theory of Cancer, The
85–6
Epigenetics 10-11, Appendix II
epithelial growth factors 250
Epsom Salts 41
Essiac 169, 170–2, 269
*Everything You Need to Know to
Help You Beat Cancer* 159, 231–8
exercise
   for boosting immune system
   282
   dieting and 50
   fat storage and 115
   for increasing blood oxygen
   levels 224–30
   in Mediterranean people 70
   overdoing 226–7
   in SE Asia 56

F
Far Eastern food 126
farmers
   better immune systems in children of 139
   cancer in 133

dangers to 22
farming methods, hydroponic 131
fast food 125–6
fat in body
   burning up visceral fat 228
   calories in 226
   oestrogen production by 195–6
   toxins and 39
fats in diet
   from animal fat 201
   bad fats 41–2, 115–16
   doctors recommending 75
   in fish 135
   hydrogenated 116–18
   limiting 93, 98
   liver function and 41–2
   Mediterranean Diet
   consumption 69
   from milk 114
   monounsaturated 119
   polyunsaturated 118–19
   saturated 116, 116–18
   toxins in 135
   trans
      see fats, hydrogenated
   unsaturated 118–19
fatty acid pool in body 209
Fell, Dr JW 168
Ferenczi, Dr 244
fertilisers as toxins 22
   loss of minerals and 131
   in non-organic food 127
feverfew 178, 311
fibre in diet 65, 216–17
Finistride 195
fish in diet 53, 55
   dioxins and 201
   GI 218

toxins in 135
fish oils 63, 119–20, 260–61
    aggression and 60
    for boosting immune system
    285
    colon cancer prevention 78
    against inflammation 211, 212,
    235
    orthodox therapies and 152
    supplements 144, 260–1
Fishbein, Morris 169
fizzy drinks 47–8
flavenoids
    in bee propolis 274
    in organic food 128
flavenols, in organic food 128
flaxseed oil 119–20
flaxseeds 102
    against inflammation 211–12
    against oestrogen 199, 201
    radiotherapy and 152
fluoride, in tap water 106–8
foetus, stem cells and 11
folate, oestrogen and 189
folic acid 154
    beneficial bacteria and 140
    deficiency 140
        oestrogen mimics and 201
foods (*general only*)
    acrylamides in 125
    acting as pro-drugs 80
    for better sleep 204
    bioactive components 81–2
    coloured 76, 243–79, 309
    containing cholesterol 121
    containing sugar 123
    contaminated vs least
    contaminated list 134

cooking tips 125, 287–8
for correct DNA copying 293–4
for decreasing free-radicals 294
denaturing oestrogen 101
eaten by teenagers 47
eating out 125–6
forbidden in Gerson Therapy 94
in French diet 66–8
in Gerson Therapy 94
GI values 218
GM 128–9
green 301
to help orthodox therapies 152
increasing antioxidants 294
increasing cellular oxygen 101
increasing HDL levels 121
against inflammation 207–12
intolerances 60
junk 47–9
to kill yeasts 234
labelling 118
for liver strengthening 41
macrobiotic 62
microwaved 126, 287–8
multi-step programme 293–7
nutritional deficiencies 146–8
against oestrogen 199
orange 300
organic 68, 93, 127–36, 283–4
pickled 123
points system in programme
303–8
polyphenol content 70
purple/blue 301
raw 93, 287, 288
red 300
refined 122–3, 126, 146
shopping for rainbow foods

299–302
sirtuins in 50
to snack on 125
sources for anthocyanins 244–5
sources for argenine 184
sources for avoiding parasites 295
sources for beta carotene 153–4, 283
sources for boosting immune system 281–5, 294–5
sources for calcium 162
sources for carotenoids 253, 254
sources for choline 156–7
sources for Coenzyme Q10 158
sources for ellagic acid 247
sources for glutathione 160–1
sources for increasing oxygen levels 296
sources for indole-3-carbinol 256
sources for isoflavenoids 269
sources for keeping alkaline body 295
sources for killing cancer cells 297
sources for lycopene 161–2, 284
sources for magnesium 99–100, 152, 162–3
sources for minimising blood pathogens 295
sources for natural progesterone 205
sources for nitrilosides 266
sources for OPCs 246
sources for phytoestrogens 197–8
sources for polysaccharides 262
sources for potassium 32–3, 99–100, 163
sources for pterostilbene 249
sources for quercitin 272
sources for reducing inflammation 295
sources for selenium 163–4, 284
sources for serotonin 204
sources for sodium 31–2, 100
sources for sulphoraphanes 257
sources for vitamin A 153
sources for vitamin B complex 154–7
sources for vitamin C 157, 283
sources for vitamin E 160, 283
sources for vitamin K 161
sources for zinc 164, 283
white/brown 301
whole 283–4
whole vs refined 122
wrapping 93
yellow 300
yin and yang 61–2
see also diet and **specific foods,** *e.g.* vegetables
formaldehyde 21, 124
Frank, Dr Benjamin 260
free-radicals
avoiding excess 294
bee propolis for 276
hydrogenated fats and 117
neutralisation 42
what are they? 10
freezing foods, vitamin loss and 132
French diets 66–71, 279, 297–8
fruit

acting as pro-drugs 80
coloured 71
fresh 63
in Gerson Therapy 94
GI 217
growing 290
home-grown 136
hydroponically grown 131
juices 93
loss of vitamins in 146
organic vs 'normal' 134
pollination 133–4
raw 93
in SE Asian diet 55
shopping for rainbow foods
299–302
toxins in 133
when to eat 289
FTO gene 46
fucoidan 273–4
fumaric acid, chemotherapy and
151
fungi, wormwood for 177

G
galactose 270
galangal 57
against inflammation 210
gallstones 39
flushing out 318–19
therapy 41, 282
garlic 55, 57, 258–9
against inflammation 210
stopping blood vessel
development to tumour 15
against yeasts 237–8
gastrointestinal cancer, chlorinated
water and 106
Gearin-Tosh, Michael 91
genetic mutations 10
bee propolis for 276
GM foods and 129
losing weight and 46
oestrogen and 189
oestrogen mimics and 201
olive oil for 253
from toxins 24
genetically modified (GM) food
128–9
trials 129–30
genistein 197–8, 198, 269, 272
Gerson, Charlotte 91, 92
Gerson, Dr Max 91, 162
Gerson Therapy 40–1, 90–6, 271
Gilbon-Garbet, Professor 263
ginger against inflammation 210
see also curcumin
glioma x–xi, 195
glucagon 214
glucorinide 267
glucose requirements by cancer cells
14, 75
glucosidase 266
glutamine, orthodox therapies and
152
glutathione 152, 160–1
increasing levels 101, 222, 224
in organic food 128
oxygenating cells with 221
glutathione S-transferases 96
glycaemic index (GI) 217–19
glycans 139
glycoproteins 261-63
goat's cheese 115
goldenseal 177, 235

Gonzalez, Dr Nicholas 85–9, 89, 297
Gonzalez diet 89
G-proteins *see* glycoproteins
Graham, Dr Roscoe 170
grains 62–3, 122
grape seed extract 95, 246, 284
grapes 128, 130
    see also red grapes; resveratrol
'grazing' 288
Green, Gerald 235, 236–8, 238
green tea 63, 251–2, 289
    curcumin with 250
    against Helicobacter pylori 235
    against inflammation 210, 211
    polyphenols in 241
grifolan 264
growth hormone 76, 135
gullet cancer, aspirin and 207

H
Hamm, Dr Caroline 242–3
Handbook of Organic Food Safety and Quality 165
happiness 57
hare's ear see thorowax
haung qi see astragalus
HDL 117, 119, 120–2
Healing -- the Gerson Way 95
heart disease
    bad fats intake and 117
    olive oil and 82
    rainbow diet for 314
heavy metals displacing 25, 294
Helicobacter pylori 177, 231, 235, 252, 258
herbal supplements 41, 43

herbicides as toxins 22, 132–3, 201–4
    in non-organic food 127
    resistance by GM foods 128–9
herbs 301, 309
    against cancer 165–80, 241
    in French diet 68
    immune system boosting 284
    Prostastol 89
    against yeasts 236–8
Herceptin 207–8
heredity of cancers 24
hermaphroditism, caused by chemicals 22
high density lipoprotein see HDL
homocysteine 161
honey 311
    see also bee propolis
hormones 181–7
    liver function and 38
household chemicals 191
Howell, Tony xii
Hoxsey, Harry M 166
Hoxsey Therapy 166–9, 269
HRT
    oestrogen levels and 193
    progestin in 205
    as supplement 146
human growth hormone 183–4
    boosting 228
human papilloma virus (HPV)
    prevention 247, 256
Hurtle's cell cancer 191
hydrogen peroxide, oxygenating cells with 221
hydrogenated fats (trans fats) 116–18, 215
hydroponic farming 131

Hyperbaric Oxygen therapy 221
hyperthermia treatment 15, 271–2
    in Gerson Therapy 95
hypothalamus changes and
    meditation 60
hypothyroidism, from fluoride 107

I
ICI 195
icon xi, xiii
IGF-1 production
    calorie restriction and 49
    melatonin and 181, 182
    reduction by natural compounds
    241
immune system
    bee propolis for 275–7
    beneficial bacteria and 137–9
    diet and 77, 281–5, 294–5
    fucoidan for 273
    herbs for 173–4, 176–7
    liver function and 38
    mushrooms for 263
    parasites and 232
    stimulation with Gerson
    Therapy 91
    sugar weakening 123
    supplements and 152–3
    vitamin C and 157
    vitamins and minerals for 157,
    238
    weakened, factors causing 10
Imupros 90
Indian rhubarb 171
indigestion 211
indole-3-carbinol 255–7, 310

chemotherapy and 151
    in foods 145
    against oestrogen 199, 201–2
    supplements 144
indoles 25, 309
infection
    causing cancer 12
    CoQ10 for 158
    eating to avoid 295
    garlic for 258–9
    see also specific infections
inflammation 207–12, 235,
250, 260
    bee propolis for 274–5
    eating to avoid 295–6
inositol, neutralising free-radicals
42
insecticides see pesticides as toxins
insulin
    calorie restriction and 49
    COX-2 and 209
    damaging cells 100
    diet for beating 213–20
    oestrogen and 189
    resistance 219–20
    surges 196
    see also diabetes
insulin receptor sites 213, 233
insulin-like growth factor 1 (IGF-1)
114
Integrated Cancer and Oncology
News see **icon**
interleukin-6 210
inulin, beneficial bacteria and 142
iodine deficiency 185
ionisation 112
iron
    chlorella and spirulina 270

for increasing blood oxygen
levels 224
irritable bowel syndrome 211
Ishizuka, Sagen 60–1
isoflavenoids 198
isoflavones 268–70
    for glioma x
    radiotherapy and 152
    stopping blood vessel develop-
ment to tumour 15
isothiocyanates 240–1

J
Jason Winter's tea 269
juicers 94, 287, 290
junk food 47–9

K
kafir lime leaves 57
Keller, Rudolf 162
Kelley, Dr William Donald 86, 319
Kelley's diet 86
kelp 171
kidney cancer 20, 133
Kim, Young S. 81
Kirlian photographs 28, 132
    of microwaved food 126, 287–8
Kopp, William 126, 287
Krebs, Ernst 266, 267
Kupffer cells 37–8

L
lactic acid production, liver function and 40
Lactobacillus
    chlorella and 271
    L. acidophilus 142, 205
    L. bifidobacteria 205
    L. shirota 205
laetrile 240, 266, 267
laughter boosting immune system
285
LDL 120–2
    hydrogenated fats raising 117
    polyphenols for 251
lead in water 108
Lee, John 193
lemon grass 57
lentinan 265
leukaemia
    carbonates and 222
    causes 22
    curcumin for 250
    dandelion for 243
    in farmers 133
    feverfew and 178
    fucoidan for 273
    grape seed extract for 246
    green tea for 252
    mushrooms for 265
    nitrates and 123
    quercitin for 272
    vitamin A and 153
    vitamin K and 161
life expectancy *see* longevity
lifestyles
    changing 58
    obesity and 48–9
lignans

bad fats intake and 42
heavy metal displacement by
145
against oestrogen 198
against toxins 25
Lilley, Roger 110
linoleic acid 118–19, 264
linseed oil 119–20
liquorice 169
lithocholic acid 210
Live Longer Diet, The 53
liver 37–43
blood detoxification by 37
in cancer patients 14
damage from GM foods
(general only) 129
detoxification 40–1, 92, 267,
281–2, 318–19
diet and 41–3
extract, in Gerson Therapy 95
fatty 38–9
magnesium needed by 35
strengthening 296
testing 37
toxins and 133
liver cancer
choline and 157
garlic for 259
vitamin B-17 therapy 267
vitamin K and 161
vitamin K supplements and 140
liver fluke 135, 231
longevity
calorie restriction and 49
in older people on Mediterranean Diet 69
in SE Asia 56
UK vs others 49

low density lipoprotein see LDL
lung cancer
bee propolis for 277
carotenoids for 254
diesel fumes and 223
garlic for 259
mushrooms for 264
quercitin for 272
radon causing 109
vitamin E and 160
lungs, toxin clearance 227
lutein 254
lycopene 161–2, 254, 310
foods for 284
lymph
cleaning up 282
moving around body 227–8
lymph node cancers
green tea for 252
mushrooms for 264
lymphoma, fucoidan for 273

M
Macrobiotic Diet 60–3, 297
macular degeneration, carotenoids
for 254
magnesium
blood oxygen levels and 222
-calcium balance 33–5
against cancer 162–3
causes of lowered levels 35
in Epsom Salts 41
increasing in diet 99–100
inhibition of uptake 33–4
liver and 35
mitochondria and 35

oestradiol and 12
reducing cholesterol levels 121
sources 34, 152
maitake mushrooms 263–5
malaria, wormwood for 177
male cancers from oestrogen 194–5
malignancy system (Kelley's) 86
Manchester, Christie 311
mannose 270
Mayer, Anne-Marie 146
meal sizes 217
meat in diet 52–4
additives in 122–3
dioxins and 201
GI 218
toxins in 135, 140, 201
meat products, additives in 122–3
meditation, hypothalamus changes
and 60
Mediterranean Diet 67–9, 297–8,
312
melanoma
AK13 and 258
Gerson Therapy 91
Hoxsey Therapy 169
quercitin for 272
suma root for 177
melatonin
depletion 23, 101, 182, 204
garlic and 260
oestrogen levels and 191
sleep and 181–3
meningitis, fucoidan for 273
menopause
in Asian women 200
Mediterranean Diet for 312
oestrogen levels and 193
menstrual cycles, breast cancer risks

from more 192
Mercola Complete Probiotics 283
Mercola multi-strain supplement
205
mercury in water 108
metabolic rate, calorie restriction
and 49
Metabolic Therapy 97, 266–7
metabolic typing 53–4, 86–7, 98
methanol, produced from aspartame 124
methyl-cobalamin 240
MGN-3 Biobran 284
microbes 231–8
microbiome 137, 140, 204–5
microwaving 126, 287–8
migraine, Gerson Therapy for 91
milk
adding to tea 113–14
diabetes and 215
lacking in SE Asian Diet 55
organic 165
toxins in 114
see also dairy foods
milk thistle, for liver strengthening
41
minerals
against cancer 143–64, 162–4
deficiency 47, 53,146–8
human growth hormone and
184
imbalances 25, 145
nitrilosides 267
in organic food 127
supplements, with orthodox
therapies 150–3
see also trace minerals
miscarriages, chlorinated water and

106
mitochondria 30, 35
mobile phone dangers 23, 182
Mohs, Dr Frederick 166–7
molecules in body, balancing 27–35
monosaccharides 262
monosodium glutamate (MSG) 124, 126
monounsaturated fats 119
Monsanto 114
Montignac, Dr Michel 214–15, 217
Moss, Ralph 150–1
mould on grapes 130
MSG *see* monosodium glutamate
muesli 290
multiple myeloma 91, 133
muscle weight 226
mushroom extract, orthodox therapies and 152
mushrooms, medicinal 263–6, 311
    enzymes from 89–90
    maitake 263–5
    in Mediterranean Diet 70
    against oestrogen 201
    Phellinus linteus 265
    reishi 266
    shiitake 265
    studies on 2
myelodysplastic syndrome 264
myeloma, causes 22
myrosinase 78, 257

N
natural birth and immune systems in babies 139
Natural Compounds in Cancer Therapy 16, 150
natural killer cells, stimulation 89–90
naturopathy 59
neem 179
Nelson, Mildred 166, 169
neochlorogenic compounds 241
neurological stimulation (Kelley's) 86
niacin 138, 154–5
nicotinic acid see niacin
nitrates causing cancers 22, 109, 123
nitrilosides 266–8
nitrites causing cancers 22, 109
nitrogen-containing compounds 240
nitrogen-free compounds 240
nitrosamine compounds 140
norepinephrine, cancer cells and 209–10
nosodes 238
nutrition *see* diet; foods
nutritional deficiencies 145–6
nutritional therapy (Kelly's) 86

O
Oasis of Hope centre 96–7
oatmeal 93
oats, fibre in 289
obesity
    cancer risk and 45–6
    in children 46–8
    risks 48–9
    statistics 46–7

oesophageal cancer
   drugs causing 20
   garlic for 259
   green tea for 252
   nitrites causing 109
oestradiol 190
   damaging cells 100, 189
   disturbing sodium and magnesium levels 12
   downgrading 198–9
   driving cancers 11–12
   lowering levels 296
   prostate gland enlargement from
195
oestrogen 189–206
   affecting liver function 38
   in cattle 135
   denaturing 101
   driving cancers 11–12, 189
   eicosanoids and 228
   exercise and 225
   from fats 115
   increased levels 101
   indole-3-carbinol for 256
   lack of beneficial bacteria and
140
   limiting in diet 77
   male cancers and 194–5
   melatonin and 181, 182
   menopausal levels 193
   menstrual cycles and 193
   mimics 110, 191, 194, 201–4
      in home 202–4
      indole-3-carbinol for 256
   production 195–6
   resveratrol for 248
   role of 190–1
   stem cells and 11

   in tap water 109
Oestrogen: the Killer in Our Midst
190
oestrogenic products 25
oestrone 190
Ohsawa, George 61
oils
   'bad' 115–16
   'friendly' 119–20, 301
   hydrogenated 116
   polyunsaturated 118–19
Okinawans' diet 49, 53, 63, 273
oleocanthal 253
oligomeric proanthocyanidins
(OPCs) 245–7
olive oil 82, 119, 252–3
   HDL and 121
   against *Helicobacter pylori* 235
   against inflammation 210, 211
omega-3 311
   aggression and 60
   for cell health 96
   cholesterol and 121–2
   colon cancer prevention 78
   in farmed fish 135
   in fish oil 260
   from 'friendly' oils 119–20
   for glioma x
   against inflammation 15, 210
   longevity and 82
   in organic food 127
omega-6 260
omega-9 260
oncologists see doctors
One Answer to Cancer 86
onions 55, 57
   beneficial bacteria and 142
   Welsh, organic 128

oral cancer, carotenoids for 254
organic food 68, 93, 127–36, 283–4
    definition 128
    Kirlian photographs and 132
osteoporosis
    avoiding 228
    in West 33, 34
ovarian cancer
    dairy foods and 113
    green tea for 252
    obesity and 45
    oestrogen and 194, 195
Over the Rainbow xiii
overweight, increasing oestrogen
levels 101, 196, 197
oxygen, low levels damaging cells
100
oxygenating cells 221–30
ozone 221

P
p21 gene 256
p53 repair gene 12
painkillers, causing cancer 20
pancreas 215–16
pancreatic cancer
    curcumin for 250
    Kelley's therapy for 87–8
    prostaglandins and 118
    vitamin K and 161
pancreatic enzymes 85
    in Gerson Therapy 95
    increasing 296
    in Metabolic Therapy 97
pancreatic hormones 214

Pandey. Siyaram 243
papain 267
papaya 57
parabens 203
paracetamol, taken with coffee 20,
124
parasites 231–8
    eating to avoid 295
    liver function and 42–3
    in water 109
    wormwood for 177
parthenolide 178
pasta, refined 122
Pasteur, Louis 239
Pau d'Arco 310
    in Gerson Therapy 95
    against yeasts 235, 238
PCBs 203
peaches, organic 128
peppermint tea 93
peppers 78
peptides, cancer patients lacking 97
perfumes 191, 194, 202–4
periwinkle 172
pesticides as toxins 22, 100, 102,
132–3, 201–4
    blood oxygen levels and 222
    GM foods and 129
    lacking in SE Asian Diet 55
    in meat products 135
    in non-organic food 127
    washing out from body 25
Pfeifer, Professor Ben 89–90, 297
phagocytosis 176
Phellinus linteus mushrooms 265
phenolics, in organic food 128
phenols 127, 210
phenylalanine, produced from

aspartame 124
phone masts 23
photodynamic therapy 224, 271
phytoestrogens 197–8, 268–70
    blocking oestradiol 12, 101, 190
phytomedicine 244–79, 315
piceatannol 80
pickling foods 123
picrocin 68
pigments in plant compounds 76, 243–79, 309
pill see contraceptive pills
pine bark 246,284
piperine 250–1
plankton, farmed fish and 135
plant hormones see phytoestrogens
Plaskett, Dr Lawrence 96
Plaskett Therapy 96, 269, 271, 297
plasticisers 110
plums, organic 127
poke root 167
pokeweed 168
policosanols 121
pollination 133–4
pollutants in tap water 103
pollution in air 223
polycystic ovary syndrome, oestrogen levels and 192
polypharmacy 19–20
polyphenols 309
    against cancer 241
    in green tea 251
    in Mediterranean Diet 70
    in olive oil 252
    in organic food 128
polysaccharides 261–2, 309
    in mushrooms 263
    sources 270, 284

polyunsaturated fats 118–19
pomegranates 241
posture 228
potassium
    blood oxygen levels and 222
    against cancer 163
    in diets 63, 93, 96, 99–100
    need for 30
    -sodium balance 29–33
    sources 32–3
potatoes
    GM, cancer risks from 129
    loss of vitamins in 146
    organic 127, 128
Potter, Gerry 79
prawns, toxins in 135
Prebiota 7 142, 205
prebiotics 142
preservatives 123
press-ups 228
prickly ash bark 167, 168
Probiota 8 283
probiotics 140–1, 283
    radiotherapy and 152
procarcinogens 249
procyanidins 241
progesten, synthetic 194
progesterone 193, 205
progestin 205
programme for eating natural compounds 291–3
    multi-step 293–7
    points system 303–8
prostaglandins
    bad fats transforming to 117–18
    causing inflammation 118, 208
    types 117–18
Prostastol 89

prostate cancer
    abiraterone for 79
    calcium and 162
    dairy foods and 113
    diet for 78
    garlic for 259
    grape seed extract for 246
    lowered zinc levels 108
    lycopene and 161–2, 254
    mushrooms for 263, 264, 265
    obesity and 45
    oestrogen levels and 191, 194–5
    Pfeifer therapy 89–90
    phytoestrogens and 200
    pomegranates for 241
    quercitin for 272
    selenium for 164
    sulphoraphanes for 258
    vitamin A and 153
    vitamin B-17 therapy 267
    zinc for 164
prostate gland enlargement from oestradiol 195
protein
    carbohydrates and 289
    digestion 211
    limiting in diet 93, 96, 98
protein uPA 13
Prozac, diabetes and 215
prunetin, against oestrogen 199
psycho-neuro-endocrino-immunology 59
PTEN gene 78, 258
pterostilbene 249, 311
ptyalin 288
pulses 63
    against cancer 241
    fibre in 289

isoflavones 269
limiting 93

Q
quercitin 271
    against oestrogen 199
    in organic food 128
    supplements 144

R
radiation around body 28
radiotherapy
    garlic with 259
    for glioma x
    herbs and 173–6
    mushrooms with 264
    supplements and 150, 152
radishes, for liver strengthening 41
radon in water 109
rain pollutants 103
Rainbow Diet, The xiii–xiv
ras gene 12
rectal cancer see colorectal cancer
red cells, in cancer patients 14
red clover 169, 171, 198, 268–9
red wine 215, 248, 289
    see also resveratrol
refining problems 122
reishi mushrooms 266
resistance training 183, 228
resveratrol 90, 247–8, 310
    chemotherapy and 151
    grape mould and 130
    against inflammation 210, 211

against oestrogen 199, 201, 248
in organic food 128
as pro-drug 79
stimulation of sirtuins by 50
supplements 144
retinoic acid 153
reverse osmosis filtration 111–12
rhodinase 267
rice, GI 217
rice bran 89–90
roasting food 125, 287
rock wool for hydroponic farming
131
Rosch, Dr Paul 88
ruscogenins 179
Ruscus aculeatus see butcher's
broom

S
saccharin 124
safflower oil 118
saffron 68
safranil 68
salad crops 131, 290
salad Niçoise 68
salicylin, reducing inflammation 15,
79
salt in diet
deficiency 55
Far Eastern food 126
Mediterranean Diet
consumption 69
salts 29
salvestrols 79–80
Sanguinaria canadensis see blood
root

sanguinarine 167
saponins 177
sarcomas, vitamin B-17 therapy
and 267
saturated fats 116–17, 116–18
seaweed 273
seeds, against cancer 241
selenium
for boosting immune system
238
against cancer 163–4
enhancing glutathione levels 222
foods for 284
in garlic 259
in Gerson Therapy 95
for glioma x
heavy metal displacement by 25,
145
neutralising free-radicals 42
radiotherapy and 152
supplements 144, 148, 284
self-empowerment in cancer
patients 73
serotonin 204, 260
sex hormone binding globulin 198
sheep sorrel 171
shiitake mushrooms 265
sirtuins 50, 248
skin cancer
BEC5 for 245
capsaicin for 255
carotenoids for 254
chlorinated water and 106
grape seed extract for 246
green tea for 252
quercitin for 272
sulphoraphanes for 257
sleep

in darkness 56, 57, 102, 182
melatonin and 181–3
oestrogen increases and 204
reducing oestrogen levels 196
slimming see dieting
slippery elm 171
Slow Poisoning of America, The
124
smoked foods 123
smoking
blood oxygen levels and 222–3
cancer risk and 45
non-smoking cutting risks of
death 70
in SE Asia 56
smoothies 123
snack food 216
snacks 125, 288
sodium
blood oxygen levels and 222
consumption 29–30
damaging cells 100
decreasing in diet 99–100
exclusion from diet 93
oestradiol and 12
-potassium balance 29–33
sources 31–2
sodium bicarbonate for alkalisation
99, 102
sodium butyrate killing cancer cells
138
sodium chloride 29
sodium fluoride 107
sodium lauryl sulphate 203
soils, depletion of minerals in 146–7
soups 290
South East Asian Diet 54–8
soya 199–201, 269

dangers of 115
GM, cancer risks from 129
milk 55
sperm count levels
decreased, from oestrogen in
water 109
oestrogen mimics and 201
spermicides 203
spices 290, 301
spinach, organic 128
spiritual healing 86, 97
spirulina 270–1
for displacing heavy metals 25
for increasing blood oxygen
levels 224
for liver strengthening 41
statins in tap water 110
stem cells
controlling 81–2, 85
oestrogen and 189
what are they? 10–11
Stern, Dr 19–20
steroids
damaging cells 100
from fats 115
inflammation from 209
in tap water 110
Stevia 238
stews 288
stillingia root 167, 168
stomach cancer
carotenoids and 254
chlorinated water and 106
fucoidan for 273
garlic for 259
Helicobacter pylori and 235
mushrooms for 264
nitrites causing 109

oestrogen and 195, 204
olive oil for 253
pickled foods and 123
salt consumption and 30
stem cells and 10–11
stomach disorders, yeasts and 233
strawberries, organic 127, 128
stress
    cortisol levels and 59–60
    damaging cells 100
    management 77
    pre-cancerous changes from
    209–10
    response, calorie restriction and
    50
sugar in diet 123, 196, 216–17
sulphoraphanes 78, 210, 240–1,
257–8
sulphuryl fluoride 107
suma root 177
sunflower oil 116, 118
sunlight
    for boosting immune system
    283
    against inflammation 211
    see also vitamin D
supercarbs 261–2
supplements 301–2
    beneficial bacteria 205
    calcium 35
    chlorella 284
    to combat soil deficiencies in
    minerals 146
    definitions 146
    Gonzalez therapy 89
    with Hoxsey Therapy 169
    magnesium 35
    melatonin 183

Pfeifer therapy 89–90
    selenium 284
    synthetic vs natural 143–4
    vitamin E 284
    zinc 284
    see also herbal supplements
survival times for glioma x–xi
sweet potatoes 78
sweetcorn milk 55
sweeteners 110, 124
swimming 228
symbiosis 140

T
Tae Woong Kim, Professor 265
t'ai chi 228
Tamoxifen
    blocking oestradiol 190
    in tap water 110
    vs indole-3-carbinol 256
Taxol 172
tea, adding milk to 113–14
telephone mast dangers 182
telomeres 261
Templeton, Al 168
testicular cancer 109, 191, 194
testosterone levels in men
    chlorpyrifos and 222
    oestrogen and 194–5
    shutting off 79
Thai people, lifestyle 54–7
Thomas, David 146
thoracic duct, clearing toxins 228
thorowax 176

throat cancer, pickled foods and 123
thyroxin 146, 184–5
T-lymphocytes, stimulation 89–90
tocopherols 160
tocotrienols 160
toiletries 191, 194, 202–4
tomatoes 78
tongue, appearance 37
toothpastes 107
toxic bodies 19–26
toxins
    affecting liver function 37–8, 38–9
    in animal products 135
    blood oxygen levels and 222
    in bloodstream 223
    chelation 138
    environmental 100, 110, 145, 191
    in milk 114
    from overexercise 227
    removing 294
trace minerals, hydroponic farming and 131–2
trans fats
    in diets 47 see fats, hydrogenated
Tree of Life, The xiii
trichloroethylene 106
Trichopoulos, Dimitrios 312
trihalomethanes 106
trophoblast cells 85
trypsin 267
tryptophan 204, 211
    in garlic 259
tuberculosis, Gerson Therapy for 91

tumours *see* cancer *(general only)*
turmeric *see* curcumin

U
UK National Cancer Plan (2000) 76
Uno de Gato (cat's claw) 175–6
    chemotherapy and 151
    immune system and 173
unsaturated fats 118–19
urine colour to test hydration 105
uterine cancer, oestrogen and 195

V
vaccines
    diabetes and 215
    killing beneficial bacteria 139–40
vaginal cancer, PCBs and 203
Vane, John 208
vanilloids 255
Varner, Julie 108
vegetables
    acting as pro-drugs 80
    alkalising 102
    against cancer 241
    coloured 71
    fibre in 289
    in French diet 68
    fresh 63
    in Gerson Therapy 94
    GI 217
    glutathione levels and 222

green, for liver strengthening 41
growing 290
home-grown 136
hydroponically grown 131
for increasing blood oxygen
levels 224
isothiocyanates in 240
juices 93
loss of minerals in 131
loss of vitamins in 146
organic vs 'normal' 134
phytoestrogens in 198
pollination 133–4
raw 93, 288
shopping for rainbow foods
299–302
toxins in 132–3
in UK diets 47
see also foods (*general only*)
vegetarian diet 98
cancer and 52–3
viral disease, bee propolis for 275
visceral fat 228
vitamin A 153
from carotenoids 254–5
nitrilosides 267
vitamin B complex 154–7
for better sleep 204
chlorella and spirulina 270
deficiency 122, 216, 232
to help orthodox therapies 152
neutralising free-radicals 42
nitrilosides 267
vitamin B-2, beneficial bacteria and
140
vitamin B-3 see niacin
vitamin B-6, reducing cholesterol
levels 121

vitamin B-7 see biotin
vitamin B-12 155, 240
beneficial bacteria and 140
chlorella and spirulina 270
deficiency 53, 140
reducing cholesterol levels 121
vitamin B-17 155–6
cyanide-containing 240
therapy 95, 97, 266, 267–8
vitamin C 157
for boosting immune system
238
chemotherapy and 151
foods for 283
loss in vegetables 132, 146–8
megadoses 97
nitrilosides 267
in organic food 127
oxygenating cells with 221
reducing cholesterol levels 121
supplements 148, 149
synthetic vs natural 143
vitamin D
for boosting immune system
283
chemotherapy and 151
chlorella and spirulina 270
for glioma x
against inflammation 210
magnesium and 34
radiotherapy and 152
from sun 69, 152, 158–9
supplements 150
vitamin E 159–60
for boosting immune system
238
chemotherapy and 151
destruction by chlorine 106

foods for 283
loss in vegetables 131, 146
neutralising free-radicals 42
nitrilosides 267
supplements 143, 148, 149, 284
vitamin K 161
for boosting immune system 283
chlorella and spirulina 270
liver cancer and 140
supplements 150
vitamin K3, chemotherapy and 151
vitamins *(general only)*
against cancer 143–64
deficiency 53, 146–8
human growth hormone and 184
liver function and 38
losses in unripe foods 132
multivitamin supplementation 148
'new' 149–50
in organic food 127
supplements, with orthodox therapies 150–3

W
Wolcott, Bill 54
walnut oil 119
Wang, Professor 10–11
Warburg, Otto 100, 221
Ward, Patricia Spain 166, 169
Wargovich, Professor 259
water
acidification 111
boiling 111

clean 103–12
for cooking 93
distillation 111
filtration 111, 290
Gerson Therapy and 93
how much to drink? 104–5
ioniser 112
overhydration 104
plastic bottled 110–11
re-mineralisation 112
reverse osmosis filtering 111–12
tap water 103, 140
oestrogen in 202
toxins in 105–10
when to drink 288
watercress 171
wheat, refined 122
wheat grass, for liver strengthening 41
white cells
in cancer patients 14
liver function and 39
phagocytosis 176
White Lies 113
whole grains 217
WiFi dangers 182
WobeMugos tablets 95
wokked food 288
Wolcott, Bill 87
womb cancer *see* uterine cancer
wormwood 177, 310
against parasites 43
against yeasts 235, 238
wound healing 275

X

xenoestrogens see oestrogen mimics

Y

Yakult 142, 205
yam, wild 176, 184, 205
yeasts 232–4
    bee propolis against 275
    diet and 236–8
    eliminating from body 101, 234
    fruit consumption and 289
    poisoning 234–6
yin and yang 61
yoga, cortisol levels and 60, 226
Your Body's Many Cries for Water
104

Z

zeaxanthan 254
zinc
    for boosting immune system
    238
    calcium inhibiting uptake of
    33–4
    against cancer 164
    lead and copper inhibiting
    uptake 108
    milk fats preventing uptake 114
    oestrogen and 189
    supplements 144, 148, 283

CANCERactive

CANCERactive is a UK Registered Charity No. 1102413. Its aims, as agreed with the Charities Commission, are 'to inform and support' cancer patients and to provide 'research' into treatments.

CANCERactive Mission:

The aim of the charity is to provide information, not just on orthodox cancer treatments but on complementary and new, alternative therapies allowing people to make more informed personal choices and so increase their personal odds of survival.

CANCERactive provides the information in a number of ways:
1. A 3,800 page website
2. A unique, free magazine called Integrated Cancer and Oncology News (**icon**) available in 640 UK hospitals, cancer clinics and health centres in libraries.
3. Downloadable prevention leaflets
4. Catherine Corners in Chichester, the Wirral, Hull and Kenilworth.
5. A series of books compiled by Chris Woollams

Books and websites
BOOKS:

All books are compiled and written for CANCERactive by Chris Woollams from information on the CANCERactive, Rainbow Diet and Chris Woollams Health Watch websites. References can be checked more fully there.

Books written by Chris Woollams and currently available include:

Everything you need to know to help you beat cancer

The Rainbow Diet

Rainbow Recipes (a recipe book based on the Rainbow Diet)

The Secret Source of your Good Health (a book about gut bacteria)

Cancer - your first 15 steps

Oestrogen - the killer in our midst

CANCERactive has neither distribution facilities, nor a sales operation. The Trustees of CANCERactive have appointed Health Issues Ltd (www.ournaturalselection.com) as the sole distributor for all CANCERactive published books and **icon** magazine in the world. Books are currently available from official wholesale points in the UK, Australia and the United States of America.

WARNING: You should never pay more than roughly £15 for the bigger books or £10 for the smaller ones. (That is roughly $25 and $16 US respectively). These are the prices through our official wholesalers.

USEFUL WEBSITES:

CANCERactive: www.canceractive.com

Tel: +44 (0)300 365 3015

Health Issues: www.ournaturalselection.com

The Rainbow Diet: www.the-rainbow-diet.com

General Health Information:
www.chriswoollamshealthwatch.com

For an impressive range of toiletry, personal care and household products see http://www.chriswoollamshealthwatch.com/Shop

Sign up for Chris' e newsletter with a message to
chrismeanshealth@gmail.com